DATE DUE

DEC 0 3 2002	
APR 2 2003	

BRODART   Cat. No. 23-221

THE FAMILY APPROACH TO EATING DISORDERS

Assessment and Treatment of Anorexia Nervosa and Bulimia

Edited by
Walter Vandereycken, M.D., Ph.D.
Elly Kog, Ph.D.
Johan Vanderlinden, M.A.

PMA PUBLISHING CORP.
New York

Library of Congress Cataloging in Publication Data

The Family approach to eating disorders / edited by Walter Vandereycken,
    Elly Kog, Johan Vanderlinden.
         p.   cm.
    Bibliography: p.
    Includes index.
    ISBN 0-89335-306-X : $45.00
    1. Eating disorders.   2. Family—Mental health.   3. Family
psychotherapy.   I. Vandereycken, Walter, 1949-   . II. Kog, Elly.
III. Vanderlinden, Johan.
    [DNLM: 1. Appetite Disorders.   2. Family.   WM 175 F198]
    RC552.E18F36   1988
    516.85'2 – dc19
    DNLM/DLD   88-39389
    for Library of Congress   CIP

Contents

iii

FOREWORD

R.A. Pierloot, M.D.

It can hardly be denied that eating disorders confront us with very complex problems. Overeating as well as starvation occur in many different illness patterns. Moreover they are often present in the same person, eventually alternating and/or combined with bizarre food manipulations such as provoked vomiting, hoarding, unbalanced dieting, compulsive cooking etc. Also psychological mechanisms assumed in persons with different eating disorders are often very similar. These problems, however, are not surprising if we look at the multiple and varied roots of eating behavior.

As an essential biological function, food intake is regulated by a large number of neural centers in the brain; the limbic system alone contains six thousand different sites influencing eating behavior. In animals, destruction or stimulation of specific parts of the thalamic and hypothalamic regions provoke specific changes in different aspects of food intake. How far can these findings be applied to eating behavior in humans? If so, how are they related to hormonal mechanisms studied in different disorders?

In man, eating as well as different food substances have a symbolic meaning. Eating behavior also has a pleasure-seeking aspect and, as such, it is connected with other libidinal activities. This implies that conflicts and defense-mechanisms in the area of sexual drives can find their expression in quantitative and/or qualitative changes in food intake. From a certain age, and especially in puberty, food intake becomes closely linked to body weight and shape. Preoccupation with body weight influencing eating behavior is a widespread phenomenon. Why this process becomes so disproportionate and almost delusional, in some persons raises many questions.

Also, eating occupies an important place in interpersonal relations. Eating obtains a significant meaning in the development of object-relations in early childhood. Feeding-activities are the most important form of interaction between mother and baby. In later stages of life eating also represents an important means of communication within the family context. It is no wonder that family interactions are considered as the ideal basis of therapeutic approach in some eating disorders.

The focus of this book is the family of patients presenting with an eating disorder. In the various chapters the importance of family variables in the genesis, the course and the therapy of this eating disorder are taken into consideration.

They illustrate the difficulties to arrive at clearcut and global formulations in this area. Conclusions have to be limited to more fragmentary and circumscribed aspects of the problem.

This is not amazing. As a system, the family consists of a number of persons connected to each other by quite divergent kinds of links: genetic connections, affective interactions, educational rules, common as well as opposite values pursued. Moreover, family patterns are determined in an important way by the general socio-cultural context. The structure of the family, the roles attributed to each of its members and the expectations connected with these roles, evolve in accordance with cultural norms. They are different in different cultures and they change with cultural evolution. The family in Western society is quite different from what it was fifty years ago.

Both eating disorders and the family system are very complex phenomena. Aware of this complexity, the authors of this book have been very cautious and critical in their conclusions. It is to their merit and it does not prevent their contributions from stimulating continuing research in this area.

PREFACE

This book is the result of many years of multidisciplinary team work at the University Psychiatric Center (U.P.C.) in Kortenberg, in collaboration with the Department of Psychology of the University of Leuven. Working in Flanders, the Flemish part of Belgium, bounded on the north by The Netherlands (we speak about the same language as our Dutch neighbors), we are situated near Brussels, the so-called capital of Europe. Both the historical background and the geographic position of our small country may explain why our scientific work is almost forced to cross the frontiers of language and nationality. Nevertheless, the reader should realize that English is not our mother tongue and, therefore, we apologize for any unevenness in our English or any lack of clarity of which we might possibly be guilty.

The scope and structure of this book are explained in the first chapter. Since the book is the product of team work, we just briefly present the different collaborators in alphabetic order. *M. Elisabeth Houben,* M.A., is a clinical psychologist and Head of the Department of Clinical Psychology at U.P.C. Kortenberg. *Elly Kog,* Ph.D. in clinical psychology, was at the time of writing a senior research assistant of the Belgian National Fund for Scientific Research, affiliated with the Department of Psychology at the University of Leuven; she is currently chief psychologist of personnel selection in one of Belgium's largest banks. *Claire Perednia,* M.A. in orthopedagogy, was at the time research assistant at U.P.C., but is currently psychotherapist and case manager in a unit for adolescents at the Psychiatric Hospital Alexianen in Tienen. *Roland Pierloot,* M.D., is psychiatrist and medical director of U.P.C. Kortenberg and Professor of Psychiatry at the University of Leuven. *Stephan Van den Broucke,* M.A. in clinical psychology, is preparing his Ph.D. as a research assistant of the Department of Psychology at the University of Leuven. *Walter Vandereycken,* M.D. & Ph.D. (Medical Sciences), is psychiatrist and Head of the Department of Behavior Therapy (including the Eating Disorders Unit) at U.P.C. Kortenberg and Associate Professor of Psychopathology at the University of Leuven. Both *Johan Vanderlinden* and *Ellie Van Vreckem* have an M.A. degree in clinical psychology, and are working as psychotherapists in the Eating Disorders Unit of U.P.C. Kortenberg. *Hans Vertommen,* Ph.D. in clinical psychology, is Associate Professor of Clinical Psychology at the University of Leuven.

All kinds of feedback from the readers, for which we would be grateful, can be addressed to Dr. W. Vandereycken, U.P.C., Leuvensesteenweg 517, B-3070 Kortenberg, Belgium.

Chapter 1

Introduction

Walter Vandereycken, Elly Kog and Johan Vanderlinden

This book originated at the intersection of two rather popular themes — family functioning and eating disorders — crossing with two major lines of force; research and practice. The inevitable narrowing of our focus in this book might be misinterpreted as if we consider this scope as the alpha and omega in understanding and treating anorexia nervosa and bulimia. Time and again, we will warn the reader throughout the various chapters that a one-sided viewpoint on etiology and treatment will lead to a dead-end. Only a *multidimensional* viewpoint of somatic as well as psychological and socio-cultural factors, including the family milieu, and their complex interplay can help solve the enigma of eating disorders (see Garfinkel & Garner, 1982; Vandereycken & Meermann, 1984). Hence, this book must be placed within the framework of modern psychosomatic medicine which attempts to elaborate — in basic research as well as in everyday clinical practice — a biopsychosocial view.

While preparing this book and having read a considerable amount of literature on our subject, we were struck by the imbalance between theoretical speculation and factual knowledge. The first part of this book addresses the ever-recurring question, *is the family victim or architect of the eating disorder?* It seems to us that many family theorists avoid the problem of etiology by dismissing the linear-causal manner of thinking. But however appealing a circular model may be, it remains to be substantiated that *specific* abnormal family interaction patterns occur in eating disorder patients and that they are *causally* related to the development of the condition (Hsu, 1983; Yager, 1982). Sociocultural and family factors may provide a context for an eating disorder, but do not explain the choice of this particular symptom (anorexia or bulimia) in this particular (predominantly female) subject. The "open systems model of psychosomatic disease" proposed by Minuchin and coworkers (1978) contains physiological, endocrine, and biochemical factors as "mediating mechanisms." They consider diabetes and asthma as "primary" psychosomatic disorders in which a physiological dysfunction is already present before becoming exacerbated by

1

emotional factors. In "secondary" psychosomatic disorders, "no such pre-
disposing physical dysfunction can be demonstrated. The psychosomatic element is apparent in the transformation of emotional conflicts into somatic symptoms. These symptoms may crystallize into a severe and debilitating illness like
anorexia nervosa" (Minuchin et al., 1978, p. 29). Aside from the fact that these
authors do not give clear evidence to support this statement, they leave it to the
imagination of the reader how this second type of symptom choice takes place.
The only specific factor they sometimes mention is that eating represents an important issue in families of anorexics. For the rest, they just emphasize characteristics of overall family functioning which would typify psychosomatic families (see Chapter 2).

Family theories do not explain the mechanisms whereby so-called typical
family patterns are translated into altered self-perceptions, desire for thinness,
preoccupation with food and weight, amenorrhea, hyperactivity and the many
other psychological and physiological features of eating disorders. "While the
family system formulations may help to explain how symptoms can be sustained
and reinforced once they appear, they do not account specifically for the occurrence of anorexia nervosa, rather than any other breakdown syndrome" (Yager,
1981, p. 264). The same criticism applies to the cybernetic theories of Selvini
Palazzoli (1974). This author has tried to bypass the question of "symptom
choice" by using a more sociological viewpoint which emphasizes the "cultural
roots" of anorexia nervosa: (a) an affluent society in which the availability of an
abundance of fad is in contrast to the fashion for thinness, especially for women;
(b) the change in the position of the child in Western family passing from a tradi-
tionally marginal to a central position which accentuates the parents' responsibility (Selvini Palazzoli, 1985). But, why is it that not all girls exposed to such
socio-cultural forces develop an eating disorder, and why anorexia in one case
and bulimia in the other?

The big issue here is the *difference in levels of abstraction*. Speaking about
family dynamics, for instance, one may analyze the emotional, ideational and
behavioral levels of interaction (Neal & Herzog, 1985). The concept of family
psychopathology, on the other hand, may be examined in many different ways
(Kalucy, 1983): as a formal psychiatric illness of an enduring nature, as a "disorder" related to developmental stages (family life cycle), as lasting interactional dysfunctioning, as intrapsychic pathology of family members, as a
pathology of the family system as a whole, etc. As a third example, observations
made about the families of eating disorder patients may reveal information at
different levels (Dare, 1985): the socio-cultural and historical perspective, the
genealogical and intergenerational perspective, the demographic and life cycle
features of the family, the structure of the family as an interpersonal network or
transactional system, and the psycho-biological characteristics of the individual
in the family. Hence, when we investigate family characteristics, which type of
information at which level are we gathering? If this is clear, we have to know

what aspect of the eating disorder (physiological, behavioral, emotional, inter-actional) we are addressing in the attempt to find (and influence) the link — if any — between a particular family and a particular syndrome. The greater the gap between the respective levels of abstraction, the greater the temptation to fill it with a chain of associations, the appeal and "truth" of which mainly de-pend on the imagination and conviction of the theorist or therapist concerned.

We will not present "innovating" theories in this book, nor advertise "success-ful" therapies. We have tried to summarize the state of the art in these areas.

Chapter 2 gives an overview of the many considerations and assumptions about the families of eating disorder patients. The vast majority of this litera-ture concerns rather personal thoughts and reflections colored by the theoreti-cal framework of the authors. Three groups may be distinguished: theories about (a) causal influences from other family members on the patient, (b) patho-genic parent-child interactions, and (c) dysfunctioning of the family system as a whole. When turning to the facts, however, solid research data which may en-dorse either theory are scarce or contradictory.

Chapter 3 critically analyzes the various investigations of family factors sup-posed to be involved in the occurrence or development of eating disorders: (a) genetic factors, (b) demographic features, (c) individual pathology in the family, (d) intrafamilial relationships; as well as family factors related to treatment out-come and prognosis. Though the list of investigations that meet minimal methodological requirements seems already quite impressive, the quality and comparability of these studies do not allow for firm conclusions.

Our discontent with the available research literature has led us to design a series of studies described in the second part on assessment.

Chapter 4 discusses the main problems with which the investigator is faced either in basic or applied family research. In fact, the following chapters are in-tended to demonstrate the many different directions in which future research can develop. Though chapters 5 and 6 illustrate a rather sophisticated approach, the following ones clearly show that less ambitious small-scale projects may yield interesting results that throw new light on some "forgotten" topics.

Chapter 5 describes the multiple problems of a multi-method study aimed at verifying Minuchin's well-known model of the psychosomatic family structure. Four interactional dimensions are investigated: (a) the intensity of intrafamil-ial boundaries, (b) the degree of the family's adaptability, (c) the degree of avoidance or recognition of intrafamilial tension, and (d) the family's way of handling conflicts. These concepts have been tested with a multitrait-multi method approach including two behavioral methods (family tasks and direct observation of interaction) and a self-report method. Concerning the latter, *Chapter 6* presents a newly developed instrument, the "Leuven Family Ques-tionnaire," designed specifically for assessing the family members' own ex-perience (the insiders' perception) of the family. This self-report questionnaire comprises three scales: conflict, cohesion, and disorganization.

Chapter 7 underlines an often neglected aspect; the educational role of the parents and their parenting behavior. This exploratory study shows the great diversity of the parents' reaction to a child with an eating disorder. The parental rearing behavior and attitudes seem to be influenced by the way the parents have been raised themselves (this transgenerational issue will also be discussed in Chapter 17).

Chapter 8 presents a comparative study (between anorexics and normal controls) about the family members' own perception of interpersonal relationships; how mother, father, and daughter experience the way they behave toward each other (as measured by Barrett-Lennard's Relationship Inventory).

Chapter 9 describes a prospective study aimed at assessing the evolution of family functioning as well as individual symptomatic and psychosocial adjustment of eating disorder patients before and after family-oriented inpatient treatment, and at follow-up after one year.

Chapter 10 contains one of the very few investigations in married patients: a systematic comparison with unmarried anorexics and an exploratory pilot study of the marital relationship in anorexics and bulimics.

The third part of the book addresses the treatment of eating disorders insofar as it concerns the various ways of dealing with family issues.

Chapter 11 presents an overview of the international literature on family therapy in eating disorders. Many schools have arisen in this rather popular field, but the "second generation" of family therapists seems to have evolved toward eclecticism and integration within a flexible framework which is governed by everyday pragmatism instead of orthodox ideology.

Chapter 12 is an example of such an approach in an outpatient setting, according to four levels of management: identification, information, intervention, and intensive therapy. This procedure may end in the decision of hospitalization, the execution of which does not exclude the family from the treatment process.

Chapter 13 discusses the dynamics of the triangular relation between hospitalized patient, the other family members, and the treatment staff. Special attention is paid to the strain on the family and the way team members can deal with it.

Chapter 14 stresses the important principle that parents must be approached at the level at which they are asking for help and to the extent they are ready to accept it. Therefore, a variety of parent counseling methods are described, gradually ranging from educational guidance to specific therapy.

Chapter 15 demonstrates, with many practical examples and an extensive case history, the way in which family therapy may be incorporated in an inpatient treatment program. A series of specific interventions is described together with the many practical problems (indications, pitfalls) involved.

Chapter 16 highlights several important issues that are virtually neglected in the current literature on family therapy: transgenerational issues (the dynamics within the extended family), broken home situations (single parent families), and chronic cases with a long-lasting and seemingly treatment-resistant problem history.

Chapter 17 describes both from a theoretical and practical viewpoint the way in which an eating disorder may have a special place within the patient's marriage. Whether or not the problems may be connected with both partners' background (the families of origin), the marital interaction itself calls for specific therapeutic attention.

Chapter 18, finally, gives a detailed account of a very interesting method of dealing with ambivalent and distressed parents. Counseling groups for these parents have special possiblities and important advantages if placed within a flexible therapeutic approach which emphasizes the necessity of working *with* instead of *against* the family system.

At the end of the book we hope the reader may be left with the idea that we did a fine job, but that there is a lot more to describe, to investigate and to discuss. We will be pleased, then, to have stimulated the reader's appetite and we offer the hungry ones an extensive, selected bibliography on the subject. Indeed, the menu we have presented was our personal choice "à la carte." We hope the reader will appreciate our taste!

REFERENCES

Dare, C. (1985), The family therapy of anorexia nervosa. *Journal of Psychiatric Research,* 19:435-443.

Garfinkel, P.E. & Garner, D.M. (1982), *Anorexia Nervosa: A Multidimensional Perspective.* New York: Brunner/Mazel.

Hsu, L.K.G. (1983), The aetiology of anorexia nervosa. *Psychological Medicine,* 13:231-238.

Kalucy, R.S. (1983), Family psychopathology and anorexia nervosa. In: Krakowski, A.J. & Kimball, C.P. (Eds.), *Psychosomatic Medicine.* New York: Plenum Press, pp. 125-141.

Minuchin, S., Rosman, B.L. & Baker, L. (1978), *Psychosomatic Families. Anorexia Nervosa in Context.* Cambridge (Mass.): Harvard University Press.

Neal, J.H. & Herzog, D. (1985), Family dynamics and treatment of anorexia nervosa and bulimia. *Pediatrician,* 12:139-147.

Selvini Palazzoli, M. (1974), *Self-Starvation. From the Intrapsychic to the Transpersonal Approach to Anorexia Nervosa.* London: Chaucer.

Selvini Palazzoli, M. (1985), Anorexia nervosa: A syndrome of the affluent society. *Transcultural Psychiatric Research Review,* 22:199-205 (reprinted in the *Journal of Strategic and Systemic Therapies,* 1985, 4(3):12-36); see also the letter by the same author in *Transcultural Psychiatric Research Review,* 1986, 23:83-85.

Vandereycken, W. & Meermann, R. (1984). *Anorexia Nervosa. A Clinician's Guide to Treatment.* Berlin-New York: Walter de Gruyter.

Yager, J. (1981), Anorexia nervosa and the family. In: Lansky, M.R. (Ed.), *Family Therapy and Major Psychopathology.* New York: Grune & Stratton, pp. 249-280.

Yager, J. (1982), Family issues in the pathogenesis of anorexia nervosa. *Psychosomatic Medicine,* 44:43-60.

Chapter 2

The Speculations: An Overview of Theories About Eating Disorder Families*

Elly Kog and Walter Vandereycken

INTRODUCTION

The role of the family in the treatment of anorexia nervosa was already mentioned in the 19th century, both in English and French literature. It mainly reflected a pragmatic attitude on the part of the physician whose major concern was to separate the patient from her family for treatment to be successful, an idea which would govern the therapeutic approach to anorexia nervosa for many decades (see Chapter 11). Although this attitude implied, at least indirectly, the conception that parents played a pathogenic part in the eating disorder, this view was not explicitly elaborated. But, in the 19th century, the influence of familial factors and interactions on the development of mental illness was rarely explored (McPeak, 1975). The recognition of the importance of interpersonal dynamics within the family unit came only after the adoption and exploration of Freud's insights. Until World War II, psychoanalytic investigators dominated the literature and, hence, the familial role in the development of anorexia nervosa was narrowed to a one-sided analysis of the pathogenic mother-daughter interaction. From the 1950's on, the scope enlarged under the influence of disciplines such as sociology and anthropology, leading to a fundamentally new movement — a paradigmatic shift — in psychology and psychiatry, namely the systematic study of the family as the primary context in which human development takes place (Jackson & Satir, 1961).

At the turning point of this evolution, one important but forgotten figure should be brought into the spotlight, Henri B. Richardson. This remarkable physician coordinated a prestigious project on "the family in sickness and health

---

* Parts of this chapter have been published in an article by the second author: "The Constructive Family Approach to Eating Disorders" (*International Journal of Eating Disorders,* 1987, 6:455-467).

7

care" at the Cornell University Medical College in New York, the results of which are published in an avant-gardist but poorly known book with the simple but all-telling title: *Patients Have Families* (1945). It was an avant-garde project both because of the multidisciplinary approach and the utilization of a cybernetic systems language. The basic idea was: "The family is the unit of illness, because it is the unit of living" (Richardson, 1945, p. 76). One is struck by the fact that, already in 1945, the concept of "the family equilibrium" was defended. As such, Richardson's book antedated by almost a decade the work of Gregory Bateson and the Palo Alto group. The book is particularly interesting because of its special attention to psychosomatic disorders: "The disease for which the personality structure is most characteristic is anorexia nervosa, and in this *family life plays a very definite part*" (Richardson, 1945, p. 73; italics added).

From the analysis of fifteen families, Richardson demonstrates very convincingly how misleading it may be to analyze medical complaints of diseases in a purely individual perspective. One of the families, analyzed in detail (the family Martin Q), had an anorexic daughter. From separate interviews with the different family members, the investigator found that all of them had gastrointestinal complaints. Father is described as an anxious-neurotic man, complaining of stomach ache and vomiting. His obese wife was found to have a peptic ulcer. The youngest daughter, Catherine, in whom some heart disease was suspected (one sister died from a reumatic heart disease), happened to have functional digestive complaints together with a tendency of overeating. Finally, her sister Agnes was diagnosed as having anorexia nervosa. The family pattern was characterized by an extremely dominating position of the mother, which corresponded with her husband's submissivity, and an important rivalry between the siblings. The mother identified with her anorexic daughter, Agnes, who symbolized the failure she herself had been in her own youth (this episode in mother's teenage years had been accompanied by a transitory phase of weight loss). Catherine, on the other hand, seemed to incorporate the success the parents were not able to achieve themselves. But the less Catherine's carreer seemed to fulfill the promises, the more she showed weight fluctuations contrary to those of Agnes, and she finally became obese, like her mother.

To quote the *interactional analysis* Richardson made of this family Q: "Mrs. Q's drive for domination, and her penchant for spending money, interfered with Mr. Q's competence as a 'provider,' which was the one means by which he could feel secure, and his only recourse was vomiting. Conversely, any attempt of his to escape from domination constituted a threat to her which reacted on her health. Mrs. Q needed Agnes as the scapegoat of her own failure; Agnes submitted to her mother's domination and any prospect of her escape was likewise a threat to her mother. Here again the chance of illness was increased on both sides. A similar system existed between the mother and Catherine based on success instead of failure with similar possibilities as to health. These systems were interrelated; the maladjustment between the parents resulted in the psychologically hazardous arrangement by which Agnes slept in the same room as her father, which exposed her to the effect of her father's vomiting, thereby interfering with her appetite and facilitating her self-starvation as a way out of her subjection to Mrs. Q" (Richardson, 1945, p. 91). Remember, when reading this citation, that these words were written during World War II!

At the end of this fascinating study, Richardson raised the important matter of research on *family typology*, especially the relationship between a certain type of family equilibrium or organization on the one hand, and a particular disease or adjustment disorder on the other. Though Richardson was certainly influenced by the then popular idea of typical personality structure connected with a particular psychosomatic disorder, the discussion of forty years ago has not lost much of its timeliness. "To put the question in a nutshell, is there just one family of Martin Q's, which is unique, or are there a great number of Martin Q families, such that if we knew one of them thoroughly we would have a very good idea of the others?...The question in the Martin Q's is not whether they are an 'anorexia nervosa family' or an 'ulcer family', but whether or not the disease is systematically related to their type of family equilibrium....If the answer is affirmative, the probability is that a similar type of equilibrium will be found in other families in which the same disease occurs" (Richardson, 1945, p. 295, 299). In fact, this is a variant of the ever recurring question whether there exists a typical "anorexigenic" family pattern.

As emphasized above, Richardson's concept of the family as the unit of illness, proved to be an avant-garde point of view because the elaboration of concrete theories about the (causal) process of family influence in anorexia nervosa started but two decades ago. Different from at least some literature on schizophrenia, most of the family theories about eating disorders are premature due to the scarce and methodologically weak family research (see Chapter 3). Therefore, we will review the current family theories on eating disorders, without taking into account their degree of empirical testing. Aside from the fact that most of the theories on familial factors in eating disorders do lack empirical support and remain fragmentary, there is also a growing amount of research on certain family variables, especially genetic factors, without any elaborated theory (see Chapter 3).

We will group the family theories under three headings. Firstly, we will discuss those authors who stress the linear causal role of certain family members in particular. The second group of theories concerns the pathogenic role of particular parent-child interactions. Thirdly, we will discuss family systems theories in eating disorders. It is striking that French literature is predominantly of the first type, German literature of the second one, while the English literature is spread over the three groups. The most influential authors are situated in the second and third type of theories.

CAUSAL FAMILY INFLUENCES

The Mother

In many papers, it is especially the mother who seemed to be held responsible for the development of the eating disorder. The recurring theme is the dyadic bonding between mother and anorexic child, characterized by its dependence on ambivalent maternal attitudes (an hypothesis also put forward in male cases of anorexia nervosa; see e.g., Albert et al., 1984; Rampling, 1980).

Boutonier (1948) considers the relationship between mother and baby as crucial from a physiological and psychological point of view because the mother is the first source of food. The satisfaction of the first care is associated with the mother. But it is unavoidable that the wishes of the child and those of the mother sometimes clash. So, the child is attached but reacts to the insecure, overprotective attitude of the mother by means of food refusal. Sours (1974) also emphasizes excessive symbiosis and maternal control. The mother needs to have a submissive, perfect child in order to fulfill her own pathologically driven wishes.

Edhouse (1975) even labels the child as "the presenting symptom of the mother." A case of anorexia nervosa in a nine-and-a-half-year-old child revealed a combination of profound regression and hypermaturity. The girl was poor in age-appropriate childishness and had been reared in mother's image of strong super-ego formation and ego control. The deficiency in mother's own personality development produced the pathological growth of the child's personality. Mother's own problem was thus presented as a problem in the child.

The Father

Far fewer authors (Launay et al., 1965; Jeammet et al., 1973; Wold, 1973) mention the role of the father in the development of anorexia nervosa. He is predominantly characterized as emotionally distant, sometimes as weak and passive, and sometimes as a dominant person. Besides the weak father acting like a child which needs protection, Launay and coworkers (1965) differentiate two other types of fathers. The second type is emotionally distant because of a serious, but secret, conflict between the parents. The daughter is either emotionally abandoned by both parents or has formed a secret alliance with her mother against her father. The third type of father is active but unreachable because he is good and intelligent and the daughter cannot come up to his requirements. So, the daughter remains infantile and considers her father as an image outside her own life.

Stressing the pathogenic role of the father, Wold (1973) noted maternal depression in the background of the anorexic's childhood, with the father being an angry, violent, rigid man, still idealizing his own mother by means of displacing her to his daughter.

In bulimic women, on the other hand, Sights and Richards (1984) noted a close father-daughter relationship during early childhood but a deterioration of this relationship with the onset of puberty.

General Parental Attitudes

Parents of anorexia nervosa and bulimic patients are described as emphasizing achievement, success, conformity and traditional concepts of femininity, and appearance. They are viewed as domineering, demanding and controlling, but they fail to negotiate separation and individuation (e.g., Boskind-Lodahl, 1976; Dally, 1969; Gensicke, 1979; Sights & Richards, 1983). Kalucy (1983) states: "It sometimes seems that they are relatively 'good' at raising children, but 'bad' at adolescence" (p. 127).

Harper (1983) called this phenomenon *parenting failure*. This is apparent in the following parental attitudes: (1) complicity in harmful self-medication by fear of their daughter's anger; (2) persistent triangulation, in intact as well as in divorced families; (3) malignant denial of the severity of the illness; (4) subversion of a clinical plan; (5) parental desertion and depression; and (6) breakdown of householding.

Andersen (1985), Israel et al. (1971), and Vandereycken and Meermann (1984) mention the parents' failure to recognize the extent of the anorexic symptomatology and its significance, in a way comparable to the patient's typical denial of illness. The parents often minimize the problems or even maintain an extreme degree of tolerance to the most obvious physical and psychological symptoms.

Although several authors mention the presence of individual pathology in the parents of eating disorder patients (see Chapter 3), its significance in the pathogenesis is quite unclear. Crisp et al. (1974) suggested a relationship between the anorexia nervosa symptoms and psychological difficulties in the parents. The majority of parents of anorexia nervosa patients appeared to become more psychoneurotic after weight restoration of their daughter, compared with the moment the inpatient therapy started. According to these authors, this may reflect the fact that the majority of family psychopathology and morbidity is displaced into the patient: "...the daughter's illness sometimes serves a protective function for one or both parents as well as the patient, especially if the marital relationship is poor and acutely threatened by the prospect of their child's independence" (Crisp et al., 1974, p. 172).

Finally, Jackson (1986) noticed a neglected issue in the pathogenesis of anorexia nervosa, which he called "the denial of death and *death themes.*" He focuses on the parental, usually maternal cross-generational transmission of morbid, violent, and depressive themes. According to this author, death fears and anxieties and a close associative linking between death and basic life (body) functions, play a central role in the dynamic etiology of anorexia nervosa. Eating is conceptualized as an encounter with death, which serves to continuously re-activate in the anorexic patient an obsessional pre-occupation with death imagery. A similar idea, but more on a symbolic level, has been recently expressed by Friedman (1985) who speaks about "suicidal guilt" in the pathogenesis of anorexia nervosa. Anorexic patients seem to be much more concerned with harming than they are with being harmed. Then, a special separation guilt may lie at the heart of the problem, namely the belief that growing up and separating from mother will damage or even destroy her. In this respect, it is interesting to note that in the discussion section of the interesting paper by Frazier et al. (1955) which we will discuss further on (see Oedipal Conflicts), the death of anorexic patients is conceived as "somatic suicides:" "One of the major issues is that the mother of each of these patients, currently or at an earlier time, chronically wished for the patient's death. This fact causes the patient such despair that it is forced into the unconscious. Driven into the unconscious, the fact still operates as to drive the patient to starve to death" (p. 242). Achimovich (1985) also criticizes the lack of attention in scientific literature for the threat of suicide in families with an anorexic member, but he considers suicidal depression of the fathers as more intensive and obvious than maternal depression. The anorexic's suicidal behavior is interpreted as metaphorically representing the parental (especially paternal) depression. This author stresses that it is necessary to engage the fathers in therapy in order to resolve this issue before the anorexic patient is willing to give up her symptom permanently.

Siblings and Grandparents

The role of the siblings in the development of anorexia nervosa is not given much attention to. Hall (1978) found an intense, ambivalent, rivalrous relationship with the nearest-in-age sibling, whether older or younger, whether brother or sister, and an expectation that the patient would relate well with a close-in-age sister who was of incompatible personality. Sights and Richards (1984) suggest a strong sibling rivalry, particularly between sisters in the families of bulimics. Weber and Stierlin (1981) speak about a secret rivalry between the sisters in an anorexic family (see Family Psychodynamics).

Sperling and Massing (1970) brought into attention the role of the maternal grandmother in the development of anorexia nervosa. There is often a powerful grandmother, who plays a dominant role in childrearing and household activities. Amdur et al. (1969) hypothesize the transmission of irrationality concerning food from one generation to the next. "The fact that in many of these families there has been a perpetuation of problems and concerns related to obesity, food and control from grandparents to parents to child would imply some importance of the family constellation in this problem" (p. 565-566). Some of these transgenerational issues will be discussed in Chapter 16.

PATHOGENIC PARENT-CHILD INTERACTIONS

In the previous group of theories the role of family members was predominantly conceived as a linear, unidirectional factor which causes the eating disorder. Other authors consider a specific type of parent-child *interaction,* isolated from the many other family interactions, as causing the illness. They stress the pathogenic influence of characteristics in the child as well as in the parents, and their mutual influence (the bidirectional nature of the relationship).

In a comment on the article of Sours (1974), Kramer (1974) underlines the contribution of the child to the disturbed mother-child relationship. The child is not only pushed by the mother, but accepts to play the perfect, submissive child. In his book *Starving to Death in a Sea of Objects,* Sours (1980) himself no longer claims that there exists something like an "anorexigenic mother," although he discusses some recurring maternal, paternal and family types. Faltus (1980) also ascertains some recurring parental attitudes but gives some attention to the patient's attitudes as well. According to this author, one of the parents is a conscious, careful and solicitous personality, always trying to guide the child and leaving it no space for independent decisions. The patients' reaction, then, is ambivalent, often averse to hostile, especially in the mother-daughter relationship.

Developmental Learning Processes

Hilde Bruch (1973) is well-known for her detailed analysis of the developmental learning process of the anorexic child in the mutual interaction between parents and child which contributed to the development of the eating disorder. She observed that anorexic children are extremely immature and clingingly dependent on their mothers, though they are advanced in physical and intellectual development. Reconstruction of the early development of the patients revealed that they had been well cared for children to whom many advantages and privileges of modern living had been offered. However, closer examination revealed that encouragement or reinforcement of self-expression had been deficient. Reliance on their own inner resources, ideas, or autonomous decisions remained undeveloped in these patients. Pleasing compliance became their way of life, which resulted in a sense of ineffectiveness when development demanded autonomy. The inability to recognize hunger and other bodily sensations, shows that the learning process of perception of one's own bodily sensations was deficient. The innate needs of the child and the environmental responses were poorly attuned to each other, resulting in a perplexing confusion in the child's conceptual awareness. The parents emphasize, however, the normality of their family life. Yet, on closer study, the egocentric atmosphere of the home becomes apparent. The parents used the child to bolster their pride. The response to the child's needs was superimposed according to what the parents, often mistakenly, felt the child needed. The mother especially is considered important in the early infancy, in which hunger and bodily sensations have to be learned. Bruch (1973) states, "In these cases, the parents' conviction of their own correctness will blind them to all signals indicating doubts and frustrations from which their children suffer. With such failure in communication, even benevolent and appropriate parental actions are apt to be experienced by the child as over-control and as disregard or rejection of anything that comes from him" (p. 86). Selvini Palazzoli (1974) initially worked out a similar conceptualization but it evolved to a family systems approach, which will be discussed in the third group of theories.

Oedipal Conflicts

Some psychoanalytically oriented therapists highlight oedipal conflicts and regard the fear of becoming a grown-up, sexually attractive girl as a crucial element in the genesis of anorexia nervosa, related to parent-child interactions during infancy. In 1955, staff members of the Section of Psychiatry at the famous Mayo Clinic in Rochester published a remarkable but generally unnoticed report on parental antecedents in five types of neurotic eating difficulties exhibited by children: (1) family obesity, (2) clinical obesity, (3) skinniness, (4) certain ulcer problems, and (5) anorexia nervosa. Frazier et al. (1955) introduced a totally new point of view, that a child would rather give parents pleasure than displeasure and thus consciously and unconsciously does the things that are in keeping with the parents' dominant wish. The child *complies with the parents' wishes and fostering,* whether it be overeating or undereating. The authors observed a relatively unhappy marriage in the parents together with an ambivalence toward the child in each of the eating problems mentioned. The hostile component in this ambivalence increases from types 1 to 5. Moreover, except for type 1, there is also a parental ambivalence about eating in all types. Again the intensity of this conflict increases from type 1 to 5. In the anorexia nervosa group, the hostility may be so marked that the child is repelled by food because of the parents' revengeful attitude about eating. The parental wish, with which the child complies, is frequently not verbalized but is conveyed by smiling, vacillating affection, or the manner of preparing food.

Frazier et al. (1955) illustrated these concepts with case examples. In a 14-year-old anorexic girl they found that the father apparently was highly flirtatious with his daughter and "that the child, entering adolescence, was far too closely tied to her father and thereby aroused her mother's destructive jealousy. It was as if her mother who formally enjoyed stuffing her daughter now revengefully wanted to starve her to death. Food was their medium of love and barter. The child complied with marked anorexia and loss of weight to the point that the physician feared for her live" (p. 235). The authors emphasize that such a rivalry between mother and daughter for the father's attention may be observed particularly in patients who alternate between obesity and states of anorexia. Finally, it is important to note that these authors, as early as 1955, pleaded for a collaborative treatment. "It is impossible to treat this girl without having both parents and the girl in collaborative psychotherapy. The parents cannot free this child to a healthy adaptation without resolution in part, at least, of their major problems, including, of course, the basic marital adjustment" (p. 235). So, in fact, Frazier et al. (1955) were not only describing rather complex family interactions but they were among the first to include parents into the treatment of anorexia nervosa patients (see Chapter 11).

Beckers and Massing (1974) give a picture of a family in which *instinct and sexuality* are considered uncontrollable and even sinful. A sense of duty, economy and tidiness are the standards in these families. The mother-daughter interaction is of great significance in this family ideology because the mother is the concrete manifestation of a sexually mature woman, representing what the daughter does not want to be. The mother is a subject of negative identification. The ideal of the patient does not correspond with reality when, while in her puberty, the first feminine body elements start to develop. This leads to an individual crisis in the girl and a repression of sexuality, psychologically as well as physically.

Kestemberg et al. (1972) interpret this refusal of an anorexic patient to become a sexually attractive girl as an oedipal conflict and stress the role of the father in this unconscious family dynamic. The pre-anorexic girl is idealized in the family. She is a unique child, who is admired for her intelligence and obedience. At the same time, however, she is overprotected and isolated from her peers, especially by the mother because of her dominant role in the family. The girl reacts passively and forms a secret alliance with her father. Together, they try to irritate the mother. The father takes on the role of "the good mother" in latent or explicit conflicts. Consequently, the father becomes an object of oedipal investment. The father experiences the anorexia nervosa, accompanied by a mental and physical destruction of his daughter, as a narcissitic injury and a legitimation of a regression to oedipal feelings. A particular family organization develops. The feeling of disappointment, which father and mother have in common, results in their unification. The father is irritated by the anorexic symptoms and mother becomes the intermediary between father and mother. But, unconsciously, the father is fascinated by the symptoms because he can keep his girl in his neighborhood and communicate with her by means of the mother go-between.

Deegener (1982) gives a very similar picture of the father-mother-daughter relationship in anorexia nervosa, emphasizing the importance of the oedipal complex. In a case example of a 17-year-old girl, he illustrates the jealousy of the mother toward her daughter because of her intimate relationship with her father. As a reaction, the mother tries to repress all sexuality in her girl, while father and daughter continue to have a quasi-incestuous relationship.

Symbiosis

For other psychoanalytic authors, a pre-genital symbiosis between mother and patient is more important than a possible superimposed oedipal conflict. Berger (1977) called this a *prolonged symbiosis,* characterized by two features:

firstly, the symbiotic developmental phase is pathologically prolonged; and secondly, the first and most important attachment figure, i.e., the mother, is pregenitally structured herself and is thus symbiotically attached to her ill child.

Ehrensing and Weitzman (1970) discuss a case in which the *interconnected pathology of mother and child* leads to anorexia nervosa in both of them. The daughter is admitted to the same inpatient service where her mother was hospitalized 24 years before. Anorexia nervosa is conceptualized by these authors as the regressive resolution of a maturational crisis in the young girl, confronted with the developmental tasks of adolescence, to which she is unable to adapt. The illness reveals a disturbed ego and psychosexual development, beginning with the earliest mother- daughter relationship. A mother-daughter symbiosis existed because of continuing maternal absence and deprivation. Successful separation-individuation was impossible because of this unsatisfactory symbiotic phase. The father, largely absent both physically and psychologically, was not able to intervene effectively. When he was present, his flagrant sexual behavior excited but frightened his daughter, making a satisfying relationship impossible.

Even a more striking case study in this respect is published by Besançon et al. (1978), and concerns three anorexia nervosa cases in the same family. The mother developed the syndrome at 30 years of age and both of her daughters at pubertal age. Since the mother's own mother, was an overprotective but controlling and unpredictable woman whereas her father was absent during her infancy, the mother herself had developed a pre-genitally structured personality. But now, she acted in the same way toward her own daughters. Moreover, both girls were separated from their mother for a long time during the first years of life, because of tuberculosis. Meanwhile, the father neglected his wife and two daughters because of marital problems.

Igoin-Apfelbaum (1985) similarly hypothesized that a history of violent separations in the family, combined with a severe denial of actual family problems, is an important etiological factor in bulimia. There exists a strong fantasy of inseparability in these families, although most patients come from broken homes or "closed families", massively hiding internal tensions. Bulimia, with the double polarity of incorporation – total love and total destruction within the same movement – expresses the dilemma between the need to identify with both parents and the perception of their incompatability.

Finally, the peculiar interconnectedness of psychological problems in members of the same family is discussed by Harju and Fried (1982). They describe three cases: an obese father and an anorexic daughter, an obese mother and an anorexic son, and an obese father and an anorexic son. One family member actually lives the role rejected by the other, and both symptoms may be unified in the same person, for which the term "dysorexia" is used. Harju and Fried (1982), therefore speak of a dysorectic family rather than of an anorectic (or bulimic) individual, emphasizing both the embeddedness of a symptom in a more comprehensive syndrome, and the social unit as the source of its members' problems.

DYSFUNCTIONING OF THE FAMILY SYSTEM

Several authors (e.g., Kalucy et al., 1977; Bruch, 1973; Hall, 1978; Garfinkel & Garner, 1982) characterize the anorexia nervosa family as a middle- or upper-class family with a success, achievement and appearance orientation and an unusual preoccupation with weight and eating. Crisp et al. (1980), however, state that an "anorexic family" does not exist. According to these authors, neither a pathological dyad (involving the patient) nor a pathological family interaction are causal factors for the eating disorder. The observed tendency to be unusually close, loyal and mutually interdependent would rather be the result of the disorder than an etiological factor. This widely discussed cause-consequence controversy (Vandereycken & Meermann, 1984) is considered irrelevant in systems theory.

With regard to anorexia nervosa, Doerr-Zegers et al. (1985) claim: "A dominant mother, a tyrannical father or a powerful grandmother, each one by themselves, do not represent 'the anorexic family', but the striking phenomena of different constellations of an interaction pattern, in which the extreme complementariness of the relations between its members does not leave space for the development of that transformation capacity, which, together with the tendency to homeostasis, characterized the dynamics of bio-systems" (p. 463). Beside this complementarity in the family interaction pattern (one dominant and one weak or ill parent), these authors stress *the family ideology of self-sacrifice.* The self-sacrifice drive has an anthropological status, greater than sexual rejection or the dynamics of social climbing. The anorexic patient appears more as a martyr than as an ill person. She experiences a hidden pleasure in the act of suffering. The patient carries out a mission to which she was pushed by the whole family and whose true sense is to maintain the threatened homeostasis.

According to White (1983), self-sacrificing is one of the role prescriptions for women in anorexic families. These families have a rigid system of implicit beliefs which are transmitted from one generation to the next and have a highly constraining effect on all family members. Women in these families, and especially certain daughters (who are the ones most likely to become anorexic), are generally expected to be sensitive, devoted and self-sacrificing. Beside this specific role prescription for the anorexic daughter, White (1983) focuses on the standard of *loyalty* in these families. They value very highly any behavior that appears to be motivated by loyalty to other family members and to family tradition. As a consequence, two-person alliances and peer relationships are discouraged and grandparents intrude in nuclear family life. Guilt induction is used to promote conformity. Finally, anorexic families are characterized by the belief of insightfulness. Family members are unable to recognize the existence of mutual influence between people because they believe all behavior is insightful and intentional. Individual integrity is evaluated according to the interpretation of one's intentions, the nature and quantity of one's feelings, and the level of understanding of needs of others. This blinds family members to the nature and consequences of their belief systems and promotes guilt-inducing transactions.

Communication and Transaction

After having elaborated a developmental model of anorexia nervosa, based on Kleinian psychodynamics and existential-phenomenological concepts, Mara Selvini Palazzoli (1974) has made a shift to a transpersonal approach inspired by cybernetics, systemic thinking and communication theory (see also Chapter 11). She identified peculiar communication patterns in anorexic families. From an analysis of blaming behaviors in these families Selvini Palazzoli (1974) concluded that family members feel guilty but cannot and may never be blamed when something goes wrong: "Precisely because every family member 'effaces' himself for the sake of the rest, no one member is really prepared to assume responsibility when something goes wrong" (p. 213). This problem of *blame-shifting* is accompanied by a problem of leadership in the family. All decisions are for the good of someone else, so decisions are never attributed to personal preferences. The parents do not accept their responsibility because of this *rejection of personal leadership*. A third characteristic, the existence of *secret alliances* in the family, constitutes the central and most serious problem, according to this author. The belief that the family is unified and cohesive may not be destroyed and thus two-person alliances are taboo. But each of the parents, deeply disillusioned with their partner, secretly encourages the patient to make up for the partner's shortcomings. Selvini Palazzoli (1974) called this *three-way matrimony*. Each member of the family is married to two persons; the mother to her husband and daughter, the father to his wife and daughter, and the daughter to both of her parents. This works fairly well for the parents but not for the daughter, who is expected to distribute her attention as equitably as possible. Consequently, she has no energy to build a life of her own, or to risk open rebellion. The parent-daughter coalitions have to be kept secret because the parents do not want to acknowledge their deep disillusionment with each other. The facade of marital unity may not be destroyed. Finally, in families in which the anorexic symptoms are complicated by other symptoms, like bulimia and violence, marked communication disorders are present too. Family members qualify their own communications coherently, verbally and non-verbally, but reject messages sent by others. They seem to be sure of what they say and of their right to say it but reject the content of what another says, even though they acknowledge the other's right to say this.

Structural Family Theory

The structural family theory of Salvador Minuchin and collaborators is undoubtedly one of the landmarks in the development of family theory and therapy (see Chapter 11). Its application to families with a psychosomatically ill

child (Minuchin et al., 1975, 1978) — anorexia nervosa, diabetes mellitu
psychosomatic asthma — had a tremendous influence on the treatment of
disorders. Their clinically derived model states that psychosomatic families are
characterized by an enmeshed, overprotective, rigid and conflict-avoiding
family structure. This typical family organization, together with the physiological vulnerability of the child, forms the basis for the occurrence of a psychosomatic symptom in the child, whose involvement in parental conflicts reinforces
the psychosomatic symptoms.

The first characteristic of the psychosomatic family organization, *enmeshment,* refers to loose boundaries between subsystems in the family. There is an
interdependence of relationships, a poorly differentiated perception of self and
other family members, and weak family subsystem boundaries, especially between parents and children. *Rigidity* is a concept that bears upon the degree of
adaptability of the family interaction. When external stress (e.g., changes in occupation) or internal family changes (e.g., children reaching adolescence) induce the need for a change of the usual transactional patterns, these families
experience great difficulty and attempt to maintain a status quo. *Overprotectiveness* is defined as a high degree of concern for each other's welfare in the family.
"In such families, the parents' overprotectiveness retards the children's
development of autonomy, competence, and interests or activities outside the
safety of the family. The children, in turn, particularly the psychosomatically ill
child, feel great responsibility for protecting the family" (Minuchin et al., 1978,
p. 31). *Lack of conflict resolution,* finally, refers to an absence of negotiation in
the family, which can take either the form of avoidance of all conflicts because
of the myth of family unity, or the form of continuous quarrelling without ever
reaching a solution because of constant interruptions and subject changes. *The
involvement of the child in parental conflicts* reinforces the symptoms, once they
occur. The authors differentiate three patterns of involvement. In the first two
patterns "triangulation" and "parent-child coalitions," the spouse dyad is in
open conflict. In triangulation, the child is put in such a position that she cannot express herself without siding with one parent against the other. In the
parent-child coalition pattern, there exists a fixed coalition with one parent
against the other. In the third pattern, "detouring," the parents hide their marital conflicts by protecting their ill child, who is defined as their only problem
but in fact is the only reason why they stay together.

Norris and Jones (1979) appreciate the contribution of Minuchin and his co-
workers to the analysis of the necessary properties within families for the emergence of the illness. Nevertheless they suggest that "Minuchin's model is an incomplete one as it does not take cognisance of processes within the sufferer herself or of involvement of the patient in dyadic subsystems" (p. 108). Some ad-
herents of Minuchin's structural psychosomatic family model seem to have realized these shortcomings. More recently, Sargent (1983) published an article
in which individual psychological and physiological mediating mechanisms in

the vulnerable child, as well as extra-marital stresses were added to the open systems model of psychosomatic disease.

Family Psychodynamics

Similarly to Minuchin's psychosomatic family model, Helm Stierlin and his associates in Heidelberg (West Germany), developed a theoretical framework for psychosomatic disorders in general (see Stierlin, 1983; Winawer, 1983; Wirsching & Stierlin, 1985). A combined psychodynamic and systemic picture of the etiology and pathogenesis of anorexia nervosa is presented by Weber and Stierlin (1981). They discuss five dynamic interaction features which reoccurred regularly in anorexic families. The first characteristic, *loose individual boundaries,* resembles Minuchin's concept of enmeshment. Weber and Stierlin (1981) compare these families with a house in which all inner doors are continuously open, even the one of the parents' bedroom, but the outer door is continuously locked. This metaphor symbolizes the family clan in which individuation is hampered. The second characteristic, associated with this lack of individual boundaries, is *emotional bonding as most important mode of interaction.* The authors differentiate an Es, Ego and Super-Ego aspect in this second feature. The Es aspect refers to the sublimation of sexuality into care for the other family members and for the family as a whole. The Ego aspect is the disencouragement of all strivings for autonomy. The Super-Ego aspect finally refers to the tie of loyalty that the anorexic girl invisibly connects with her both parents. The third characteristic, *delegation,* further elaborates this loyalty bond. The anorexic girl is the enormously duty- and prestation-minded delegate, who is willing to pay any price in order to realize even the most excessive parental expectancies. Fourthly, the loyalty bond and the self-sacrifice drive overlap generations. They are transgenerational strivings. *The status of reciprocity,* as final characteristic, is transgenerational too. It is based upon the myth that there is not enough for everyone in the family. Consequently, giving is better than taking, and someone who dares to take somewhat more than the others (maybe enjoys somewhat more) loses control. There exists a hidden rivalry between the sisters in the family. The mother of the anorexic patient constantly felt destituted, compared with her sister. The pre-anorexic girl was identified with this sister. So, she was driven in an act of complete self-sacrifice in order "to give rather than to take." In fact, one or more of the siblings is benefited and the pre-anorexic daughter feels a big lack of attention. But this differentiation in the family is not accepted. On the contrary, equality is stressed.

Then, Weber and Stierlin (1981) discuss four characteristics in order to explain the *vicious circle* in which the family gets entangled once the anorexic syndrom starts.

1. The separation during adolescence is complicated because of the fear of the parents to have nothing left anymore; a fear which they verbalize

frequently. The children, and especially the anorexic daughter, also worry about their parents because they feel they indeed have nothing in common but their children.

2. The anorexic girl tries to get the approval and attention by means of playing the perfect child. But, sooner or later, father or mother is more interested in someone else and the anorexic girl feels betrayed.

3. The complementarity changes in symmetry. All the patient's pride, frustration and revenge are mobilized against her family. She will live her own life and decide what she wants from now on.

4. The communicative meaning of the starvation, finally, is a dramatic appeal (I die, I need food) but a refusal at the same time. It is as if the anorexic girl wants to say, "I need something but not that what you want to give me; I need attention and acknowledgement." However, the starvation results in attention and she chooses the safest way. Staying ill guarantees further attention which she might loose by getting better. Moreover, the family is unified again because of the illness.

These are the motors that drive the illness, according to Weber and Stierlin (1981).

DISCUSSION

The preceeding overview is far from exhaustive since there are maybe as many theories as there are authors who have been fascinated by the "enigma of anorexia nervosa" (Bruch, 1978). And that number keeps on growing! Through the recent bulk of publications, anorexia nervosa got the reputation of being *the* paradigmatic psychosomatic disorder in which a family dysfunction is expressed by the symptomatology of the child. The anorexic patient is no longer a piteous victim but a kind of misunderstood hero who acts as the secret family rebel, challenging patriarchal, collectivist, and self-sacrificial values and morals of traditional families who are caught in the whirlpool of postindustrial civilization. Anorexia nervosa is thus conceived as an escape from (or a protest against) our affluent, overnourished and materialistic society with its conflicting changing attitudes toward (female) sex role, and its overaccentuation of efficiency and achievement (Vandereycken & Meermann, 1984a).

But, neither the researcher nor the practitioner can expect progress from vague and unspecific slogans. Practically all theories we have reviewed are based on clinical observations and impressionistic explorations rather than on methodologically reliable research (Kog et al., 1983). Moreover, many etiological theories are post-factum constructs usually inspired by a small or selected sample of patients. Regardless its appealing character, Bruch's (1973, 1978) conceptualization for instance, of the anorexic's family background and related deficiency in ego-development is an etiological model typically based on (a) a non-specific stereotyped overgeneralization, (b) a clinical-impressionistic, retpective reconstruction, (c) relying on the patient's actual perception of her past, and (d) as evoked in a psychotherapeutic context (Vandereycken & Meermann, 1984b). This criticism applies to most of the theories mentioned above.

It seems that many theorists are still looking for the "typical" family profile. Even when they defend their etiological or pathogenic constructs by referring to empirical data (see Chapter 3), they usually overlook the basic fault of mistaking statistical or clinical correlation for causality. We must, therefore, be particularly aware of the danger of presenting "old" psychosomatic personality typologies in a "new" dress. Otherwise, this may lead to stereotyped interpretations with a certain risk of abusing theoretical concepts as, for example in the case of "psychohistory" wherein psychoanalytic ideas are often misused for the reinterpretation of historical events or figures. The same danger as to family theories is not imaginary. Lewis (1982), for instance, diagnosed the Victorian poet Elisabeth Barrett Browning as having anorexia nervosa because her family showed "abundantly" the typical structural features described by Minuchin more than hundred years later! To put our discussion in a nutshell, let's turn *from myths to facts* (Vandereycken, 1980). Then, theories must always be regarded as a set of hypothetical constructs waiting for empirical verification. The proverbial saying, that "there's nothing so practical as a good theory" may guide us in the choice of a theoretical framework. As advocated (Chapter 1), we prefer a multidimensional perspective in eating disorders which we like to investigate and to treat in a "scientist-practitioner" spirit.

In this sense, family theories can and should inspire further research. As an example of such an approach, we like to mention the working hypotheses Sights and Richards (1984) offered in the case of bulimic women, of whom they speculated (in comparison with normal females) that:

1. their parents are more demanding;
2. their mothers maintain higher than average expectations for their daughters' academic and social success;
3. their parents foster high levels of sibling rivalry by comparing their children more openly;
4. their mothers exhibit more problems related to behavioral control (e.g., domineering, drinking, overeating, etc.);
5. their fathers exhibit such characteristics as depression, rigidity, excessive self-discipline, and emotional distance from others;
6. a great deal of mental conflict occurs in their families;
7. their parents' sexual relationships are problematic;
8. there exist high levels of tension in their homes;
9. there exist high levels of parent-daughter stress in these families;
10. their fathers are likely to become increasingly distant over the course of development.

One may, of course, propose with as much or little probability another series of hypotheses. Each theoretical proposition, however, must be judged on two questions: Is it verifiable? Is it clinically relevant? Therefore, we expect fruitful answers from a constructive dialogue between the scientist and the practitioner. But who will bridge the gap between them?

REFERENCES*

Berger, M. (1977), Zur Psychodynamik der Mutter-Kind-Beziehung bei psycho-somatischen Er-krankungen von Sauglingen, Kindern und Juchendlichen (About the psychodynamics of mother-child relationship in psychosomatic diseases in infants, children and adolescents). *Zeitschrift fur Kinder- und Jugendpsychiatrie*, 5:151-154.

Boskind-Lodahl, M. (1976), Cinderella's stepsisters: A feminist perspective on anorexia nervosa and bulimia. *Signs, Journal of Women in Culture and Society*, 2:342-356.

Bruch, H. (1973), *Eating Disorders. Obesity, Anorexia Nervosa, and the Person Within*. New York: Basic Books.

Bruch, H. (1978), *The Golden Cage: The Enigma of Anorexia Nervosa*. Cambridge (Massachusetts): Harvard University Press.

Crisp, A.H., Hsu, L.K.G., Harding, B. & Hartshorn, J. (1980), Clinical features of anorexia ner-vosa. A study of a consecutive series of 102 female patients. *Journal of Psychosomatic Research*, 24:179-191.

Dally, P.J. (1969), *Anorexia Nervosa*. London: William Heinemann.

Friedman, M. (1985), Survivor guilt in the pathogenesis of anorexia nervosa. *Psychiatry*, 48:25-39.

Garfinkel, P. & Garner, D. (1982), *Anorexia Nervosa. A Multidimensional Perspective*. New York: Brunner/Mazel.

Jackson, C.C. (1986), The anorexic patient as a survivor: The denial of death and death themes in the literature on anorexia nervosa. *International Journal of Eating Disorders*, 5:821-835.

Jackson, D. & Satir, V. (1961), A review of psychiatric developments in family diagnosis and family therapy. In: N. Ackerman, F. Beatmen & S. Sherman (Eds.), *Exploring the Base for Family Therapy*. New York: Family Service Association of America, pp. 29-51.

Kestemberg, E., Kestemberg, J. & Decobert, S. (1972), *La Faim et le Corps. Une Etude Psycha-nalytique de l'Anorexie Mentale* (The hunger and the body. A psychoanalytic study of anorexia nervosa). Paris: Presses Universitaires de France.

Kramer, S. (1974), A discussion of the paper by John A. Sours on "The anorexia syndrome." *International Journal of Psycho-Analysis*, 55:557-579.

McPeak, W.R. (1975), Family interaction as etiological factors in mental disorders: An analysis of the *American Journal of Insanity*, 1844-1848. *American Journal of Psychiatry*, 132:1327-1329.

Richardson, H.B. (1945), *Patients Have Families*. New York: The Commonwealth Fund. (Chapter Four, *The family equilibrium*, has been reprinted, with an editorial introduction, in *Family Systems Medicine*, 1983, 1(1):62-74).

Sargent, J. (1983), The family and childhood psychosomatic disorders. *General Hospital Psychiatry*, 5:41-48.

Stierlin, H. (1983), Family dynamics in psychotic and severe psychosomatic disorders: A comparison. *Family Systems Medicine*, 1(4):41-50.

Sours, J.A. (1974), The anorexia nervosa syndrome. *International Journal of Psycho-Analysis*, 55:567-572.

Sours, J.A. (1980), *Starving to Death in a Sea of Objects. The Anorexia Nervosa Syndrome*. New York: Jason Aronson.

Vandereycken, W. & Meermann, R. (1984a), *Anorexia Nervosa. A Clinician's Guide to Treatment*. Berlin/New York: Walter de Gruyter.

---

* This list contains only secondary literature, whereas the other references are mentioned in the final section of this book: "Bibliography on Family Aspects of Eating Disorders."

Vandereycken, W. & Meermann, R. (1984b), Anorexia nervosa: Is prevention possible? *International Journal of Psychiatry in Medicine,* 14:191-205.

Wirsching, M. & Stierlin, H. (1985), Psychosomatics. I. Psychosocial characteristics of psychosomatic patients and their families. *Family Systems Medicine,* 3:6-16.

Winawer, H. (1983), The Heidelberg concept: An introduction to the work of Helm Stierlin and his associates. *Family Systems Medicine,* 1(4):36-40.

Chapter 3

The Facts: A Review of Research Data on Eating Disorder Families*

Elly Kog and Walter Vandereycken

INTRODUCTION

Among the many etiological theories on anorexia nervosa and bulimia, considerations about the pathogenic role of the family have attracted much attention in recent years (Hsu, 1983). A review of the research literature on this issue may focus on different family variables that are supposed to play a role in the development and course of eating disorders (Garfinkel & Garner, 1982; Kalucy, 1983; Rakoff, 1983; Yager, 1981, 1982; Yager & Strober, 1985):

1. genetic variables,
2. demographic variables,
3. different forms of individual pathology in the family,
4. specific types of family relationships, and
5. family factors related to treatment and prognosis.

Although the methodological weakness that affected the greatest part of the family research is often stressed in previous reviews, its impact upon the existing (lack of) knowledge in this area has been overlooked. However, one may obtain totally different results when using even slightly different methods for the study of the same family variables, as is illustrated by Walker et al. (1984) and Oliveri and Reiss (1984). Moreover, the research purpose of studies investigating the same variables may differ fundamentally, an issue which applies especially to family interaction data (the linear-circular causality controversy; see Kog et al., 1983).

---

* This chapter is a revision of a previously published article: "Family characteristics of anorexia nervosa and bulimia: A review of the research literature" (*Clinical Psychology Review,* 1985, 5:159-180).

25

For these reasons, we critically analyzed the available literature with respect to research methodology. We do not discuss single-case studies or purely descriptive investigations of an undifferentiated group of eating disorder patients. At the least a systematic intergroup comparison is required for the incorporation of the study in this analysis, except for some publications concerning variables 1 and 5. Detailed technical information on the design of the selected investigations – concerning variables 2, 3, 4 and 5 – are summarized in the Appendix. We differentiated four types of studies. The *clinical studies* use data, gathered from hospital records, personal interviews, or questionnaires (on personality or general psychosocial functioning). When such studies compare different eating disorder families with normal families or other psychiatric families, we call them *intergroup comparisons* (type I). Systematic comparisons between various eating disorder families are categorized as *intragroup comparisons* (type II). The *self-report studies* (type III) investigate the viewpoint of the family members themselves with regard to certain family relations, or the family interaction in general, on the basis of specific family questionnaires. In the *observational studies* (type IV), intrafamilial interaction is directly observed and assessed by independent observers. Finally, *therapy studies* (type V) investigate family factors related to the therapeutic process in general or study the outcome of family therapy in eating disorder patients.

Our discussion of the state of the art and the perspectives for the future of family research in this area is organized around five types of variables:
1. genetic factors (concordance rates for eating disorders in twins);
2. demographic characteristics (social class, parental age at the time of patient's birth, incidence of broken homes, patient's birth order);
3. individual pathology in the family (weight and eating problems, somatic illnesses, psychiatric disorders);
4. family relationships (family interaction characteristics as experienced by the family members themselves or analyzed by external observers);
5. family factors related to treatment and prognosis.

The very few studies on married patients are mentioned in Chapter 10 and 17.

A major methodological problem concerns the lack (at least before the 1970s) of generally accepted *diagnostic criteria* for anorexia nervosa and related eating disorders such as bulimia. For research purposes, the criteria of Feighner et al. (1972) have been used quite often, but they are rather restrictive by excluding the older and the less emaciated patients (Rollins & Piazza, 1978; Vandereycken & Meermann, 1984a). In recent years, the DSM-III criteria (American Psychiatric Association, 1980) are preferred, but they exclude the milder cases of anorexia nervosa in children because of a too high standard of weight loss (Irwin, 1981). Halmi (1983) criticized the DSM-III criteria as to the relationship between anorexia nervosa and bulimia. The latter is described both as a symptom (binge eating) in anorexics and as a separate syndrome to be distinguished from anorexia nervosa. It is still unclear if binge eating, which is usually alternated with periods of vomiting/purging and/or fasting, has to be interpreted as a sub-type of anorexia nervosa or as a distinct eating disorder (Schlesier-Stropp, 1984). That is why we summarize the family research on three types of eating disorders as either the restricting anorexics ("pure" dieters), the bulimic ano-rexics (those who also binge, vomit and/or purge; cf. Vandereycken & Pierloot, 1983b), and the normal-weight bulimics (with or without a previous history of anorexia nervosa; i.e., "bulimia nervosa" according to G. Russell, 1979).

GENETIC FACTORS

From the biological point of view, there seems an ever-increasing interest in conducting research to adduce arguments in support of some innate predisposi-tion to anorexia nervosa (Vandereycken & Meermann, 1984a). First, in this re-spect, there is a bulk of literature on the question of primary or secondary hy-pothalamic dysfunction in anorexics. Next, some controversy was raised by a series of reports on the coincidence of anorexia nervosa and gonadal dysgene-sis, especially Turner's syndrome. Finally, the issue of inheritability is currently receiving much attention, particularly with regard to the fact that families of an-orexia nervosa and bulimia patients appear to show a higher than expected oc-currence of eating disorders, affective disorders and substance use disorders (see further individual pathology in the family). Such association of disorders within a family, however, does not automatically imply a genetic link or hered-itary predisposition since the disorders may be shaped by a common en-vironmental pathogenesis. The same applies to the finding of mother-child con-cordance for anorexia nervosa or an overrepresentation of anorexia nervosa in siblings (see Garfinkel & Garner, 1982; Fichter, 1985).

The best known method for determining whether an eating disorder has a genetic component is the comparison of homozygous versus heterogous twins or, even better, the comparison of homozygous twins reared together versus those reared apart. Several reports have been published on twins with anorexia nervosa (for review see: Askevold & Heiberg, 1979; Vandereycken & Pierloot, 1981; Garfinkel & Garner, 1982; Nowlin, 1983; Schepank, 1981, 1983; Fichter, 1985). The following recent case reports have not been included in these re-views: Elbadawy et al. (1985); Hsu et al., 1984; Moskovitz et al. (1982) and Steinberg (1982). Depending on the strictness of selection (especially the cri-teria for diagnosis and zygosity) 30 to 50% of the reported homozygotic twins were found to be concordant for anorexia nervosa. But a comparison of these cases is hampered by many shortcomings. First of all, the literature may be biased by an underreporting of discordant cases. Indeed, a concordance of an-orexia nervosa in twins is so unusual and striking for the clinician that he may be more probably inclined to report such cases while neglecting the discordant ones. Moreover, different criteria have been used for diagnosing anorexia ner-vosa and confirming homozygosity. Most of these methodological problems

have been avoided in a collaborative study between St. George's and the Maudsley Hospitals in London (Crisp et al., 1985; Holland et al., 1984). These researchers identified 34 pairs of twins and one set of triplets in which the proband had anorexia nervosa. They found a concordance rate of 9/16 in the homozygotic and 1/14 in the heterozygotic female twin pairs.

An unusual concordance of anorexia nervosa in twins may be considered as
an argument in favor of the "genetic predisposition theory", a presumed genetic
vulnerability as to psychiatric illness in general (particularly affective disorder),
a specific personality type, a disturbance of body image, or a hypothalamic dysfunctioning. But a "psychosocial induction theory" cannot be ruled out, i.e., that
common psychological processes and environmental influences may explain the
occurrence of anorexia nervosa in more than one member of the family. Hence,
the old *"nature versus nurture"* debate remains unsolved. Only the adoptive
method of research (a comparison of homozygous twins reared apart) seems
appropriate to allow any conclusion about the role of inheritance in anorexia
nervosa or other eating disorders.

DEMOGRAPHIC CHARACTERISTICS

These data are usually based on a retrospective analysis of hospital records
(e.g., Kay & Leigh, 1954). The information is mostly unreliable and not comparable because of a considerable variability in diagnostic criteria over time,
and because the investigated variables themselves are historically determined
(e.g., the incidence of broken homes has changed strikingly during the last decades). The clinician-researcher should collect data on the basis of information
obtained from the patients and/or their families by means of a well-structured
interview or a questionnaire, and over a limited time period (e.g., Kalucy et al.,
1977). But even this information has little significance if it is not compared with
an appropriate control group. Theander (1970), Hall (1978), Halmi (1974a),
Halmi and Loney (1973), Mester (1981a), and Morgan and Russell (1975) did
compare some of their findings with data on the general population, but this
control is too general. For these reasons, we confine our analysis to a series of
well controlled studies.

Social Class

The over-representation of the higher social class, as reported by descriptive
clinical studies, has been validated by well controlled research. Askevold (1982)
compared a group of 112 anorexia nerosa patients with 54 female physically ill
inpatients and a sample of 354 psychosomatic patients. Significantly more anorexia nervosa patients belonged to the higher social classes than in the control
groups. The findings of Heron and Leheup (1984) do not support the previous
results, but their groups were very small. The 16 anorexia nervosa patients came

from families of all social classes and there was no significant difference within the group of 40 problematic adolescents.

Nevertheless, there seems to be some variability when various subgroups of eating disorders are compared. Bruch (1973) subdivided her sample in primary anorexia nervosa and atypical anorexia nervosa and noted more upper-class families in the primary anorexia nervosa group, 56.9% versus 26.3% in the atypical group. Garfinkel et al. (1980) found no significant difference between restricting and bulimic anorexics. Vandereycken and Pierloot (1983b), on the other hand, note that bulimic anorexics tended to come more frequently (61.9%) from the lower social class than did the pure dieters (35.4%). Herzog (1982) and Casper et al. (1980) found conflicting results. Bulimia patients without a previous history of anorexia nervosa appeared to have a higher family income compared with anorexic patients (Herzog, 1982). Anorexia nervosa patients who vomited (which is usually related to bulimia) showed a higher social class background than pure restricting anorexics (Casper et al., 1980). The different geographical situation of these studies (Belgium, United States, and Canada), the divergent definition and classifications of social classes as well as the use of different diagnostic criteria could account for these discrepancies.

Comparing male and female anorexics, Vandereycken and Van den Broucke (1984) found no difference in social class, but a cluster analysis of the male cases revealed that social class might be an important discriminative factor. Three variants could be distinguished: (a) a lower-class variant, the patients of which are characterized by very serious weight loss whereas their siblings often show psychiatric problems and in a considerable number one parent is deceased; (b) a middle class variant, in which less pronounced anorexia nervosa symptoms are combined with family problems, namely a broken home situation, and a high incidence of eating/weight problems in the siblings; (c) a (pre)pubertal variant, in which the patients are fairly young at the onset of the disorder and stem from all social classes and from families without apparent psychiatric disorders or eating/weight problems.

Parental Age at the Patient's Birth

Several descriptive studies (Bruch, 1973; Hall, 1978; Halmi, 1974a; Theander, 1970) reported a higher parental age at the time of the proband's birth. But Weiss and Ebert (1983) found no significant difference between normal-weight bulimics and normal controls.

The parent's age did not differ between bulimic and restricting anorexics (Casper et al., 1980; Garfinkel et al., 1980). Moreover, the significance of this variable may be questioned since a higher parental age seems to apply to several psychiatric disorders (Hare & Moran, 1979).

Patient's Birth Order

As to the variable of birth order, no consistent pattern is found in the descriptive literature, although in the first reports of large samples, firstborns as well as lastborns were observed more frequently than children occupying a middle position (Bruch, 1973; Crisp et al., 1980; Halmi, 1974a; Theander, 1970). A recent descriptive study of a large sample of anorexia nervosa patients (Gowers et al., 1985) revealed, however, no systematic birth order of the patient. But there are very few comparative studies on this subject. Weiss and Ebert (1983) found no significant differences in birth order between normal-weight bulimics and controls.

Regarding the same variable, bulimic and restricting anorexics do not differ (Garfinkel et al., 1980; Vandereycken & Pierloot, 1983), nor do normal-weight bulimics versus anorexics (Herzog, 1982).

Incidence of Broken Homes

This factor seems to vary considerably among the studies, probably because of sociocultural influences. Bruch (1973) mentioned but two cases of parental separation in her sample, which is an unusually low incidence (3%), given the divorce rate in the United States. Halmi (1974a) noticed that even an incidence of 18% in her sample is still significantly lower than in the general U.S. population. Similarly, Heron and Leheup (1984), in Great Britain, reported 18% incidence of broken homes for the anorexia nervosa group, which was lower than 32% for the problematic adolescent control group, but this difference was not significant because of the small sample sizes.

Halmi (1974b) compared two subgroups of anorexic patients as to this variable, those who were of normal weight before emaciation and those who were premorbidly obese. A broken home situation due to loss of one or both parents prior to illness was significantly more frequent in the first (22%) than in the second subgroup (10%).

INDIVIDUAL PATHOLOGY IN THE FAMILY

Weight and Eating Problems

The higher incidence of weight and eating problems in anorexic families, as mentioned in descriptive reports (e.g., Bruch, 1973; Crisp et al., 1980; Theander, 1970), is confirmed by some controlled studies but not by others. Strober et al. (1985) state: "However, in the absence of equivalent methods of cohort sampling, case ascertainment, and diagnosis of relatives, it is hardly surprising that there is marked inconsistency between studies in the reported incidence of eating disorders in relatives of affected individuals, ranging from 3 to 27%" (p.

239). Gershon et al. (1983) found significantly more eating disorders (anorexia nervosa or bulimia) in first-degree relatives (fathers, mothers, brothers, and sisters) of patients with anorexia nervosa or bulimia in comparison with medical patients, but groups were not matched for social class. Though anorexics often state they fear to become overweight like some close relative, usually the mother, Halmi et al. (1978) could not find a significant difference in the weight of their parents compared with control parents, although a significant relation existed between educational status, the higher the parental weight. Strober et al. (1985) did match anorexic and control probands (psychiatrically ill patients) for age and social class and they found significantly more cases of anorexia nervosa and other eating disorders (except bulimia nervosa) in first- and second-degree relatives of the anorexics. Garfinkel et al. (1983) compared the families of restricting and bulimic anorexics with control families, matched for social class. No differences were found as to the parents' actual weight, body size estimates, and body satisfaction. The study by Hall and Brown (1983), however, revealed a significant difference in the attitude toward thinness between the mothers of anorexia nervosa patients and mothers of normal controls. The patients' mothers rated thinness for themselves as worse than did the control mothers. In a recent study, Hall et al. (1986) compared weight history and attitudes toward weight-related matters in mothers of anorexia nervosa patients and mothers of schoolgirls of similar age and socioeconomic status. No differences were found, and mothers of anorexics even showed a lower concern about weight-related matters. This may, however, reflect a certain denial or minimization. Looking for problems in the sisters, Maloney and Shepart-Spiro (1983) compared the eating attitudes and behaviors of the closest-in-age sister with those of the anorexic patient and of normal controls. The scores on the Eating Attitudes Test for the sisters differed significantly from the patients but not from those of normal controls.

When different eating disorder groups are compared, there is cumulative evidence that the incidence of obesity is greater in the parents of the bulimic subgroups (bulimic anorexics and normal-weight bulimics) than in the parents of the restricting anorexics. In the study of Garfinkel et al. (1980), a history of obesity is observed in 48% of the mothers of bulimic anorexics and in 28% of the mothers of their restricting counterparts (a significant difference at the .05 level). Though Strober (1981) reported similar findings, the difference of 40% versus 18% was not significant. Paternal obesity is also more common in bulimic than in restricting anorexics, although the difference did not reach significance in Strober's study (1981), nor in that of Garfinkel et al. (1980). Herzog (1982) compared bulimia patients (without a previous history of anorexia nervosa) with anorexia nervosa patients and noted obesity in at least one parent in 37% of the bulimics and 10% of the anorexics (a significant difference at the .01 level). Strober et al. (1985) also noted more first- and second-degree relatives with an eating disorder in bulimic anorexics, compared with their restricting counterparts. Moreover, there seemed to be a specificity of transmission of bulimia within the families of bulimic anorexics because in 7.6% (an age-corrected percentage) of the female relatives, bulimic anorexics manifested bulimia (with or without anorexia nervosa) compared with 1.1.% of the female relatives of restricting anorexics. However, Gershon et al. (1984) found no significant difference in the incidence of eating disorders in the first-degree relatives of the following groups: anorexia nervosa patients with (7.3%) and without bulimia (5.9%), or patients with (6.4%) and without self-induced vomiting (6.6%). Nevertheless, there seemed to exist a certain specificity for the occurrence of bulimia in the group of patients with bulimic anorexia nervosa and with self-induced vomiting, because their relatives showed bulimic rather than purely anorexic symptoms, while relatives of anorexia nervosa patients without bulimia and without self-induced vomiting showed as much anorexic as bulimic symptoms.

Somatic Illnesses

The data on this topic are difficult to interpret. Sperling and Massing (1970) found a highly significant difference between the 25% incidence of chronic illnesses in the fathers of anorexic patients, compared with 2.4% in a normal control group. Chronic illness was defined as being in continuing medical care for a disease, but it remains unclear what kind of illness (physical or psychiatric) this concerned. Moreover, these results are based on a retrospective analysis of hospital records. Weiss and Ebert (1983) noted no statistically significant difference between normal-weight bulimics and normal-weight controls in the number of hospitalizations for physical illness in their families, nor in the incidence of allergic disorders and asthma. Hall and Brown (1983) reported a significantly more favored attitude toward illness (feeling sick, having pain in the stomach) in anorexic patients and their mothers, compared with normal controls and their mothers.

Although this variable has not been compared so often among eating disorder subgroups, the existing evidence shows a similar tendency. Strober (1981) noticed significantly more serious physical illness at some point during the proband's childhood in bulimic anorexics (45%) than in restricting patients (14%). Gastro-intestinal illness was not found to be a discriminative factor, although tending to be more prevalent in parents of bulimics, 14% versus 5% in the mothers and 32% versus 14% in the fathers. Similarly, Herzog (1982) found that 50% of the bulimic patients had at least one parent with serious morbidity or mortality due to physical illness, versus only 23% of the anorexics.

Psychiatric Disorders

General Psychopathology
Although psychopathology in the parents is considered an important etiologic element for the development of the disorder (see Chapter 2), the existence of psychopathologic features in the parents has hardly been confirmed by

controlled research. Weiss and Ebert (1983) found no difference in the number of hospitalizations for psychiatric disorders between normal-weight bulimics and normal-weight controls. Similarly, Garfinkel et al. (1983) could not establish any significant difference between the mothers of bulimic or restricting
anorexics and normal controls on a series of psychological tests. Only the anorexics' fathers scored higher on conscientiousness. Whatever the significance
of this finding, it remains a tentative one in view of the fact that a few fathers
did not complete the questionnaire and, therefore, may have biased the results
toward an increased obsessionality in the fathers who participated. The overall
conclusion is that, according to the psychological test results, there is little psychopathology evident in the parents of anorexia nervosa patients. Similar results were obtained by Crisp et al. (1974). They compared the parents of anorexic patients with a series of normal parents on the Middlesex Hospital Questionnaire. The parents of the patient group only scored lower on the somatic
scale and higher on the hysteria scale and even these differences were not great.

The results of studies comparing different subgroups of eating disorders are
inconsistent. Garfinkel et al. (1980) found no differences in terms of history of
parental mental illness between bulimic anorexics and their restricting counterparts. Strober (1981), however, reported significant differences between these
groups: 50% of the mothers and 50% of the fathers of bulimic anorexics evidenced some manifestation of psychiatric disorder versus 18% and 14% in the
group of restricters. On the MMPI, the fathers of bulimic anorexics showed
more signs of a personality disorder (hostility, immaturity, impulsiveness and
dyscontrol), whereas fathers of restricters were characterized by greater reserve
and passivity. Mothers of bulimics exhibited more pronounced depression,
hostility and emotional dissatisfaction with intrafamilial problems, while emerging as less socially introverted, submissive and neurotically tense.

Affective Disorders

Several investigators found considerable evidence for presence of affective
disorder in relatives of patients with anorexia nervosa or bulimia. Hudson et al.
(1983), studying the incidence of affective disorder in first-degree relatives, reported an incidence of 27% in the eating disorder groups versus 12% for the
bipolar affective disorder group, 1% for the schizophrenic group, and 3% for
the borderline personality disorder group. The difference was not significant
between the first two groups, but highly significant between these two and the
latter two. Winokur et al. (1980) compared anorexic patients with normal
women. Twenty-two percent of the first- and second-degree relatives of the
patients had a clear history of primary affective disorder versus only 10% in the
control group. This incidence appears to be similar to that reported in family
studies of probands with primary affective disorders, suggesting some (perhaps
genetic) relationship between anorexia nervosa and affective disorders, according to these authors. However, any direct biological-genetic link has not been

demonstrated. There was no specific distribution in terms of generation or relationship, but more female (30%) than male relatives (13%) had a history of
primary affective disorder. Rivinus et al. (1984) found a lower frequency of affective disorders. Ten percent in the first-degree relatives of anorexia nervosa
patients and 2.0% in the first-degree relatives of controls. These findings are
consistent with these of Gershon et al. (1983) who also calculated age-corrected
percentages. The morbid risk of depression in the parents is then 21.6%. Gershon et al. (1983) studied first-degree relatives of patients with anorexia nervosa or bulimia, in comparison with medical patients. They found significantly
more affective disorders in the relatives of the patient group (22%) than in the
controls (7%). In contrast with the previously reported authors, Stern et al.
(1984) noted a nonsignificant difference between the lifetime prevalence of affective disorder in first- and second-degree relatives of normal-weight bulimics
(10%) and normal controls (9%). This contrasting result is the more interesting because the authors used a sound methodology: i.e., independent personal
interviews with mother and proband by interviewers who were blind to the proband's diagnosis. The previously mentioned studies also used personal interviews where possible, but interviewers were not blind to the probands' diagnoses.

Eating disorder subgroups seem to differ with regard to this variable. Piran
et al. (1985) noted a significant difference between the percentage of bulimic
patients who had at least one first-degree relative either hospitalized for depression or receiving anti-depressant medication (61%), and the percentage of
restricters with a positive family history of depression (23%). Strober (1981)
found a similar difference but his percentages are lower in both groups, maybe
because he only investigated the parents. However, when the mothers and the
fathers are considered together, the difference in the proportions of bulimic
and restricting anorexics with a positive family history of affective disorder (41%
and 14%, respectively) proved significant at the .10 level. In another investigation, Strober et al. (1982) found an incidence of affective disorder in first- or
second-degree relatives of 13% of the bulimic and 6% of the restricting anorexics (significant at the .01 level). The same authors noted a fourfold difference
in the prevalence of maternal affective disorder: 23% of the mothers of bulimic
anorexics versus 6% of the mothers of restricters. Likewise, affective disorders
were more prevalent in fathers of bulimic anorexics, but it did not yield a significant difference. Hudson et al. (1983) reported a high prevalence of affective
disorder in the first-degree relatives of all eating disorder groups and did not
find any significant difference between the three subgroups, anorexia nervosa
(31%), bulimia (26%), and both together (28%). The authors consider these
results as growing evidence that anorexia nervosa and bulimia are closely
(geneticly?) related to affective disorder. But how could one explain the following results? Dally (1977) differentiated three subgroups according to the age at
onset, 11-14, 15-18, and 19 onwards. He found a highly significant difference in

the occurrence of depression in the mothers. Three quarters of the youngest anorexia nervosa patients had depressed mothers. This was significantly greater than in other age groups, which did not differ from one another on this variable. Depression in the fathers was found in a quarter of the youngest patients, and this was also more common than in the other age groups. Although these results are based on hospital records and thus less reliable, they draw attention to the possible significance of interactional problems, related with the patient's age, as a discriminative factor.

Substance Use Disorders

Some uncontrolled studies (Halmi & Loney, 1973; Collins et al., 1985) suggest a higher than expected rate of familial alcoholism in (bulimic) anorexia nervosa patients. But Winokur et al. (1980) found a lower incidence of alcohol abuse in relatives of anorexic patients (4%) than in relatives of normal controls (7%). On the contrary, Rivinus et al. (1984) observed a substance use disorder in at least one of the relatives of 12.5% of the patients and in 8% of the controls. The most consistent results were obtained from comparison of the pooled diagnosis of depression, alcoholism and drug use disorders, which occurred significantly more frequently in the first- and second-degree relatives of anorexia nervosa patients.

The investigators who compared different eating disorder subgroups noted a higher incidence in the bulimic patients' relatives. In the study of Hudson et al. (1983), alcohol use disorders were second in prevalence to affective disorders and accounted for respectively 5.7%, 9%, and 17% of the first-degree relatives of anorexia nervosa patients, bulimia patients, and both groups mixed. Strober et al. (1982) found a prevalence of alcoholism in first-degree relatives of 16% of the bulimic anorexics (comparable with Hudson's mixed group) and in 4% of restricting anorexics (comparable with Hudson's first group). Thus, findings of both studies support each other. Strober et al. (1982) also reported a significant difference (.05 level) for prevalence of alcoholism in the fathers of bulimic anorexics, compared with their restricting counterparts. For the mothers, no significant difference was found. These results confirm the findings of an earlier study (Strober, 1981). Concerning the comparison between anorexia nervosa and bulimia patients, Herzog (1982) noted a high incidence of alcoholism in first-degree relatives of both groups, 20% and 33% respectively; a difference which is not significant. Piran et al. (1985) found a similar nonsignificant tendency for bulimic patients to show a higher frequency of alcoholism in first-degree relatives: 32% versus 15% of the anorexia nervosa patients.

Drug use disorders seem to be far less prevalent than affective disorders and alcoholism. Their occurrence in first-degree relatives is not significantly different among eating disorder subgroups: 6% for bulimic anorexics and 1% for restricting anorexics in the study of Strober et al. (1982); 3% for anorexia nervosa,

1% for bulimia, and 2% for mixed anorexia nervosa/bulimia in the study of Hudson et al. (1983).

FAMILY RELATIONSHIPS

Clinicians often observed a too tightly knit family structure and a poor parental relationship in anorexia nervosa families, but the methods used to study these variables (mostly information from medical records) were inadequate in a great number of these studies. In most cases we can only speak from clinical impressions. Many of the newer concepts and measurement techniques in the field of family theory are just now beginning to be applied to eating disorders. Crisp et al. (1980) found a disturbed premorbid relationship between patient and parents in over half of their 102 anorexia nervosa cases, and this was often related to a disturbed parental relationship. In the presence of a poor parental relationship, the relationship between patient and one or both parents often became enmeshed, with the mother in 22% of the cases, with the father in 11% of the cases, and with both of them in 3% of the cases.

But, as Kalucy (1983) stated: "With respect as to why such families should produce illness in their adolescent children, it is important to note that the most commonly described functional and operational problems within such families (e.g., enmeshment) are also described as background factors for a wide range of disorders which frequently show an unusual upsurge and incidence and prevalence in the adolescent phase of development" (p. 132). Even if specificity has been proven, by means of comparative research, one still does not know whether these interaction features are the cause or the consequence of the illness unless one studies highly vulnerable families before the onset of the illness. Up until now, this prospective type of research is totally lacking in eating disorders.

Some clinicians carried out systematic comparisons between eating disorder familes and other types of families, but they studied family relationships indirectly. Using a retrospective analysis of hospital records, Heron and Leheup (1984) tried to specify the *family dynamics* of anorexics compared with problematic adolescents. The anorexics seemed to come significantly more often from an exclusive family, with few external stresses and in which the patients professed to be happy. Sperling and Massing (1970) compared the *role structure* in the family of anorexics and matched normal controls. They noted that in the anorexia nervosa group, the dominant role is situated in more than 50% of the cases outside the nuclear family. It concerned the maternal grandmother in 31% of the cases and in 20.5% of the cases another woman living in the household. In the remaining cases, the mother herself is the dominant person in the family. Significant too, is the percentage of mothers who worked outside the family, 60% of the mothers of anorexics, versus 30% of the control mothers. Moreover, in 25% of the cases, the father was chronically ill. Thus, Sperling and

Massing (1970) observed a marked female dominance in virtually all anorexia nervosa families.

Selvini Palazzoli and coworkers (1974, 1976) studied the family interaction patterns by direct, but uncontrolled observation. She compared the interaction patterns in the families of anorexia nervosa patients and schizophrenics in order to reveal the relationship between anorexic or schizophrenic behavior and the family transaction pattern, within the scope of a noncausal interaction model. She did not use, however, a comparative research design with matched groups and independent observers checked for interobserver reliability to score the interaction pattern. Therapy sessions with anorexic families and schizophrenic families were analyzed by four experienced family therapists in order to formulate some hypotheses about the role or function of the symptoms within the transactional pattern of the family system. The clinical interpretation of the anorexic families generated four major *interactional hypotheses* (see Chapter 2):

(a) there exists an extremely rigid symmetrical type of relation definition in which the anorexic symptom is an ultimate refuge; (b) there is no leading figure in the family and the anorexia nervosa patient does not take the responsibility in this family interaction pattern. Her behavior is out of personal control ("she is ill"); (c) coalitions of two persons against a third one are not accepted; and (d) responsibility for own mistakes is rejected. The anorexic symptom is accepted because the patient cannot help it. The approach by Selvini Palazzoli (1974) has to be regarded as impressionistically explorative, but the clinical hypotheses have to be investigated further by a systematic study of interaction, using a matched control group and a methodologically appropriate assessment procedure.

Family relationships seem to be troublesome for bulimics as well as for anorexics. Johnson and Berndt (1983) compared the results on the *Social Adjustment Scale* of bulimia patients with those of depressed, alcoholic and schizophrenic patients as reported in the literature. The bulimic women exhibited a tendency toward less social impairment than the depressed women, but more impairment than the schizophrenic patients. The bulimics' general pattern of social adjustment was most comparable to that of the alcoholic sample, except for the scale of the adjustment within the family unit, on which the alcoholics scored higher (poorer adjustment). Compared with a normal community sample described in the literature, bulimics scored significantly higher on all the scales, including the relationship with the family, indicating poorer adjustment.

Studying a complex phenomenon such as family interaction will be determined both by theoretical viewpoints and concrete research procedures. We focus the following discussion on the latter, making a distinction between self-report studies addressing the internal perception of family interaction (*the insider's view*) and observational studies assessing the external observation of family interaction (*the outsider's view*). For practical reasons, we further distinguish between intergroup comparisons (eating disorders versus other psychiatric groups or normals) and intragroup comparisons (various subgroups of eating disorders compared with each other).

Internal Perception of Family Interaction

Intergroup Comparisons

Wold (1985) compared 9 bulimic, 8 unipolar depressed patients and 9 normal controls on their *perception of their family's attitude toward weight*. The three groups did not differ in their report of the presence of an overweight family member. However, the bulimic patients differed significantly from the depressed and the control probands on questions dealing with ridiculing overweight people and distress of a family member about being overweight. Since both the control groups and the bulimic group were largely college students, it seemed unlikely that these differences relate to social class or age. This author interpreted her results as an evidence for the hypothesis that the attitude of the family toward weight, an extension of the cultural emphasis on thinness as a beauty ideal, is crucial for the development of an eating disorder, but this investigation requires a replication with larger patient samples.

Hall and Brown (1983) studied the *attitudes toward sickness, arguments, tension, social isolation, thinness, growing up, and being grown-up* in young anorexia nervosa patients and their mothers versus nonpatient schoolgirls and their mothers. The majority of significant differences were found between the total group of the anorexic patients and their mothers, on the one hand, and the total control group of daughters and mothers on the other. Sickness was rated as better and thinness as worse by both anorexic patients and mothers, although the second difference was predominantly due to the mothers' attitude. Patients and mothers seemed to consider arguments in the family and tension as more favored and social isolation as less desired. When the authors compared all the ratings of the daughters with all the ratings of the mothers, both the patient and nonpatient daughters valued thinness more, while to be grown up was valued better by the mothers. When predicting each others' responses, neither the group of mothers nor daughters consistently misjudged each other. The only variable on which mothers and daughters in the patient and nonpatient group differed significantly was on the growing-up variable; the nonpatient daughters believed their mothers would have rated growing up as worse than it actually was. So, these results apparently reject the well known opinion (e.g., Bruch, 1973; Sours, 1980) that anorexic patients are misunderstood by their mothers, who are supposed to hamper the development of personal autonomy in their daughters.

Houben (1981) and Houben, Pierloot and Vandereycken (see Chapter 8) also noted that anorexic daughters experience their relationship with their parents as similar to normal daughters. They compared anorexic triads (father, mother and patient) with normal triads. Using the *Barrett-Lennard Relationship Inventory,* father, mother and daughter had to report their own attitude toward each other and how they experience the attitude of both of the others toward themselves. In general, no statistically significant differences were found between the anorexic group and the normal control group with regard to the way the daughter described her own attitude toward her parents and her parents' attitude toward herself. But anorexic patients do experience a greater empathy from their mothers than normal girls do. Anorexics also show more transparency toward mother than toward father who is perceived as less empathically understanding toward them. In the normal group, fathers show significantly more openness and positive feelings toward their wives than toward their daughters whereas such differentiation is far less obvious in anorexics' families. The latter may reflect a kind of emotional enmeshment in these families.

In a study of *projective identification,* Owen (1973) used the semantic differential method in order to compare young anorexia nervosa patients and their parents with a control group of schoolgirls and their parents. The mothers of anorexic patients seemed to be overidentified with their daughters, which was not the case for the fathers.

Garfinkel et al. (1983) also noted similar results between the response pattern of anorexic daughters and their mothers on the *Family Assessment Measure* (FAM), a self-report questionnaire. They compared the FAM results of anorexic triads with normal controls. Both anorexic daughters and mothers reported more difficulty in the family regarding task accomplishment, role performance, communication, and affective expression. They also scored lower on the social desirability scale. The fathers of anorexics did not report any significant abnormalities on the FAM and scored similar to normal fathers.

Ehle and collaborators (Ehle & Ott, 1981; Ehle et al., 1982; Ehle, 1984) observed that some anorexia nervosa patients perceived the relationship with their parents during their early childhood as extremely negative and that others did not. These authors studied a sample of 65 subjects (35 anorexia nervosa patients and 30 females with postpill-amenorrhea) on various biological, intrapsychic and social characteristics. They differentiated three clusters of patients by means of an hierarchical *cluster analysis.* The three clusters differed on a range of characteristics but we will only mention the results regarding the patients' perception of their relationship with both of their parents during childhood (they used a questionnaire similar to the one described in Chapter 7). Cluster A, comprising 25 patients with postpill-amenorrhea and 6 patients with anorexia nervosa, did not experience any difficulties in their family and manifested the least severe symptoms in general. Cluster B, grouping 21 anorexia nervosa patients and 3 patients with postpill-amenorrhea, denied difficulties in the parent-daughter relationship during childhood. Cluster C, comprising but 10 cases, 8 anorexia nervosa patients and 2 with postpill-amenorrhea, finally noted severely disturbed family relationships. The latter group was the most disturbed in general. They characterized their mother as anxious, overprotecting, uncharitable and neurotic. These characteristics stress the dominance of the mother. The father was experienced as anxious, neurotic and pseudostabile. Finally, the marital relationship of the parents was said to be poor.

Leon et al. (1985) compared a group of adolescent anorexics with a normal weight control group by means of the Moos *Family Environment Scale (FES)*. There were no differences among the youngsters in their perception of the family environment, nor were there differences between the bulimic and restricter subgroups. The group of control parents rated the family system as more conductive to the expression of feelings, and as engendering a greater degree of closeness and warmth. Further, compared with the anorexics' mothers, the group of control mothers viewed the family atmosphere as more accepting of strivings for independence.

Kog, Vertommen and De Groote (1985) investigated families of (restricting or bulimic) anorexia nervosa patients, normal-weight bulimics, and normal controls using the *Leuven Family Questionnaire,* measuring conflict, cohesion, and disorganization (see also Chapter 6). When they compared the average scores of mother, father and daughter of the eating disorder families (a total of 235 subjects) with those of normal family triads (837 subjects), the former reported significantly more conflict and more disorganization, but did not differ from control families with regard to perceived cohesion in the family. A separate comparison of each of the three eating disorder subgroups with the normal control sample revealed that each subgroup reported more conflict and more disorganization. However, restricting anorexics showed a response pattern which was most similar to that of the normal control families on the three scales. Bulimic anorexics and normal-weight bulimics showed a mutually comparable, more differing response pattern.

The results of Johnson and Flach (1985), on the family characteristics of normal weight bulimics, only partially sustain the previous results. These authors compared the perceptions of the family environment by 105 bulimia patients and 86 normal control subjects, who had to fill in the *Family Environment Scale* (FES). The bulimic subjects experienced a great deal of conflict and anger (high conflict) in their family interaction while open, direct expression of feelings was discouraged (low expressiveness). This is consistent with the results on the conflict-scale of the aforementioned Kog et al. study (1985), when taking into account only the data of the daughters. But the bulimic patients in the study by Johnson and Flach (1985) did not report significantly less organization (or more disorganization) and did report less cohesion in their family. These results are not consistent with those of Kog et al. (1985), but the latter included restricting and bulimic anorexics as well as normal-weight bulimics. Johnson and Flach

(1985) further reported that the achievement expectations were not significantly different between the two groups of families, but there was significantly less emphasis in the bulimic patients' families on intellectual and social activities and participation in recreational activities. Finally, bulimic patients did not report significantly more control in their family. Peculiarly, although "achievement orientation" and "organization" were the two scales that did not discriminate between groups (besides the scale "control"), these two Family Environment Subscales were selected in a stepwise regression analysis as predictor variables for the severity of illness.

Intragroup Comparisons

Strober (1981) compared the attitudes toward family interaction between restricting and bulimic anorexics. The results on the *Family Environment Scale* (FES), ratings of the emotional relationship with parents, and the *Locke-Wallace Marital Scale* (for the parents) were, in general, less favorable for the bulimic than for the restricting subgroup. On the FES, the family environment of bulimics was characterized by significantly higher levels of conflicting interactions and expression of negativity among family members (conflict), whereas marital support and concern among family members (cohesiveness) and clarity of structure, rules and division of responsibility (organization) were more strongly associated with families of restricting anorexics. The emotional relationship with both father and mother was worse for bulimic anorexics, and there was significantly greater alienation from father than from mother in these patients, a difference which was absent in the restricting counterparts. Marital discordance seemed to be present in both groups, but significantly higher levels of discordance were reported by both mothers and fathers of the bulimic subgroups.

Kog et al. (1985), yielded convergent results comparing the answers of restricting anorexics, bulimic anorexics, and normal-weight bulimics on the *Leuven Family Questionnaire* (see Chapter 6). The families of restricting anorexics reported significantly less conflict, more cohesion, and less disorganization than the families of bulimic anorexics and normal-weight bulimics. The latter two did not show significant differences.

Using the FAM as in the aforementioned study by Garfinkel et al. (1983), Garner et al. (1985) also noted significantly more family pathology as perceived by bulimic anorexics and normal-weight bulimics, compared with restricting anorexics. The patients in the first two groups showed pathologic scores on task accomplishment, role performance, communication, affective expression, affective involvement, control and values and norms, while restricting anorexics scored within the normal range, indicating an absence of perceived family pathology by the patient.

Humphrey (1983) compared one family triad of a normal-weight bulimic patient with one family triad of an anorexic patient, using *Structural Analysis of*

Social Behavior (SASB). When used as a self-report instrument, it concerns the dimensions of affiliation and interdependence, which have to be rated on three levels; other, self, and introjection. By far, the majority of average cluster profiles for self and other ratings were friendly and autonomous. The important exceptions to this were the introjection profiles ("how I treat myself") for both the anorexic and bulimic daughter. The anorexic patient's introjection rates best fit the control pattern (helping and protecting, belittling, and blaming) as well as the attack pattern (self-rejecting and destroying). The bulimic patient's introjection profile best fit the attack pattern (self-indicating and oppressing, self-rejecting and destroying). The anorexic's view of her mother's attitude toward her showed a significant control profile, and both parents perceived the anorexic daughter's reaction to them as submissive. The bulimic daughter saw only her father as controlling toward her. There was no evidence for perceived parental attack toward the daughter in either family. The findings of Humphrey's (1983) study should be regarded as hypotheses to be tested on a large sample, preferably with a between-groups design.

Finally, Kagan and Squires (1985) compared 105 male and 195 female college students who tended to overeat compulsively or dieted restrictively; in fact, no real clinical cases of eating disorder. They applied Olson's *Family Adaptation and Cohesion Scales (FACES II)*. Neither the scale for family cohesion nor the one for adaptability were correlated with dieting behaviors, among both males and females. Compulsive eating among females was associated with only one of the hypothesized family variables but in the opposite direction, i.e., lack of family cohesion. Compulsive eating among males was strongly related to family variables. Males who scored high on compulsive eating perceived their family as relatively rigid and uncohesive. It is hypothesized that in females dieting and compulsive eating are reactions to social pressure rather than to family stress or lack of family support, which play a role in males. Because eating is an unusual way for normative males to express negative emotion, when it does occur it may be symptomatic of much more profound and pervasive disturbances than in the case of females.

External Observation of Family Interaction

Intergroup Comparisons

Minuchin et al. (1975; 1978) compared the family interaction of three psychosomatic groups (anorexics, asthmatics and diabetics) and two non-psychosomatic control groups. Their clinically derived model stated that psychosomatic families are characterized by an enmeshed, overprotective, rigid and conflict-avoidant family structure (see Chapter 2). In order to test this model, they compared the psychosomatic groups with the non-psychosomatic control groups on certain behavioral parameters of family interaction. The authors operationalized the four interactional characteristics in behavioral categories, which were coded and scored, using videotapes of the family interaction, while the family was carrying out semistructured tasks. The clinical hypotheses were confirmed for all psychosomatic groups but most significantly for the anorexic group. A detailed analysis and methodological criticism of Minuchin's concepts have been published elsewhere (Kog, Vandereycken & Vertommen, 1985).

Caring behavior and poor differentiation between patient-parent dyads have also been observed by Goldstein (1981). This author compared the family triads of hospitalized anorexics, hospitalized non-anorexic patients, and pre-schizophrenic adolescents (disturbed adolescents who are supposed to be at great risk for developing schizophrenia). The study was intended to test some presumedly etiological family factors in schizophrenia. Therefore, Goldstein analyzed two interactional attitudes in the families with a disturbed adolescent offspring, which are supposed to be risk indicators for the development of schizophrenia in the offspring, i.e., parental attitudes of *communication deviance* (CD) and *negative affective style* (NAS). The attitude of CD was not measured on actual family interaction data, but was coded on verbal records of the transaction between a parent and a tester, using the Thematic Apperception Test (TAT). The measure of NAS was based on the occurrence of certain verbal and non-verbal behaviors during directly observed interaction between parent and child. The prospective part of the study showed that a combined attitude of CD and NAS was a very good predictor for the appearance of schizophrenia-spectrum disorder in the offspring five years later. Goldstein (1981) also carried out a second test by comparing the sample of pre-schizophrenic adolescents with a sample of hospitalized anorexics. Half of the parents in the anorexic sample revealed CD but not single parent manifested an overt NAS in direct interaction with his or her daughter. In order to test whether the anorexic parents relate in any distinctive way with their daughter compared with a sample of non-anorexic inpatients, Goldstein examined parental behaviors of dependency/insecurity, interpersonal boundary problems, and cross-generational blurring as manifested in the triadic interaction between mother, father, and index offspring. The highest score on the total of these behavioral features was shown for the anorexic family units, which differed significantly from the disturbed adolescent (out-patient) group and the non-anorexic (inpatient) group. This difference cannot be accounted for by the impact of having a hospitalized, psychiatrically disturbed child because the scores of the anorexic group also deviated from the non-anorexic inpatients. When the components of the total score were analyzed separately, scores for a combined index of dependency/insecurity (requests for support, protectiveness of others, tentative speech and backing down when statements are countered by another) most consistently discriminated families of anorexics from the other groups both at the level of the total family system, the parent subsystem, and the offspring.

Sights and Richards (1984) gave a different picture of the parental and parent-daughter relationship in bulimic patients. They compared the mothers and fathers of 6 bulimic and 6 nonbulimic college women by means of separate and joint structured interviews in which they were asked about their marriages, spouses and relationships with their children. The interviews were audiotaped and the verbatim transcripts were scored independently by two judges, who were blind to the diagnostic status of the probands. The observation instrument, the *Parental Characteristic Rating Scales,* consists of 44 items, grouped according to 11 topical areas. On the basis of these data, bulimic mothers were judged to be more domineering, controlling and were seen as holding higher expectations for their daughters than their nonbulimic counterparts. Fathers of bulimic women were seen as close to their daughters during the early childhood years, but distant during adolescence. This deterioration of the father/daughter relationship was not observed in the control groups. The parents of bulimic women were more demanding and more inclined to compare siblings openly and there was more parent/daughter stress in the patient group. There was little evidence, however, that the two groups differed in any important way as far as their "sexual attitudes" and "quality of life scores" are concerned.

Intragroup Comparisons

Beside the self-report part of the study discussed above, Humphrey (1983) also compared the family triad of an anorexia nervosa patient with the family triad of a bulimic patient on interactional categories that are behavioral operationalizations of the dimensions of *affiliation and interdependence.* Videotaped family interaction during two 10-minute role-plays were coded verbatim from transcripts. The results of this detailed intrafamilial analyses suggested that both families were struggling with conflicts over control and autonomy. The parents of both the anorexic and bulimic patient were highly controlling and intrusive toward their daughter during family interactions. This parental behavior was often combined with the opposite message of affirming and understanding on behalf of the daughter. The hypothesis that the bulimic family would show more hostility than the anorexic family received only support from the daughter. However, such a comparative question is difficult to address with a single-subject design. A controlled between-groups design is needed here. The same applies to the interesting findings that the parents rarely showed direct verbal interaction, and when they did (which was the case for the anorexic's parents once in a while), it was in the same controlling way as they treated their daughter. Humphrey (1983) considered these findings comparable to Minuchin's ideas about a lack of conflict resolution and a focus on the child, factors which might suggest an absence of marital intimacy in parents of psychosomatic patients.

Some of Minuchin's concepts have also been tested in the study by Kog et al. (1986). Beside the self-report portion of the study discussed above, Minuchin's four family characteristics were operationalized by way of direct observational measures (see also Chapter 5). The final result of the semistructured interaction tasks — on the basis of written information — as well as the interaction process — on the basis of videotaped observation of verbal and non-verbal behaviors — was studied. A pilot study of three families with a restricting anorexic, five families with a bulimic anorexic, and two families with a normal-weight bulimic patient did not sustain Minuchin's statement that all anorexic families are characterized by an enmeshed, overprotective, rigid and conflict-avoidant family structure. For each of these characteristics, there seemed to exist a great variability among anorexic/bulimia nervosa families, thus rejecting the notion of a "typical" family structure. These findings were supported by a study on a larger group of patients, which will be discussed extensively in Chapter 5 of this book.

FAMILY FACTORS RELATED TO TREATMENT AND PROGNOSIS

We will differentiate two family related issues in the treatment of eating disorders. On the one hand, we discuss empirical evidence with regard to family related phenomena in the *process* of family treatment. On the other hand, we discuss family factors in the *outcome and prognosis,* which we further subdivide as prognostic relevant family factors and the outcome of family therapy as treatment modality in eating disorders.

Family Issues Related to Therapy

Vandereycken and Pierloot (1983b) carried out a therapy evaluation study on their strict behavioral therapy program and concluded that their program proved to be very efficient for short-term weight restoration but that it also induced considerable side-effects. The rule of "parentectomy," i.e., strictly isolating the patient from her family — no mail, no phone calls, no visits — for several weeks until the target weight was reached, had especially negative effects on the relationship between the doctor and nurses on the one hand and patient and parents on the other, even resulting in a high dropout rate. This was one of the reasons why these authors adapted their program to a more family-oriented treatment regimen (Vandereycken, 1985).

Crisp et al. (1974) even found considerable evidence for the emergence of more psychoneurotic symptoms in the parents during weight restoration of their daughter. Both mother and father scored higher levels on the 6 scales of the *Middlesex Hospital Questionnaire* (MHQ), a self-rating inventory of psychoneurotic symptoms, after than before restoration of weight to a normal level. The anxiety and phobic scales were especially elevated. When the parents were subdivided according to the quality of their marital relationship, parents whose relationship was judged to be poor, showed greater overall change with increased morbidity as measured by the MHQ. The mothers with a poor marital relationship were found to change significantly more with respect to anxiety and somatic complaint and the fathers showed significantly more depression. Moreover, when the patients were divided into those who habitually overate and vomited as distinct from those who habitually abstained from eating, the fathers of the first group revealed more psychoneurotic morbidity after weight restoration, especially more anxiety, obsessionality and depressin. Finally, the 6-month outcome of the patient's illness was importantly related to the initial levels of psychoneurotic morbidity in the parents. On the basis of these findings, the authors conclude that "...the daughter's illness sometimes serves a protective function for one or both parents as well as the patients, especially if the marital relationship is poor and acutely threatened by the prospect of their child's independence" (Crisp et al., 1974, p. 172).

Amdur et al. (1969) noted especially more dynamic family issues in the interactions and verbalizations of patients and family during the second phase of hospitalization, once weight was no longer a critical problem. They analyzed the family interactional patterns of 10 families with an anorexia nervosa patient by means of direct observation of family treatment sessions. The emerging dynamic family issues were related to, (1) *dependency,* (2) *separation,* and (3) a pattern of *changing alliances* within the family. Patients as well as parents verbalized a desire for independence but their behavior indicated the reverse. The parents controlled many areas of the patient's life and only allowed the patient to control food intake. Similarly, patients performed in a manner that resulted in maintaining a dependent relationship with their parents even if geographically separated from them. The majority of patients had an extremely close relationship with their father during childhood, who however, withdrew at the onset of adolescence although some seductive teasing continued. The families tended to overlook this behavior despite the patients' obvious discomfort with such interactions.

The single subject study of Ben-Tovim et al. (1977), using the Repertory Grid technique, also revealed a *sexual tinge in the relationship between father and anorexic daughter.* Three weeks after admission, a 14-year-old female anorexic patient and her parents were interviewed individually to elicit their respective attitudes toward various body shapes (shape grid). Moreover, they were set the task of estimating their own body widths at various defined levels. The parents also made various estimates of their daughter's width. In the week prior to the patient's discharge from the hospital, the parents were presented with 19 measurements. Eight were widths across the subject's own body parts, 2 each for face, bust, waist and hips. The parents were presented with both the actual measured width across the body part, and their own prior estimate of this body part width. The remaining 11 measurements presented to each parent were widths relating to their daughter, 8 of them being estimates across her body at the 4 described levels, derived, as above, from the actual dimensions and from their own previous estimates. The other 3 widths were the parents' concepts of ideal measurements at bust, waist and hips. The results revealed that for both parents, decreasing width lead to a more favorable evaluation of their daughter. The father's grid showed this particularly. Though he had been comparativity accurate when estimating the actual widths of his daughter, he had slightly over-estimated her face, her bust and her hips. He responded, however, more favorably to the actual smaller widths of these body parts. Curiously, the father under-estimated the width of his daughter's waist, and when asked to evaluate its larger, actual size at the end of treatment he saw it as clearly "odd" and "unattractive" in comparison to the smaller, estimated, waist. This is especially noteworthy because from her initial assessment interview onwards, the patient had shown a particular fear of putting on weight at the waist. Mother also responded more favorably to the smaller of the two widths but this was less striking because her own initial judgment of her daughter's were greater over-estimates than her husband's responses. The authors conclude that "...one could speculate that parental sensitivity to increasing body size acts as a feed-back mechanism to the child, and is at least involved in the disorder's prolonged and relapsing course" (Ben-Tovim et al., 1977, p. 255).

A similar complex, methodologically impressionistic study was presented by Foster and Kupfer (1975). Their study reports on the application of *telemetric mobility* to the assessment of family interaction and hospital-ward events. The investigation uses a single subject design, recording nocturnal telemetric activity on 122 subsequent nights in an anorexia nervosa patient, coming from a family with a father, mother, elder sister and monozygotic twin sister concordant for anorexia nervosa. They examined the impact of various types of daytime family visits (female dominated meetings, mother-father dominated meetings and father-twin dominated meetings) on psychomotor activity observed 8 to 12 hours later during sleep. There was an activating effect of the patient's slightly elder female sibling and mother on the patient's nocturnal arousal which can be understood in terms of Oedipal competition or competition for attention. There was a neutral effect of the mother-father constellation on the patient's nocturnal arousal system which is interpreted by the parent's complementarity, neutralizing the impact of their coalition on this particular child. Finally, the patient's nocturnal behavior after contact with the father-twin configuration was withdrawn, suggesting an episode of depersonalization.

Family Issues Related to Outcome and Prognosis

Prognostic Family Factors

Although Morgan and Russell (1975) did not use family therapy in their treatment program, they studied family characteristics as predictors of long-term prognosis. Forty-one anorexia nervosa patients were scored on a number of individual and familial prognostically relevant characteristics at the time of weight restoration, after their first admission to the Maudsley Hospital. After 4 years, a follow-up study was conducted by means of a structured interview which covered the psychiatric, nutritional, physical, and socio-economic status of the patient. The latter aspect included, among other things, family relationships and establishment of independence from the family. Each of them were scored on a 4-point scale. On admission, the families were characterized as higher social class families, with a history of mental illness in first- or second-degree relatives in 51% of the patients and a disturbed relationship between the family and the patient before the onset of illness in 54% of the cases. The latter characteristics proved to be crucial for the outcome of the illness. A poor outcome correlated significantly with a disturbed relationship between the patient and other members of the family before the onset of the illness. No significant association with outcome was found in the case of a history of mental illness in the family, social class, anomalous family structure, or sibling rivalry.

Family Therapy Outcome
    The frequently cited outcome study of Minuchin et al. (1978) focuses on the effect of *structural family therapy* in anorexia nervosa. They studied 53 restricting anorexics first at admission, then after an average of 6 months treatment predominantly out-patient family treatment. Some patients were hospitalized during a period of a few weeks at the beginning of treatment, and finally after a follow-up period of 1-1/2 to 7 years. Eighty percent of the sample was followed for 2 or more years). The outcome criteria included both the medical aspects of anorexia nervosa, predominantly weight restoration, and psychosocial functioning of the patients in relation to home, school and peers. The psychosocial evaluations were based not only on the patient's condition at the termination of therapy but also on the information obtained through follow-up contacts with the patients, families and pediatricians. Outcome criteria with regard to family functioning were not included! The results from the two assessments — immediately after treatment and at follow-up — revealed that 86% of the cases recovered from both the anorexia and its psychosocial component. This is an unusually high success rate, which, as Yager and Strober (1985) claim, "should be regarded with interest, but also with caution" (p. 496). First, there exists a selected bias in their patients sample. They studied younger patients, with a short duration of food refusal, coming from intact families. Each of these selection criteria are shown to be prognostically favorable factors. Secondly, outcome evaluations are carried out by members of their own clinical team, who cannot impartially judge the effect of their treatment program (Yager, 1981, 1982; Eisler et al., 1985). Thirdly, no specific assessment of family functioning at follow-up was carried out, a remarkable omission for a team emphasizing a family model. Finally, this study did not systematically compare the outcome of various treatment programs in eating disorder patients. A discussion of the only two existing outcome studies which use this latter form of control follows.

Hall and Crisp (1981) randomly allocated 30 patients with anorexia nervosa to either 12 weekly sessions of *outpatient dietetic advice* or 12 weekly sessions of a mixture of *outpatient individual psychodynamic therapy and family therapy,* and studied the outcome after one year follow-up. The dietetic advice focused on discussing diet, mood and daily behavior patterns. The family was seen with the patient on some occasions. In the psychotherapeutic situation, attention was focused on the role anorexia nervosa played in the relationship of the patient with her family and others. On admission and one year after the initial assessment interview, all the patients and their families were interviewed by an independent assessor, who was blind to the treatment condition, in order to to judge the patient's progress in terms of her anorexia nervosa and her social and sexual development. The patient completed the Crown-Crisp Experiential Index. There was little difference in outcome between the two treatment groups on individual measures, and there were modest improvements in terms of weight, menstruation, eating patterns, sexual and social adjustment. The two groups differed, however, significantly in outcome on three measures. The dietary advice group showed significant weight gain, whereas the group given psychotherapy made significant improvements in sexual and social adjustment. Moreover, the two groups showed different patterns of weight change. The dietary advice group showed more uniform gains which were sustained between treatment and follow-up, whereas the psychotherapy group showed a larger weight gain during treatment, and the patients tended either to continue to improve or to deteriorate when treatment was discontinued.

Szmukler et al. (1985) carried out a particularly interesting and well-controlled study on factors associated with *dropping-out from treatment* in anorexia nervosa or bulimia patients, randomly allocated to either family therapy or individual (supportive) psychotherapy, carried out by the same therapist (Szmukler, 1983). Fifty-one consecutive admissions to the weight-restoration unit at the Maudsley Hospital entered this outpatient program after a period of 1 to 3 months inpatient treatment. At the beginning of the outpatient treatment, the patient was interviewed in order to gather detailed clinical and social information, as well as ratings on anorexia symptomatology, psychosexual adjustment, family relations and social functioning. Moreover, each patient completed a range of psychological tests. Both parents were interviewed with the abbreviated form of the Camberwell Family Interview. The audiotapes of the individual interviews were scored according to 5 main components of *expressed emotion:* (1) critical comments about the patient; (2) hostility to the patient; (3) emotional over-involvement; (4) warmth; and (5) positive comments about the patient. The therapists were blind to the expressed emotion evaluation of the parents and had not been involved in the inpatient treatment. Dropping-out was defined as a premature termination of treatment against the therapist's advice within three months of commencing follow-up therapy. Fourteen of the 51 patients (27%) dropped out of treatment; somewhat more in the family therapy group; nine as compared with 5 in the individual therapy group. However, but the difference was not statistically significant. The only measures which differed significantly between the drop-outs and the engaged patients was the higher *critical comment* score of both parents and the higher *emotional over-involvement* score of the fathers. Moreover, there was a correlation between parents' critical comment scores, the type of therapy and the symptomatology on the one hand, and dropping-out from treatment on the other. Defaulting was likely in the case of a critical mother in family therapy, but not for individual therapy. This relationship did not hold for fathers, but there was a tendency for patients with a critical father to dropout of individual therapy. Furthermore, a highly significant association was found between parents' critical comment scores and a diagnosis of bulimia nervosa. Patients with bulimia were also more likely to drop out from family therapy, but not from individual therapy. The relative contributions of these influences could not be further investigated because of the relatively small number of patients in the subgroups.

CONCLUSION

The majority of studies on family characteristics of anorexia nervosa and bulimia patients can be labeled as clinically descriptive. Such accounts of family-related characteristics in a large patient sample have limited significance unless appropriate control groups are used, and the data are gathered in a well-structured way; e.g., standardized interview with patient and parents. Most of the clinical studies do not meet these criteria. As to the first condition, we need systematic comparative studies of clinical characteristics: (a) intergroup comparison between an eating disorder group and normal controls and/or various psychiatric group; or (b) intragroup comparisons between various eating disorder subgroups. Such comparative investigations on a clinical level may yield results to answer the following questions:

a. whether the clinical information concerning an eating disorder family differentiates from a normal family. These differences might be important causal variables, but they have to be further tested by a prospective research design;
b. whether an eating disorder family differentiates from another psychiatric family with regard to certain clinical variables. These might concern important specific pathogenic variables, which have to be further tested by a prospective research design;
c. whether a restricting anorexic family differentiates from a bulimic anorexic family and/or a normal-weight bulimic family. These clinical differentiations might be important diagnostic variables, but they have to further investigated by a controlled between-groups design.

Clinical comparisons only yield correlational findings between an eating disorder and family features. If one finds a specific family pattern in relation to an eating disorder, this typical family organization could be a general reaction to an existing stress situation, e.g., the eating disorder itself, as well as an etiologic element for the occurrence of the disorder (Yager, 1981, 1982). We are faced here with the cause-effect controversy. Yager (1982) stressed the need for prospective studies on highly vulnerable but, as yet, unaffected children in order to test the hypotheses that are based on clinical studies. Also, adoptive studies are needed to study the genetic/environmental influences.

Self-report studies are scarce, although rather easy to carry out. The paucity of family self-report questionnaires up until a decade ago presumably explains the lack of this type of research. Intra- and intergroup comparisons, as described above, are not so essential in studies focusing on the insiders' subjective perception of intrafamilial relations. Intrafamilial comparisons are more relevant in order to study different views among the family members as to their mutual interactions. A pitfall of this type of study may be the issue of "social desirability." That is, family members do not give their personal opinion, but what they feel they are expected to answer. The tendency to deny problems — not uncommon among anorexia nervosa patients/families (Vandereycken & Vanderlinden, 1983) — might completely distort the response pattern. Consequently, the perception of one's own family organization may diverge considerably from the observation of trained researchers (Kramer, 1986).

Observational studies are still very scarce because of the considerable amount of time needed to investigate family interactions by way of direct observation techniques. Moreover, it is sometimes extremely difficult to synthesize the abundance of information in a systematic and replicable way, and the available methods have not been sufficiently validated at this point in time. For this kind of study it is important that non-verbal as well as verbal interaction be investigated. Otherwise, the family interaction data will be fragmentary and difficult to interpret so that the inordinate amount of time investment required may prove worthless. Besides many methodological problems, the critical issue in these observation studies concerns generalization. Does the observed interaction reflect what is really happening in the natural situation at home?

Because each type of study has its advantages and disadvantages, it is useful to combine different methods simultaneously in order to judge the methods' most appropriate use, taking into account research goals and time investment (Kog et al., 1983). This *multitrait-multimethod design* has been used recently by Walker et al. (1984) and Oliveri and Reiss (1984), as it is in our own research project (see Chapter 5).

Regardless of the quality of the varying methodology of the available research we have described, there is some convergent evidence for certain features of families with an anorexia nervosa or bulimia patient.

With regard to the *nature-nurture* issue, a critical examination of the available data concerning anorexia nervosa in twins does not, up to the present, substantially support the assumption that genetic factors play a determining role in the etiology of this syndrome. This issue of genetic predisposition or heredita-bility of anorexia nervosa awaits well-controlled and unbiased comparisons of homozygotic and heterozygotic twins as well as, most importantly, studies of twins raised apart.

With regard to *demographic* characteristics, anorexics and normal-weight bulimics seem to come from families of higher social class, when compared with the general population and with other psychosomatic disorders. An older age of the parents at the time of the patient's birth is probably not as typical, since it has also been found in other psychiatric disorders as well. Moreover, these two demographic variables are interrelated. When the comparison is control-led for social class, the latter variable is no longer significant. The incidence of broken homes and the patient's birth order do not significantly differ from the general population.

With regard to *individual pathology* in the family, the higher incidence of weight problems in families of anorexics and normal- weight bulimics seems to be connected to social class as well, although the mothers of bulimic anorexics and normal-weight bulimics appear to show a higher incidence of obesity, com-pared with the restricting anorexics' mothers. Serious physical illness in the family seems to be common, especially for the bulimic anorexics and normal-weight bulimics. As to psychiatric illnesses in the family, the incidence of affec-tive disorder (depression), especially for bulimics, is significantly higher than in the general population and comparable to the incidence in families of patients with major affective disorder. Alcohol abuse, especially in the fathers, is the sec-ond most prevalent psychiatric disorder.

With regard to *family relationships,* a pattern of control and interdependence seems to emerge. Such interdependence is, in the majority of the studies, not acknowledged by the patient, or, when experienced, is judged ambivalently. The anorexic child seems to react predominantly with submission and the bulimic child with hostility, although this is but a preliminary finding to be further ex-plored. The parents appear to control each other, but at the same time they live in marital discordance and seem to use the child to avoid their marital conflicts. The higher amount of conflict in bulimic anorexics compared with their restrict-ing counterparts, as reported by the families themselves, is invalidated by ob-servational research, at least for the overt behavior of the parents. Bulimic an-orexics and normal-weight bulimics seem to live in the same sort of controlling and too tightly knit family as do the restricting anorexics. The first two groups, however, experience more conflict and react to it, although the observable in-teraction in the family does not demonstrate more overt conflicts.

Finally, regarding *treatment and prognosis,* much has still to be done. There is some evidence supporting the interconnection between parental and family problems on the one hand, and individual prognosis of the patient on the other. Disturbed family relationships before the onset of illness correlate with a poor outcome and weight restoration is associated with an increase in parental problems when the parents' marital relationship was poor before the onset of the illness. However, we need some further comparative studies in order to plan a research-guided treatment which can successfully challenge this interconnectedness. In this regard, a combination of individual and family therapy was shown to yield better results than dietary advice (Crisp et al. 1981). But the data from Szmukler et al. (1985) stress the need for a careful selection (contra-indications?) of family therapy in bulimia nervosa patients and cases with a *critical* parent, since they show a higher risk of dropping-out from treatment.

In the future, family research in the area of eating disorders has to focus on the following points. Concerning the variable of individual pathology in the family, the relation between eating disorder and affective disorder in the family has to be further investigated in longitudinal research. Also, adoptive studies are required to determine genetic versus environmental influences. Concerning family relationships, (a) different eating disorder subgroups have to be further investigated by well-controlled between-groups design (presently, only paired comparisons between restricting and bulimic anorexics or between anorexics in general and normal-weight bulimics are available); (b) the observational method has to be combined with the self-report method in order to enable direct comparison between what is reported by the family members themselves and what is perceived by external observers; (c) further research has to include all family members because the blurring of generational boundaries is the most consistent finding of the three types of family studies — how the other children play a role in this transactional pattern is still totally unclear; (d) prospective research with repeated assessments after several time intervals is needed to study the interplay between certain family features and the development or maintenance of the eating disorder; (e) therapy outcome studies should study the relationship between parental/familial and individual characteristics and the outcome of different types of treatment. Thus, there is still a large unexplored field which has urgently to be worked up into a field of research.

Finally, we would like to address briefly, from the clinician's point of view, the *cost-benefit issue* related to family research in the clinical area of eating disorders. Anorexia nervosa is a multifactorial syndrome, and, as such, only a multidimensional approach, both in research and treatment, seems appropriate (Vandereycken & Meermann, 1984a; see also Chapter 1). This implies that family patterns may play a co-determining role in the etiology and pathogenesis of eating disorders, but does not explain the intermediate mechanisms whereby these family patterns are translated into altered self-perceptions, desire for thinness, amenorrhea, and other features of the syndrome (Yager, 1981; Kalucy, 1983). Hence, family research may elucidate only some part of the problem but never its entire complexity. Nevertheless, knowledge about family functioning might be of special importance with regard to at least secondary prevention (Vandereycken & Meermann, 1984b). Further research might also illuminate the possibly prognostic significance of certain family characteristics (Steinhausen & Glanville, 1983). Finally, the increasing popularity of family therapy in these patients, especially since the reports by Minuchin et al. (1975, 1978), requires a more systematic assessment of family functioning regarding indications and contraindications of this type of approach. Moreover, the possibilities and limitations of family therapy in eating disorders have still to be investigated. Claims about treatment efficacy are usually based on a large variety of personal beliefs, while research data are sparse.

REFERENCES*

American Psychiatric Association (1980), *Diagnostic and Statistical. Manual of Mental Disorders (DSM-III).* Washington: Author.

Askevold, F. (1982), Social class and psychosomatic illness. *Psychotherapy and Psychosomatics,* 38:256-259.

Askevold, F. & Heiberg, A. (1979), Anorexia nervosa — Two cases in discordant MZ twins. *Psychotherapy and Psychosomatics,* 32:223-228.

Ben-Tovim, D.I., Hunter, I. & Crisp, A.H. (1977), Discrimination and evaluation of shape and size in anorexia nervosa: An exploratory study. *Research Communications in Psychology, Psychiatry and Behavior,* 2:241-257.

Bruch, H. (1973), *Eating Disorders: Obesity, Anorexia Nervosa, and the Person Within.* New York: Basic Books.

Cantwell, D.P., Sturzenberger, S., Burroughs, J., Salkin, B. & Green, J.K. (1977), Anorexia nervosa: An affective disorder? *Archives of General Psychiatry,* 34:1087-1093.

Casper, R., Eckert, E., Halmi, K., Goldberg, S. & Davis, J. (1980), Bulimia: Its incidence and clinical importance in patients with anorexia nervosa. *Archives of General Psychiatry,* 37:1030-1035.

Crisp, A.H., Hsu, L., Harding, B. & Hartshorn, J. (1980), Clinical features of anorexia nervosa: A study of a consecutive series of 102 female patients. *Journal of Psychosomatic Research,* 24:179-191.

Crisp, A.H., Hall, A. & Holland, A.J. (1985), Nature and nurture in anorexia nervosa: A study of 34 pairs of twins, one pair of triplets, and an adoptive family. *International Journal of Eating Disorders,* 4:5-27.

Ehle, G. (1984), Das Wechselspiel sozialer, innerpsychischen und biologischen Faktoren fur die Aetiopathogenese der Anorexia Nervosa. (The interplay of social, intrapsychic and biologic factors in the etiology of anorexia nervosa). *Schweizerisches Archiv fur Neurologie, Neurochirurgie und Psychiatrie,* 134:81-91.

Ehle, G. & Ott, J.(1981), Das Syndrom der Anorexia nervosa (The syndrome of anorexia nervosa). *Psychiatrie, Neurologie und Medizinische Psychologie,* 33:577-588.

Ehle, G., Wahlstab, A. & Ott, J. (1982), Psychodiagnostisch Befunde bei Anorexia nervosa und postpill Amenorrhoe. (Psychodiagnostic findings in anorexia nervosa and postpill amenorrhea). *Psychiatrie, Neurologie und Medizinische Psychologie,* 34:647-656.

Elbadawy, M.H.F., Cliffer, M.J. & James, P.T. (1985), A monozygotic twin pair discordant for anorexia nervosa. *Canadian Journal of Psychiatry,* 30:544-545.

Feighner, J.P., Robins, E., Guze, S.B., Woodruff, R.A. jr., Winokur, G. & Munoz, R. (1972), Diagnostic criteria for use in psychiatric research. *Archives of General Psychiatry,* 26:57-63.

Fichter, M.M. (1985), *Magersucht und Bulimia* (Anorexia Nervosa and Bulimia). Berlin: Springer-Verlag.

---

*   This list contains only secondary literature, whereas the other references are mentioned in the final section of this book: "Bibliography on Family Aspects of Eating Disorders."

Garfinkel, P. & Garner, D. (1982), *Anorexia Nervosa: A Multidimensional Perspective.* New York: Brunner/Mazel.

Garfinkel, P., Moldofsky, H. & Garner, D. (1980), The heterogeneity of anorexia nervosa: Bulimia as a distinct subgroup. *Archives of General Psychiatry,* 37:1036-1040.

Garner, D., Garfinkel, P. & O'Shaughnessy, M. (1985), The validity of the distinction between bulimia with and without anorexia nervosa. *American Journal of Psychiatry,* 142:581-587.

Hall, A. & Crisp, A.H. (1983), Brief psychotherapy in the treatment of anorexia nervosa. In: Darby, P., Garfinkel, P., Garner, D. & Coscina, D. (Eds.), *Anorexia Nervosa: Recent Developments in Research.* New York: Alan R. Liss, pp. 427-439. Also in: Krakowski, A.J. & Kimball, C.P. (Eds.), *Psychosomatic Medicine.* New York: Plenum Press, pp 703-717.

Halmi, K. (1974a), Anorexia nervosa: Demographic and clinical features in 94 cases. *Psychosomatic Medicine,* 36:18-26.

Halmi, K. (1974b), Comparison of demographic and clinical features in patient groups with different ages and weights at onset of anorexia nervosa. *Journal of Nervous and Mental Disease,* 158:222-225.

Halmi, K. (1983), Classification of eating disorders. *International Journal of Eating Disorders,* 2(4):21-26.

Hare, E.H. & Moran, P.A. (1979), Raised parental age in psychiatric patients. *British Journal of Psychiatry,* 134:169-177.

Herzog, D. (1982), Bulimia: The secretive syndrome. *Psychosomatics,* 23:481-487.

Holland, A.J., Hall, A., Murray, R., Russell, G.F.M. & Crisp, A.H. (1984), Anorexia nervosa: A study of 34 twin pairs and one set of triplets. *British Journal of Psychiatry,* 145:414-419.

Hsu, L.K.G. (1983), The aetiology of anorexia nervosa. *Psychological Medicine,* 13:231-238.

Hsu, L.K., Holder, D., Hindmarsh, D. & Phelps, C. (1984), Bipolar illness preceded by anorexia nervosa in identical twins. *Journal of Clinical Psychiatry,* 45:262-266.

Irwin, M. (1981), Diagnosis of anorexia nervosa in children and the validity of DSM-III. *American Journal of Psychiatry,* 138:1382-1383.

Johnson, C. & Berndt, D. (1983), Preliminary investigation of bulimia and life adjustment. *American Journal of Psychiatry,* 140:774-777.

Kay, D.W.K. & Leigh, D. (1954), The natural history, treatment and prognosis of anorexia nervosa, based on a study of 38 patients. *Journal of Mental Science,* 100:411-431.

Kog, E., Vandereycken, W. & Vertommen, H. (1985), The psychosomatic family model: A critical analysis of family interaction concepts. *Journal of Family Therapy,* 7:31-44.

Leon, G.R., Lucas, A.R., Colligan, R.C., Ferdinande, R.J. & Kamp, J. (1985), Sexual, body-image, and personality attitudes in anorexia nervosa. *Journal of Abnormal Child Psychology,* 13:245-258.

Moskovitz, R.A., Belar, G. & Gingus, C.M. (1982), Anorexia nervosa in identical twins. *Hospital and Community Psychiatry,* 33:484-485.

Nowlin, N.S. (1983), Anorexia nervosa in twins: Case report and review. *Journal of Clinical Psychiatry,* 44:101-105.

Oliveri, M. & Reiss, D. (1984), Family concepts and their measurement: Things are seldom what they seem. *Family Process,* 23:33-48.

Piran, N., Kennedy, S., Garfinkel, P.E. & Owens, M. (1985), Affective disturbance in eating disorders. *Journal of Nervous and Mental Disease,* 173:395-400.

Rollins, N. & Piazza, E. (1978), Diagnosis of anorexia nervosa: A critical reappraisal. *Journal of the American Academic Child Psychiatry,* 17:126-137.

Russell, C.S. (1979), Circumplex model of marital and family systems: III. Empirical evaluation with families. *Family Process,* 18:29-45.

Russell, G. (1979), Bulimia nervosa: An ominous variant of anorexia nervosa. *Psychological Medicine, 9:429-448.*

Schepank, H. (1981), Anorexia Nervosa, Zwillingskasuistik über ein seltenes Krankheitsbild (Anorexia nervosa: Cases of twins). In: A. Heigl-Evers & H. Schepank (Eds.), *Ursprünge Seelisch Bedingter Krankheiten* (Origins of psychologically determined illnesses). Göttingen: Vandenhoeck & Ruprecht.

Schepank, H. (1983), Anorexia nervosa in twins: Is the etiology psychotic or psychogenic? In: Krakowski, A.J. & Kimball, C.P. (Eds), *Psychosomatic Medicine. Theoretical, Clinical, and Transcultural Aspects.* New York: Plenum Press, pp. 161-169.

Schlesier-Stropp, B. (1984), Bulimia: A review of the literature. *Psychological Bulletin,* 95:247-257.

Sours, J.A. (1980), *Starving to Death in a Sea of Objects: The Anorexia Nervosa Syndrome.* New York: Jason Aronson.

Steinberg, R. (1982), Anorexia nervosa und Schizophrenie bei einem eineiigen Zwillingspaar (Anorexia nervosa and schizophrenia in a pair of monozygotic twins). *Psychiatria Clinica,* 15:184-205.

Steinhausen, H.C. & Glanville, K. (1983), Follow-up studies in anorexia nervosa. *Psychological Medicine,* 13:239-249.

Strober, M., (1981), The significance of bulimia in juvenile anorexia nervosa: An exploration of possible etiologic factors. *International Journal of Eating Disorders,* 1(1):28-43.

Strober, M., Salkin, B., Burroughs, M. & Morrell, W. (1982), Validity of the bulimia-restricter distinction in anorexia nervosa. Parental personality characteristics and family morbidity. *Journal of Nervous and Mental Disease,* 170:345-351.

Theander, S. (1970), Anorexia nervosa: A psychiatric investigation of 94 female cases. *Acta Psychiatrica Scandinavica,* Supplement 214.

Vandereycken, W. (1985), Inpatient treatment of anorexia nervosa: Some research-guided changes. *Journal of Psychiatric Research,* 19:413-422.

Vandereycken, W. & Meermann, R. (1984a), *Anorexia Nervosa: A Clinician's Guide to Treatment.* Berlin-New York: Walter de Gruyter.

Vandereycken, W. & Meermann, R. (1984b), Anorexia nervosa: Is prevention possible? *International Journal of Psychiatry in Medicine,* 14:191-205.

Vandereycken, W. & Pierloot, R. (1983a), Drop-out during in- patient treatment of anorexia nervosa: A clinical study of 133 patients. *British Journal of Medical Psychology,* 56:154-156.

Vandereycken, W. & Pierloot, R. (1983b), The significance of subclassification in anorexia nervosa: A comparative study of clinical features in 141 patients. *Psychological Medicine,* 13:543-549.

Vandereycken, W. & Van den Broucke, S. (1984), Anorexia nervosa in males. A comparative study of 107 cases reported in the literature (1970 to 1980). *Acta Psychiatrica Scandinavica,* 70:447-454.

Vandereycken, W. & Vanderlinden, J. (1983), Denial of illness and the use of self-reporting measures in anorexia nervosa patients. *International Journal of Eating Disorders,* 2(4):101-107.

Walker, N., Thomson, N. & Lindsay, W.R. (1984), Assessing family relationships: A multimethod, multi-situational approach. *British Journal of Psychiatry,* 144:387-394.

Weiss, S. & Ebert, M. (1983), Psychological and behavioral characteristics of normal-weight bulimics and normal-weight controls. *Psychosomatic Medicine,* 45:293-303.

Appendix 1. Summary of the Studies According to Research Design

	Type*	Subjects**	Matched Variables	Investigated Variables	Data Gathering Method	Data Analysis	Results
Amdur et al. (1969)	V	10 families with AN	-	Family interaction during hospitalization	Direct observation of family therapy sessions	Qualitative interpretation, Incidence ratings	After weight restoration, more dynamic family issues were discussed, relating to (1) dependency, (2) separation, and (3) a pattern of changing alliances with in the family
Askevold (1982)	I	112 AN, 354 psychosomatic P, 54 female psychiatric P	Sex	Social class	Hospital records	Frequency distribution	AN come from higher social class families
Ben-Tovim et al. (1977)	V	One family triad of an AN	-	Discrimination and evaluation of shape and size	A "shape" and a "width" grid	Comparison between the actual measured and the estimated width	For both parents, but especially for the father, decreasing width leads to a more favorable evaluation of their daughters
Casper et al. (1980)	II	566 fasting versus 49 bulimic AN, 38 vomiting versus 67 non-vomiting AN	None	Parents' age at patient's birth, Social class and education of the father	Personal interview with the patient	Means, Standard deviations	Parents' age is not significantly different between groups, Higher social class and more highly educated fathers in vomiting AN
Crisp et al. (1974)	I	36 mothers and 32 fathers of 44 AN, 240 normal triads	Age, Sex, Marital status of probands	Psychoneurotic characteristics of parents	Middlesex Hospital Questionnaire	Means, Standard deviations, T-tests	AN parents show lower scores on the somatic scale, higher scores on the hysteria scale

* A distinction is made between 4 types of study: I = clinical study: intergroup comparison; II = clinical study: intragroup comparison; III = self-report study; IV = observational study; V = therapy study (see text: "Introduction")

** AN = anorexia nervosa patients, BN = bulimia nervosa patients or normal-weight bulimics, P = patients

Appendix 1. Summary of the Studies According to Research Design (continued)

	Type	Subjects	Matched Variables	Investigated Variables	Data Gathering Method	Data Analysis	Results
Dally (1977)	II	132 AN: 11-14 yrs (34), 15-18 ys (66), 19 yrs or older (32)	None	Depression in the parents	Hospital records	Incidence ratings and percentages, Chi-square tests	More depressed mothers and fathers in the youngest group, the two remaining groups did not differ on any of the variables
Ehle et al. (1981; 1982; 1984)	III	35 AN and 30 females post-pill-amenorrhea	None	Experience of the relationship with both parents	Questionnaire	Cluster-analysis	Cluster A did not experience difficulties; cluster B denied difficulties; cluster C noted severely disturbed family relationships
Foster & Kupfer (1975)	V	One family with AN	-	The impact of various types of day-time family visits on nocturnal psychomotor activity	Telemetric assessment	Means, Percent change in subsequent nonturnal activity, T- tests	Activating effect of female-dominated meetings, neutral effect of mother-father visits and inhibiting effect of father- twin dominated meetings
Garfindel et al. (1980)	II	73 restricting versus 68 bulimic AN	None	Social class, Patient's birth order, Parental age at patient's birth, Obesity, Parental psychiatric disorder	Personal interview with the patient	Incidence ratings and percentages, Chi-square test, Chi-square tests	Only significantly more obesity in the mothers of bulimic AN

Author (year)		Sample		Variables	Measure	Analysis	Results
Garfinkel et al. (1983)	I, III	23 AN with 23 mothers and 16 fathers, 12 controls triads	Social	Attitudes to weight control and dieting, Psychological functioning, Body size estimates body satisfaction, Perception of family relations	Eating Attitudes Test, Personality questionnaire, Distorting, photograph, Family Assessment Measure	Means, Standard deviations, T-tests	Fathers scored higher on conscienciousness; mothers and daughters scored more family problems
Garner et al. (1985)	III	32 restricting AN, 33 bulimic AN, 39 BN	None	Experience of family relations	Family Assessment Measure	Means, Standard deviations, ANOVA, T-tests	Bulimic AN and BN scored significantly more family pathology than restricting AN
Gershon et al (1983)	I	99 first-degree relatives of 24 AN, 265 first-degree relatives of 43 normal controls	None	Eating disorders, Major affective disorders	54% of the relatives were interviewed, Data on the rest came from family history information	Incidence ratings, Age-corrected percentages, Chi-square tests	Significantly more eating disorders and major affective disorders in the relatives of patients
Gershon et al. (1984)	II	First-degree relatives of AN with/without major affective disorder, First-degree relatives of AN with/without bulimia, First-degree relatives of AN with/without self-induced vomiting	None	Eating disorders, Major affective disorders	54% of the relatives were interviewed, Data in the rest came from family history information	Incidence ratings, Age-corrected percentages, Chi-square tests	No significant differences between subgroups
Goldstein (1981)	IV	Family triads of: 11 hospitalized AN, 5 hospitalized non- anorexic P,	None	Family interaction: communication deviance, negative affective style,	Verbal records of the transaction between a parent and a tester	Scoring of verbal protocol	Parents of pre-schizophrenic P showed significantly more communication deviance and negative affective style

Appendix 1. Summary of the Studies According to Research Design (continued)

	Type	Subjects	Matched Variables	Investigated Variables	Data Gathering Method	Data Analysis	Results
		52 pre-schizophrenic P		dependency/insecurity, interpersonal boundary problems and cross-generational blurring	Directly observed interaction	Incidence ratings of behavioral parameters by way of videotape	Parents of AN showed significantly more dependency/insecurity, interpersonal boundary problems and cross-generational blurring
Hall & Crisp (1983)	V	30 female AN and their families	Randomization	Outcome after one year follow-up of dietary advice versus psychotherapy (individual psychodynamic and family therapy)	Interview with P and families, Medical records, Crown-Crisp Experiential Index	Global Clinical Score, Means, Standard deviation T-tests	The dietary advice group showed significant weight gain, whereas the psychotherapy group made significant improvements in sexual and social adjustment; the two groups showed different patterns of weight change
Hall & Brown (1983)	I, III	20 females AN (13-23 yrs) and their mothers, 32 non-patient schoolgirls and their mothers	None	Attitudes towards: sickness, arguments, tension, social isolation, thinness, growing up and grown up	A questionnaire based on the Semantic Differential and Repertory Grid Method	Contrast analysis of variance of the mothers and the daughters	Greatest differences between AN and their mothers a group versus control girls and their mothers
Hall et al. (1986)	I, III	58 mothers of AN, 204 mothers of schoolgirls	Age, Social status	Weight history, Attitudes towards weight-related matters	Food Fitness and Looks Questionnaire, Family Health Questionnaire	Means, Standard deviations, T-tests	No significant differences in weight history; less concern about weight-related issues in AN mothers

Study		Sample	Matched for	Variables	Data source	Statistics	Results
Halmi (1974b)	II	61 AN with normal premorbid weight, 22 previously obese AN	None	Broken home	Hospital records	Incidence ratings and percentages	More broken home situations prior to illness in the first group
Halmi et al. (1978)	I	Parents of 30 AN, 30 control parents	Fathers were matched for height, age, level of education, occupation and salary	Weight of the parents	Height and weight measurements	Means, Standard deviations, T-tests, Analysis of covariance	No significant difference with respect to weight, Education level is related to weight
Heron & Leheup (1984)	I	16 adolescent AN, 40 adolescents with behavioral disorders	Sex, Admission status	Social class, Broken home, Family dynamics	Retrospective analysis of hospital records	Incidence ratings Chi-square tests	No significant differences as to social class and incidence of broken home, AN came significantly more from an exclusive "happy" family with few external stresses
Herzog (1982)	II	30 BN without previous AN, 30 AN	None	Patient's birth order, Incidence of obesity and somatic illness in the parents	Interview with patient if older than 30 years, Otherwise interview with parent	Incidence ratings, Chi-square tests	Significantly more obesity and somatic illness in the parents of BN patients
Houben (1981) Houben et al. (1986, see Chapter 8)	III	Family triads of 43 AN, Family triads of 18 normal controls	Age, social status, educational level of P	Family members' own perception of interpersonal relationships	Barrett-Lennard Relationship Inventory	Means, Standard deviation, Mann-Whitney U-tests, Willcoxon tests, Correlations	AN experienced their relationship with their parents as rather similar to normal daughters. In contrast to normal controls fathers of AN do not clearly differentiate between their attitude towards their partner and towards their daughter

Appendix 1. Summary of the Studies According to Research Design (continued)

	Type	Subjects	Matched Variables	Investigated Variables	Data Gathering Method	Data Analysis	Results
Hudson et al (1983)	I, II	First-degree relatives of 14 AN, 55 BN and 20 AN + BN, First-degree relatives of 33 P with affective disorder, 39 schizophrenics and 15 borderline P	None	Affective disorders, Alcoholism, Drug-use disorders	Experimental groups: 1/6 of the relatives was personally interviewed, remaining information came from the patients, Control groups: retrospective study of hospital records	Incidence ratings and percentages, Chi-square tests	Affective disorders in relatives of eating disorder P were first in prevalence and were found significantly more frequent than in relatives of schizophrenic and borderline P but comparable to the frequency in affective disorder relatives. Eating disorder subgroups did not differ significantly on any of the variables
Humphrey (1983)	III, IV	One AN family triad, One BN family triad	None	Family interaction: affiliation and interdependence	Structural Analysis of Social Behavior (rating scale and observation of interaction during role-plays)	Scoring from verbatim transcripts	AN perceived her mother and BN her father as controlling Both parents perceived AN as submissive
Johnson & Berndt (1983)	I	8- BN, Normal community sample, Clinical sample of depressed P, alcoholic P, and schizophrenic P	None	Social adjustment	Social adjustment Scale	Means, Standard deviations	BN scored poorer adjustment within the family unit than normals but better adjustment than the other psychiatric P

Study	Design	Sample	Covariates	Construct	Instrument	Statistical analysis	Results
Johnson & Flach (1985)	III	105 BN, 86 normal controls	Age of subjects and parents, number of siblings, years of education, religion, race and marital status	Proband's perception of family environment	Family Environment Scale	Means, Standard deviations, T-tests, Stepwise regression analysis	BN reported significantly more conflict, less cohesion, less expressiveness, less intellectual-cultural, active-recreational orientation and moral-religious emphasis. Organization and achievement orientation are predictor variables for the severity of the illness
Kagan & Squires (1985)	III	105 male versus 195 female college students who tended to overeating or restrictive dieting	None	Perception of cohesion and adaptability in family interaction	FACES II	Pearson-correlations, Standard deviations, Multiple-regression analysis	No significant correlation between cohesion or adaptability and dieting behaviors among males and females. Compulsive eating related to lack of cohesion among females and to rigidity and lack of cohesion among males
Kog et al. (1985)	III	50 families with an eating disorder patient, 210 normal families	Stage of the family life cycle	Experience of family relations	Leuven Family Questionnaire. (see Chapter 6 in this book)	T-tests, ANOVA	All eating disorder subgroups scored significantly more conflict and more disorganization
Kog et al. (1986)	IV	Total family of: 3 restricting AN, 5 bulimic AN and 2 BN	None	Family interaction: enmeshment, rigidity, overprotectiveness, and lack of conflict resolution	Semi-structured interaction tasks (see Chapter 5 in this book)	Scoring of final results of the interaction tasks	Greater variability on each of the four interaction features
Leon et al. (1985)	III	31 AN and parents, 37 normal females and parents	Age, Socioeconomic status	Proband's perception of family environment	Family Environment Scale	Means, Standard deviations, T-tests	No differences in youngsters' perception. Normal parents scored significantly

Appendix 1. Summary of the Studies According to Research Design (continued)

	Type	Subjects	Matched Variables	Investigated Variables	Data Gathering Method	Data Analysis	Results
							higher on cohesion and expressiveness. Normal mothers, compared to AN mothers, scored higher on the independence scale
Maloney et al. (1983)	I	21 closest-in-age sisters of 21 AN, normal controls described in literature	Age, Height	Eating attitudes	Eating Attitudes Test	Means, Standard deviations, T-tests	Sisters differed significantly from patients but not from normals
Minuchin et al. (1978)	IV	3 psychosomatic groups: 11 families with AN, 10 families with asthmatic child, 9 families with a psychosomatic diabetic child 2 control groups: 7 families with a non-psychosomatic diabetic child, 89 families with a behavioral problem child	None	Family interaction: enmeshment, rigidity, overprotectiveness and lack of conflict resolution	Wiltwyck Family Task	Incidence rating of behavioral parameters by way of videotape	All psychosomatic groups were significantly more characterized by the four hypothesized interaction characteristics
Minuchin et al. (1978) (idem)	V	53 families with AN	-	Outcome and follow-up after 2 years	Weight of AN, Interview with P and her family	Qualitative interpretation, Incidence ratings and percentages	The results immediately after treatment and at follow-up revealed that 86% of the

from both anorexia and its psychosocial aspects

Study	Level	Sample	Controlled	Variables studied	Method	Statistics	Findings
Morgan & Russell (1975)	V	41 AN (38 females, 3 males)	-	Long-term outcome (4 years follow-up)	Structured interview at follow-up, Medical records on admission	Incidence ratings and percentages, Means, Standard deviations, Correlations, T-tests	Poor outcome was significantly correlated with a disturbed family relationship before the onset of the illness
Owen (1973)	III	9 AN and parents, 15 schoolgirls and parents	None	Projective identification	Semantic Differential	Incidence ratings and percentages, Means, Standard deviations, T-tests	AN mothers were overidentified with their daughters
Piran et al. (1985)	II	First-degree relatives of 33 BN versus 14 restricting AN	None	Family history of affective disorder and alcoholism	Independent psychiatric interview with P and at least one family member	Incidence ratings and percentages, Chi-square tests	Significantly more BN had a positive family history of depression
Rivinus et al. (1984)	I	First- and second-degree relatives of 40 AN and 23 normal females	Sex, Age	Family history of depression, substance use disorder	Interview with the parents	Incidence ratings, Age-corrected percentages, Chi-square tests	Significantly more AN had a positive family history of depression and substance use disorder
Selvini Palazzoli (1974, 1976)	I	35 families with AN, 15 families with a schizophrenic P	None	Communication patterns	Observations during family therapy sessions	Qualitative interpretation	Schizophrenic families disqualify their own and other messages on another level
Sights & Richards (1984)	IV	Parents of 6 BN and 6 non-bulimic college women	None	Parental functioning, Parent-child relationships	Structured, separate and joint interviews with fathers and mothers. Independent and blind scoring of verbatim transcipts	Means, Standard deviations, Reliability coefficients, T-tests	BN mothers were more domineering, controlling and holded higher expectations for their daughters. BN fathers were close to their daughter during childhood but distant during adolescence
Sperling & Massing (1970)	I	15 female AN, 15 normal females	Age, occupation, number of sisters, religion, social status	Individual pathology in the family, Family relations	Hospital records, Interview	Qualitative analysis, Incidence ratings and percentages	More chronic illnesses in fathers of AN. Female dominance in AN families

Appendix 1. Summary of the Studies According to Research Design (continued)

	Type	Subjects	Matched Variables	Investigated Variables	Data Gathering Method	Data Analysis	Results
Stern et al. (1984)	I	First- and second-degree relatives (excluding children) of 27 female BN versus 27 normal women	Sex, race and age of the probands	Lifetime prevalence of affective disorder in relatives	Independent and blind semi-strucutural interviews with proband and mother	Incidence ratings and percentages, Chi-square tests	No significant difference
Strober (1981)	II, III	22 restricting AN and 22 parents, 22 bulimic AN and parents	None	Physical or psychiatric problems in the parents, Emotional closeness between patients and parents, Experience of family relations, Experience of parents' marriage	Personal interview with the patient and her parents, Family Environment Scale, Locke Wallace, Marital Scale	Means, Standard deviations, T-tests, Chi-square tests	More maternal and paternal obesity and a family history of affective disorder in bulimic AN. More problematic family environment, a worse parent-daughter relationship and more marital problems in bulimic AN
Strober et al (1982)	II	First- and second-degree relatives of 35 restricting versus 35 bulimic AN	Age, duration of illness, percentage of weight loss, social class	Parental personality characteristics, affective disorder, alcoholism and drug use disorder in relatives	MMPI of parents, Structured interview with relatives	Means, Univariate tests, Incidence ratings, Age-corrected percentages, Chi-square tests	More affective disorders and alcoholism in first- and second-degree relatives of bulimic AN
Strober et al. (1985)	I	First- and second-degree relatives of 60 AN and 95 psychiatric P	Age, social class of the patients	Lifetime prevalence of eating disorders	Semi-structured interview with all relatives, predominantly by phone	Incidence ratings and age-corrected percentages, Chi-square tests	Significantly more AN and nonsignificantly more BN in the relatives of AN

Study	Level	Sample	Matching/Control	Variables	Method/Instruments	Statistics	Results
Szmukler (1983) Szmukler et al. (1985)	V	51 AN (96 females, and 5 males) and their parents	-	Factors associated with dropping out of treatment in individual (supportive) versus family therapy	Patient: clinical interview and questionnaires, Parents: audiotaped interview with each parent	Means, Standard deviations, Incidence ratings, T-tests, Chi-square tests	A high "critical comment" score of the mother and the father was significantly associated with defaulting in respectively family and individual psychotherapy
Vandereycken & Pierloot (1983)	II	65 restricting, 21 bulimic and 55 vomiting/purging AN	None	Social class, Position in the family	Hospital records	Chi-square tests	Bulimic AN stem from lower social class families
Vandereycken & Van den Broucke (1984)	II	107 male AN, reported in the literature, 148 inpatient female AN	Diagnostic criteria	Social class, Family size, Position in the family, Individual pathology in the family, Absent parent	Standardized analysis of published case-reports (males), hospital records (females)	Incidence ratings and percentages, Chi-square tests, Cluster-analysis	Three clusters in male AN: a lower class variant, a middle class variant and a (pre)pubertal variant
Weiss & Ebert (1983)	I	15 BN, 15 normal controls	Age, I.Q., Socioeconomic status	Demographic variables, Individual pathology in the family	Structured interview with the patient	Means, Standard deviations, Chi-square tests	No significant differences
Winokur et al. (1980)	I	First- and second-degree relatives of 25 AN versus 25 normal controls	Age and sociodemographic of proband	Primary affective disorder and alcoholism in the relatives	Independent semi-structural interview with proband and at least one relative	Incidence ratings and percentages, Chi-square tests	Significantly more primary affective disorder in the relatives of AN
Wold (1985)	I	9 BN, 8 unipolar depressed P, 9 normal controls	None	Perception of the family's attitude toward weight	Questionnaire	Incidence ratings, Chi-square tests	BN differed significantly on ridiculing overweight people and distress of a family member about being overweight

Chapter 4

Family Assessment: Research-Based or Practice-Oriented?

Elly Kog, Walter Vandereycken and Johan Vanderlinden

In the previous section, we underlined the urgent need to evolve from "myths to facts" in the field of family theory and therapy. We now present a state-of-the-art and outline some perspectives for the future of family assessment. In the following chapters, we discuss our own efforts in research-based as well as practice-oriented family assessment.

RESEARCH-BASED FAMILY ASSESSMENT

We differentiate two broad categories of studies according to the governing epistemological model (Kog et al., 1983): those based upon either the classic linear causality paradigm (the medical "disease" model) or the circular inter-action paradigm (the ecological "systems" model).

Linear Causality Paradigm

Family research started within this first research tradition. The cause of psychopathological behavior was no longer searched *within* the individual (e.g., a typical psychosomatic personality) but in the unidirectional maladaptive influence of the mother or both parents. This tradition is reflected by terms such as "schizophrenogenic mother" (Fromm-Reichmann, 1948) and "anorexigenic mother" (Sours, 1980). The majority of studies compare parents of a schizophrenic child with parents of a neurotic or normal child on certain relational characteristics. The parental attitudes are studied indirectly by means of projective identification (e.g., Singer & Wynne, 1963, 1966) and by means of self-report of the child (e.g., Parker, 1984), or directly by means of behavioral observation (e.g., Blakar, 1979).

The main problem with this type of research is the already mentioned *cause-consequence controversy*. Whether parental attitudes (communication style, affective style) are the cause or the consequence of psychopathology in the child is not proved by a comparative research design. Reiss (1976) holds that this requires prospective research on highly vulnerable but as yet unaffected children. This type of research has only recently been established. Liem (1980), for example, reviewed the family studies of schizophrenia, including prospective research on a vulnerable population.

Goldstein and his colleagues (Goldstein, 1981; Doane et al., 1981a; Doane et al., 1981b) are well known for their combination of comparative and prospective research. Goldstein (1981) compared the parents of 52 pre-schizophrenic adolescents (adolescents who were vulnerable to developing schizophrenia on the basis of their problem behavior) with the parents of 11 hospitalized anorexia nervosa patients and 5 hospitalized behaviorally disturbed adolescents, on the parental attitudes of "communication deviance" and "negative affective style" (*comparative part*). Moreover, in order to study the causal nature of the parental attitudes of communication deviance and negative affective style, Doane et al. (1981b) compared the results of the tests on pre-schizophrenic parents with the psychiatric diagnosis of the vulnerable child established 5 years later (*prospective part*). This study is well controlled because it fulfills all requirements for causal family research, according to Reiss (1976). Nevertheless, Goldstein (1981) himself states the limitations of his study. The studied parental attitudes can be caused by the problem behavior of the child, because they only became a subject of study from the moment that the child already showed behavioral problems. So, longitudinal research on a vulnerable population, from birth until adulthood, will prove a sounder form of control.

Another methodological issue in the search for linear causality is the need for *multivariate* research. Important relational variables have to be studied together in order to trace interaction effects. Moreover, relational variables should be studied in combination with sociological or individual variables. Social class could, for instance, interact with relational variables to cause a psychopathologic problem. This issue has been neglected up to the present. Further intra-group comparisons are needed to study this interaction effect (Liem, 1980). On the other hand, the genetic predisposition of the child could interact with relational characteristics of its parents. Twin studies and the adoptive method are very useful as a means of controlling this issue. Tienari et al. (1981) compared two matched groups of adoptive children in their "Finnish Adoptive Family Study": one group of children had a schizophrenic mother and the other group had non-schizophrenic biologic parents. The children of both groups were adopted before the age of four. After 15 years, the adoptive families, the adoptive parents and the adopted child were examined in order to determine their mental state. Genetic predisposition as well as psychosocial factors were shown to be causally related to schizophrenia.

Circular Interaction Paradigm

Family assessment, according to the circular interaction or systems model, focuses on the mutual influence between family members and on the organization and evolution of the family system with regard to developmental tasks with which the family is faced. Within this framework, the individuals and the family system itself develop and change over time in an interdependent fashion. This type of family research is called "transactional" (Anderson, 1981; Fisher et al., 1985). Transactional research does not focus on the causal influence of certain family members but on structural characteristics of the family, in order to carry out its developmental functions. Helmersen (1983) formulated it as follows: "We therefore seem to have two *parallel processes:* firstly, the traditional studies of the relationship between family interaction/communication and various categories of individual deviance/psychopathology (studies of familial pathology with a psychopathological point of departure) and, secondly, attempts to devise a genuine family-based typology with only a secondary interest in the diagnostic status of individual family members. This approach is an extension of the non-pathology oriented approach to family interaction which seeks to describe families as units using concepts relevant to systems rather than carry-overs or altered individual oriented terms. Again, it is a matter of both/and rather than either/or, however" (pp. 61-62).

The major problem of this type of research is developing a *family typology* which is no longer based on individual problems (e.g., the anorexic family), but on crucial interaction dimensions (e.g., an enmeshed family). Research, consistent with the systems model, still is in the phase of demarcating important dimensions of family functioning. Bowler (1981) differentiated three system notions: structure, process and activity. These notions return under modified forms in family literature. "Family structure" comprises the aspects "boundaries," "coalitions," and "leadership." "Family process" concerns itself with "time forms," "consistency," and "variability" over time and situations. "Family activity," finally, refers to family functions such as problem solving and conflict resolution. When operationalizations for these concepts are tested in a heterogeneous group of families in the future, research has to focus on the study of patterns of interaction, or "transaction," and their relation with effective or satisfactory family functioning.

This implies a *fit between methods and theories.* Fisher (1982), Miller et al. (1982) and Kog et al. (1983) criticize the leading theoretical framework in that it is not always reflected in the chosen methodology. Measurement validity has been a neglected area in family research. The linear causality model addresses the interactional behavior of the parents in a unidirectional way. As a reaction, researchers also studied the behavior of the child(ren), but in the majority of studies simple frequencies of parents' and children's behaviors have been recorded, without connecting them sequentially (Hughes & Haynes, 1978). One of the better methodologies to study the "interaction" between parents and (problem) child(ren) was developed by Patterson and his colleagues (Patterson, 1976; Jones et al., 1975). They studied patterns of reciprocal influence within the family by means of naturalistic observation. Limited periods of verbal and non-verbal interaction were observed and subsequently scored with the "Behavioral Scoring System." Afterwards, patterns were sought in sequences of behaviors, on the basis of qualitative interpretation. Patterson (1976) ascertained a reciprocal reinforcement of the behaviors of parents and child(ren). Families with one or more aggressive children showed a set of aversive behavior patterns and normal families were characterized by a set of positive behavior patterns between parents and child(ren).

The evaluation of family functioning within the scope of systems theory also demands the study of structural and functional interaction characteristics. In our view, the detailed micro-analysis of the verbal communication between family members is not always holistic enough to fulfill this requirement. *Verbal and non-verbal communication should be studied integrally* in order to grasp important systems aspects, such as coalition patterns in conflict resolution and leadership patterns in problem-solving. However, only qualitative clinical interpretation was used to study family transaction in this more holistic way. Harris and Lahey (1982) showed that such a macro-analysis of observable data yields unreliable results. In our concept validation study of Minuchin's structural family characteristics (Chapter 5), we used a mesoanalysis, i.e., observation and subsequent scoring of the verbal and non-verbal interaction, during a limited time period (minimum is 3 minutes; maximum is 7 minutes) on a 3-point scale. This procedure yielded a reasonable degree of interobserver reliability for concrete interaction categories. The reliability was, however, much lower for more abstract interaction categories. Future research has to focus on the concretization of non-verbal family transaction categories, in order to improve their reliability. Gottman (1979), for instance, coded verbal as well as non-verbal transaction of couples, with satisfyingly reliable methods.

Nevertheless, the continuous change of the family organization implies that the observer gets but one out of so many possible pictures of family organization, which is dependent upon his relationship with the family system. *A multimethod approach* (which is illustrated in the next chapter) seems appropriate to face this problem. The comparison between the evaluation by an investigator (an outsider to the family system) by means of observation, and the evaluation by a family member (an insider to the family system) by means of self-report, appears to be particularly relevant. Huston and Robins (1982) called this the interconnection between "behavioral interdependence," as measured through actual interpersonal behavior, and "psychological interdependence," as measured through the attitudes and beliefs about the relationship. Reiss and his colleagues (Oliveri & Reiss, 1984; Sigafoos et al., 1985) compared the results of the self-report questionnaires "Family Environment Scale" (Oliveri &

Reiss, 1984) and "Family Adaptability and Cohesion Evaluation Scales" (Sigafoos et al., 1985) with the results of the behavioral observation method "Card Sort Procedure." According to their theoretical definitions, certain scales of the self-report questionnaires had to correspond with certain measures of the Card Sort Procedure. However, the correlations did not prove this predicted association.

Olson (1985) explained the observed divergence by means of the different frame of reference of the two methods. The insiders' perspective, or what family members tell about themselves, and the outsiders' perspective, or what a therapist or another observer tells about the family, often do not correlate sufficiently. Sigafoos and Reiss (1985) themselves explain this divergence by means of the different social setting that is established by the research context. The self-report method creates a transaction between the investigator and each individual family member in which the meaning of the subjects' answers and what is being measured are clearly defined to the subject. The observation method creates a transaction between the investigator and the family group in which the purpose of the task and what is being measured remain ambiguous. In our view, these two explanations do not differ in essence because they both refer to the research context. Self-report methods ask for the individual's view of a social system in which he or she takes part. The individual family member is a subject and part of the object at the same time. This creates a very typical research context which is totally different from a subject (investigator) studying an object (family system) for its own purpose.

In order to study to what extent the research context or the frame of reference (insider/outsider) and the research task (observation/global evaluation) explain the correlations between the operationalizations of the same dimension, we have to compare a behavioral outsider method (e.g., a standardized observation procedure) and an experiential outsider method (e.g., a global evaluation by the therapist), a behavioral insider method (e.g., self-monitoring), and an experiential insider method (e.g., a self-report questionnaire), each time operationalizing the same dimension. Recent advances in statistics (i.e., parameter fitting models) make it possible to weigh the relative contribution of trait- and method-variance in the obtained results. Miller et al. (1982) state that these confirmatory methods of data analysis await their application in family research.

Another problematic issue concerns the *family unit* to be studied. Hodgson and Lewis (1979) were critical in that only a minority of family studies — published between 1969 and 1976 in three specialized family journals — investigated the family (15.1%) while the majority investigated the individual family member (56%). Family research, consistent with systems theory, has to study the total family or the transacation in various subsystems (e.g., parents, children) but the results about the subsystems may not be added to draw conclusions about the total family system.

Longitudinal research appears to be interesting within this model because, as mentioned above, family functioning changes over time. According to Anderson (1981), "observation of individuals in an interaction at a single point in time is inadequate for revealing developmental processes or outcomes" (p. 39). Therefore, transactional models explicitly add the dimension of time to the interactional model. Gottman (1982) also defines a relationship as "the temporal forms that are created when two people are together" (p. 943). He suggests "that the apprehension of temporal form implies its possible metamorphosis. The next time the temporal form arises, it can be changed" (p. 951). The notion of *time* is incorporated in the study of the family life cycle. Duvall (1971) published a well-known study on family development and its relation to the development of the child, which was updated several times. Family therapists have also become interested in the family life cycle (Carter & Mc Goldrick, 1980; Bentovim et al., 1982; Combrinck-Graham, 1985). Research on family development is, however, scarce. Riskin (1982) published a pilot study on two "nonlabeled" families which were interviewed over a period of 4 years (monthly during 2 years, then twice a year). Both families were followed during the adolescent phase of the family life cycle (starting from pubertal stage to launching stage). The semi-structured interviews were scored quantitatively by means of the "Family Interaction Scales" and analyzed with regard to clinical-qualitative aspects. Riskin used this in-depth analysis of family transaction in order to generate explicit hypotheses regarding the family transaction style of nonlabeled families and test them on a larger sample afterwards. Curiously, hypotheses about the evolution of family functioning through the studied adolescent stage are lacking. The hypotheses are static (e.g., "nonlabeled" families speak quietly, but not so clearly) or dynamic (e.g., "nonlabeled" families manifest variations in expressed affect; intensity fluctuates during interviews and from one interview to the next) but they never pinpoint the evolution of the interaction during the studied stage of the family life cycle.

Olson and Mc Cubbin (1983) tried to grasp the essence of the various stages of the family life cycle with a *cross-sectional research* design. They studied 1140 married couples and families, situated in one of the following stages: (a) young couples without children; (b) childbearing stage; (c) families with school-age children; (d) families with adolescents; (e) launching families; (f) empty nest families; and (g) families in retirement. Beside both parents, one of the children was investigated in the adolescent and launching group. These authors found that a medium degree of cohesion and adaptability, as measured by the self-report questionnaire "Family Adaptability and Cohesion Evaluation Scales," is experienced as most satisfactory in all stages of the family life cycle. However, the perceived degree of cohesion and adaptability differed for the various groups. Young couples without children reported a high degree of cohesion and adaptability. Families with young children scored either high or low on both dimensions. Families with adolescents and launching families scored the lowest on both dimensions. Finally, empty nest families and couples in retirement reported a high degree of cohesion and a low degree of adaptability. This cross-sectional research design yields a global picture of the family life cycle in a large sample. In our view, cross-sectional and longitudinal research supply one another, because cross-sectional research on a large population yields more global hypotheses about the family life cycle while longitudinal research yields more details on family development in a more restricted group.

We mentioned above that transactional research incorporates the dimension of time. In our view, this does not necessarily mean that this type of research demands a longitudinal research design, as stated by Anderson (1981). Another way to incorporate the notion of time in the research is to study *sequential patterns* of data, gathered in a limited time period (e.g., during a single day). Gottman (1982) studied patterns of emotion in a couple, including data on the couple's perception of their interaction in video-recall sessions, measures of their videotaped behavior, as well as physiological reactions during the interaction. These data are combined sequentially, in order to create a convergent picture of patterns of interaction. These temporal forms were powerful in a set of studies, discriminating the problem solving processes of satisfied and dissatisfied couples. An interesting finding, which supports our idea that non-verbal interaction is very important in the study of transaction, is that without the use of the non-verbal codes, the two groups of couples were indistinguishable. Family systems research needs this way of approaching its subject.

A final suggestion for future family research is the use of *secondary analysis of extant data*. On the one hand, there is a negative reason for turning away from primary data collection because it is extremely time consuming and expensive, especially when the whole family is investigated. On the other hand, there are positive reasons for the use of secondary analysis, namely: larger sample size, greater representation, and a possibility to focus one's energy either on data collection or on data analysis (Miller et al., 1982).

PRACTICE-ORIENTED FAMILY ASSESSMENT

As this book tries to demonstrate, it is important that the practitioner has a research-minded attitude in order to study family issues which are more directly linked to clinical practice. In this respect, Eisler et al. (1985) carried out a particularly interesting study on *the compatability of systematic observation and clinical insight*. The authors (experimenters) constructed a range of statements concerning family interaction in four families with an anorexia nervosa patient. These statements contained varying degrees of clinical inference and were made by the experimenters because they felt them to be clinically meaningful. Observers with varying degrees of clinical and research experience had to score, after a video-demonstration of one of the anorexic families, which statements applied to the family they had observed and which did not. The authors differentiated two observation and scoring conditions. In the first condition, the observers were shown a 30 minute videotape of a family with an anorexic daughter having a picnic lunch. During and/or after the observation, they had to score individually the 54 statements, which were made on three levels of abstraction. In the second condition, three groups of three or four observers carried out the task, viewing the tape for 15 minutes and then being required to reach a preliminary consensus agreement as to their ratings on the three levels. They next had the opportunity to review the tape and to discuss their subsequent observations. Then they viewed the second 15 minutes of the tape and reached a final consensus as to their ratings. Although the judgments required a discrimination between clinically similar families (all anorexia nervosa families), the observers were able to recognize the target statements and to reject the control statements on a significant level (2/3 of the target statements were correctly chosen and 1/3 of the control statements were wrongly chosen). The results were not better for statements on a lower level of abstraction nor for observers with longer clinical or research experience. The results were, however, better in the second situation which comprised group discussion in order to make consensus judgments. This is a promising effort to bridge the gap between clinicians and researchers. Therefore, we fully agree with the authors' final conclusion: "We cannot at this stage say how far our results could be generalized to other types of clinical descriptions or to different perhaps similar families. However, it is clear that the results have important implications for observational research. Many of the limitations of interaction research are directly derived from an acceptance of a narrow definition of reliability and, by implication, of what is 'objective'. Our results show that objective research does not have to be restricted to a narrowly defined, fixed observational framework but can include apparently subjective elements of clinical observation and judgments" (Eisler et al., 1985, p. 185).

The issue of the *outcome of family therapy* is also a crucial but almost totally neglected research topic in the area of eating disorders. Wells and Dezen (1978) reviewed all kinds of family therapy outcome studies and concluded that comparative studies did not yet prove the superiority of family therapy in comparison with other therapeutic approaches to a wide series of psychiatric problems. Several studies proved the superiority of a combination of family therapy with other therapeutic interventions, such as medication and hospitalization, in adolescent and adult psychiatric patients. However, these studies did not investigate the pure effect of family therapy. More recently, in a well controlled study of drug addicts, Stanton and Todd (1982) proved an exclusively positive effect of structural-strategic family therapy on the amount of drugs taken and on the percent mortality. In the care of eating disorders, family therapy outcome studies are almost absent. Moreover, the few existing studies, even that of Minuchin et al. (1978) with its high success rates, are uncontrolled (see Chapter 3). In order to determine the exclusive effect of family therapy, we judge a comparison with a non-treatment program inadequate because of ethical reasons (one cannot let someone starve to death for the sake of one's research design!). We suggest instead a comparison between an outpatient family therapy program and a self-help group for eating disorders, the latter representing a non-professional treatment condition, in order to prove the effectiveness of family therapy. In order to prove its superiority, a family therapy program has to be compared with another type of professional treatment, for instance, individual psychotherapy (Szmukler et al., 1985).

Another important question which is neglected in the research literature is *the indication/contra-indication of family therapy in certain subgroups of anorexia nervosa patients*. Garfinkel and Garner (1982) and Yager and Strober (1985) claim that family therapy is especially indicated in young anorexia nervosa patients, but this statement is based on clinical impressions and as such not supported by empirical research evidence. A systematic comparison of family therapy outcome on various levels (symptomatic, psychological and social functioning of the patient, and family functioning) in younger and older eating disorder patients and in various symptomatological subgroups seems especially relevant for planning a research-guided treatment (Szmukler et al., 1985; see also Chapter 9).

Thus, we need a *selection of outcome criteria* in order to judge the effectiveness of family therapy. Minuchin et al. (1978), surprisingly enough for family therapists, only evaluated the psychosomatic child on the symptom level and on its psychosocial functioning. But the symptom is supposed to have a function in the broader family context. So, changes in family functioning as well as a possible shift of symptoms — symptom substitution within the family system — have to be detected in the outcome evaluation. Crisp et al. (1974) found for instance that weight restoration in anorexic patients was correlated with increased depression in the parents (though these authors did not rule out the impact of the child's hospitalization itself upon the parents). Gurman and Kniskern (1978; 1982) claim that family therapy outcome evaluation has to focus on the following three units: (1) the identified patient, (2) the parental dyad, and (3) the whole family. Shift of symptoms or a negative outcome on one system level results in a carefully balanced appraisal which can guide the therapeutic process. The above mentioned results of Crisp et al. (1974) may, for instance, be an indication for a parallel therapeutic process engaging the parents (see Chapter 4).

Up until the present, practically all *outcome evaluation measurements* are based on a clinical judgment of the therapist himself. However, the therapist was shown to systematically over- or underestimate the effects of his therapy (Wells & Dezen, 1978). Thus, the therapist should never be the only source of outcome-information; different points of view have to be compared. A variation on the insider-outsider dimension (Olson, 1981) seems to us essential in order to judge the outcome of family therapy. In Chapter 9, we discuss an outcome study which combines a self-report method (based on the insider-view) and a clinical judgment of the therapist (based on the outsider-view). Beside the insider-outsider variation, Gurman and Kniskern (1981) underline the importance of a variation as to the level of inference (objective-subjective) in the outcome measures. Symptom behavior in eating disorders can, for instance, either be evaluated by means of an objective measure such as the amount of weight restoration or by means of a subjective evaluation of the change in attitudes toward weight (see Chapter 9).

Finally, only a minority of outcome studies evaluate the criterion behaviors before the start of the therapeutic process in order to create *a baseline*. Minuchin et al. (1978) did collect a baseline measure but only of the symptom behavior. A carefully balanced appraisal of the family therapy as a whole or of particular parts of it requires baseline measures of all the outcome variables, as is shown by Hall and Crisp (1983) and Vanderlinden and Vandereycken (Chapter 9).

CONCLUSION

In general, the quality of family research varies considerably and methodologically appropriate studies are scarce. The linear causality model is the oldest one and has thus been studied more intensively than the circular interaction or systems model. Some supportive research evidence of this model is well controlled, but other studies do not fulfill the requirements for causal family research. The circular causality model was developed in response to criticisms of unidirectional parental research, but the methodology of studying the mutual influence between parents and child(ren) is often an inadequate adoption of individual-oriented methodologies. Systems research has first to define important concepts of family functioning and develop system- oriented operationalizations, before it can study family transaction throughout the family life cycle. Practice-oriented assessment, moreover, struggles with the problem of combining a therapeutically relevant and justifiable research purpose with a methodologically adequate and ethically acceptable research strategy.

REFERENCES*

Anderson, W. (1981), Parent-child relationhips: A context for reciprocal developmental influence. *The Counseling Psychologist,* 9:35-44.

Bentovim, A., Barnes, G. & Cooklin, A. (Eds.) (1982), *Family Therapy: Complementary Frame-Work of Theory and Practice. Vol. 2.* London: Academic Press.

Blakar, R.M. (1979), *Studies of Familial Communication and Psychopathology: A Social-Developmental Approach to Deviant Behavior.* Oslo: Universitetsforlaget.

Bowler, T. (1981), *General Systems Thinking: Its Scope and Applicability.* New York-Oxford: North Holland.

---

* This list contains only secondary literature, whereas the other references are mentioned in the final section of this book: "Bibliography on Family Aspects of Eating Disorders."

Carter, E. & Mc Goldrick, M. (Eds.) (1980), *The Family Life Cycle: A Framework for Family Therapy*. New York: Gardner Press.

Combrinck-Graham, L. (1985), A developmental model for family systems. *Family Process*, 24:139-150.

Doane, J.A., West, K.L., Goldstein, M.J., Rodnick, E.H. & Jones, J.E. (1981a), Parental communication deviance and affective style: Predictors of subsequent schizophrenia spectrum disorders in vulnerable adolescents. *Archives of General Psychiatry*, 38:679-685.

Doane, J.A., Goldstein, M.J. & Rodnick, E.H. (1981b), Parental patterns of affective style and the development of schizophrenia spectrum disorders. *Family Process*, 20:337-349.

Duvall, E. (1971), *Family Development (4th Ed.)*. Philadelphia: J.B. Lippincott.

Eisler, I., Szmukler, G. & Dare, C. (1985), Systematic observation and clinical insight. Are they compatible? An experiment in recognizing family interactions. *Psychological Medicine*, 15:173-188.

Fisher, L. (1982), Transactional theories but individual assessment: A frequent discrepancy in family research. *Family Process*, 21:313-320.

Fromm-Reichmann, F. (1948), Notes on development of treatment of schizophrenics by psychoanalytic psychotherapy. *Psychiatry*, 11:263-273.

Garfinkel, P.E. & Garner, D.M. (1982), *Anorexia Nervosa. A Multidimensional Perspective.* New York: Brunner/Mazel.

Gottman, J.M. (1979), *Marital Interaction: Experimental Investigations.* New York: Academic Press.

Gottman, J.M. (1982), Temporal form: Toward a new language for describing relationships. *Journal of Marriage and the Family*, 44:943-962.

Gurman, A.S. & Kniskern, D.P. (1978), Deterioration in marital and family therapy: Empirical, clinical and conceptual issues. *Family Process*, 17:3-20.

Gurman, A.S. & Kniskern, D. (1981), Family therapy outcome research: Knowns and unknowns. In: Gurman, A.S. & Kniskern, D. (Eds.). *Handbook of Family Therapy.* New York: Brunner/Mazel, pp. 742-775.

Hall, A. & Crisp, A.H. (1983), Brief psychotherapy in the treatment of anorexia nervosa: Preliminary findings. In: Darby, P., Garfinkel, P., Garner, D. & Coscina, D. (Eds.), *Anorexia Nervosa: Recent Developments in Research.* New York: Alan R. Liss, pp. 417-425.

Harris, F. & Lahey, B. (1982), Recording system bias in direct observational methodology: A review and critical analysis of factors causing inaccurate coding bahavior. *Clinical Psychology Review*, 2:539-556.

Helmersen, P. (1983), *Family Interaction and Communication Psychopathology: An Evaluation of Recent Perspectives.* London: Academic Press.

Hodgson, J.W. & Lewis, R.A. (1979), Pelgrim's progress III: A trend analysis of family theory and methodology. *Family Process*, 18:163-173.

Hughes, H.M. & Haynes, S.N. (1978), Structured laboratory observation in the behavioral assessment of parent-child interactions: A methodological critique. *Behavior Therapy*, 9:428-447.

Huston, T.L. & Robins, E. (1982), Conceptual and methodological issues in studying close relationships. *Journal of Marriage and the Family*, 44:901-925.

Jones, J.E. (1977), Patterns of transactional style deviance in the TAT's of parents of schizophrenics. *Family Process*, 16:327-337.

Liem, J.H. (1980), Family studies of schizophrenia: An update commentary. *Schizophrenia Bulletin*, 6:429-455.

Miller, B.C., Rollins, B.C. & Thomas, D.L. (1982), On methods of studying marriage and families. *Journal of Marriage and the Family*, 44:851-875.

Oliveri, M. & Reiss, D. (1984), Family concepts and their measurement: Things are seldom what they seem. *Family Process*, 23:33-48.

Olson, D.H. (1981), Family typologies: Bridging family research and family therapy. In: Filsinger, E.E. & Lewis, R.A. (Eds.), *Assessing Marriage: New Behavioral Approaches.* Beverly Hills-London: Sage Publications, pp. 74-89.

Olson, D. (1985), Commentary: Struggling with congruence across theoretical models and methods. *Family Process*, 24:203-207.

Olson, D.H. & Mc Cubbin, H. (1983), *Families: What Makes Them Work.* Beverly Hills-London:Sage Publications.

Parker, G. (1984), The measurement of pathogenic parental style and its relevance to psychiatric disorder. *Social Psychiatry,* 19:75-81.

Patterson, G.R. (1976), The aggressive child: Victim and architect of a coercive system. In: Mash, E.J. Hamerlynck, L.C. & Handy, L.C. (Eds.), *Behavior Modification in Families.* New York: Brunner/Mazel.

Reiss, D. (1976), The family and schizophrenia. *American Journal of Psychiatry,* 133:181-185.

Sigafoos, A. & Reiss, D. (1985), Rejoinder: Counterperspectives on family measurement: The pragmatic interpretation of research methods. *Family Process,* 24:207-211.

Sigafoos, A., Reiss, D., Rich, J. & Douglas, E. (1985), Pragmatics in the measurement of family functioning: An interpretive framework for methodology. *Family Process,* 24:189-203.

Singer, M. & Wynne, L. (1963), Differentiating characteristics of parents of childhood schizophrenics, childhood neurotics and young adult schizophrenics. *American Journal of Psychiatry,* 120:234-243.

Singer, M. & Wynne, L. (1966), Principles for scoring communication defects and deviances in parents of schizophrenics: Rorschach and TAT scoring manuals. *Psychiatry,* 29:260-289.

Sours, J.A. (1980), *Starving to Death in a Sea of Objects. The Anorexia Nervosa Syndrome.* New York: Jason Aronson.

Stanton, M. & Todd, T. (1982), *The Family Therapy of Drug Abuse and Addiction.* New York: Guilford Press.

Tienari, P., Sorri, A., Naarala, M., Lahti, I., Boström, C. & Wahlberg, K.E. (1981); The Finnish adoptive family study. Family-dynamic approach on psychosomatics: A preliminary report. *Psychiatry and Social Science,* 1:107-115.

Wells, R.A. & Dezen, A.E. (1978), The results of family therapy revisited: The non-behavioral methods. *Family Process,* 17:251-274.

Chapter 5

Multimethod Investigation of Eating Disorder Families*

Elly Kog, Walter Vandereycken and Hans Vertommen

e carried out a multimethod investigation of Minuchin's psychosomatic family model in eating disorder families (Minuchin et al., 1975, 1978). The psychosomatic family model claims that a typical family organization, together with a special physiological vulnerability of the child, are underlying the occurrence of a psychosomatic symptom in the child. The involvement of the child in parental conflicts, either as an avoider or as a coalition partner, reinforces the symptom (see also Chapter 2 and 3). Families with an anorexic patient were characterized most significantly by this psychosomatic family organization. This model, and especially the investigation which was carried out to empirically support the clinical theory, resulted in two opposite reactions in family literature. Clinicians underlined the high percentage of therapeutic success that resulted from the structural family therapy, based on this model. The negative reactions predominantly refer to the research methodology. We will try to give a carefully balanced appraisal of this model by taking into account both its strengths and its weaknesses.

CRITICAL ANALYSIS OF THE PSYCHOSOMATIC FAMILY MODEL

We differentiate three types of critical parameters: the first type concerns the research design, the second one the research methodology, and the third type focuses on the investigated family concepts.

Research Design

Minuchin et al. (1978) claim they proved (on the basis of the comparative research discussed in Chapter 3) that psychosomatic families are characterized

---

*   Portions of this chapter have been published in: E. Kog, H. Vertommen & W. Vandereycken, "Minuchin's psychosomatic family model revised" *(Family Process, 1987, 26, 235-253.)*

Table 1: Research design of the study by Minuchin et al. (1978)

	Number of families	Age of the patient	Duration of illness
Psychosomatic groups			
Anorexia nervosa	11	13-16	average of 6 months
Psychosomatic diabetes	9	-	1 to 4 years
Asthma	10	10-14	-
Control groups			
Non-psychosomatic diabetes	7	-	-
Behavioral problems	8	-	-

by four typical structural interaction features — enmeshment, rigidity, overprotectiveness and lack of conflict resolution — which, together with the physiological vulnerability of the child, form the basis for the development of a psychosomatic symptom in the child. But the research design was inadequate to prove the hypothesized specificity of the model for psychosomatic families as well as the pathogenic nature of the typical family organization.

In order to prove the *specificity* of the model, experimental and control groups have to be matched for important individual and familial variables, such as age of the parents and the children, number of children, and social status of the family (Blakar, l1979; Jacob, 1975). Minuchin et al. (1978) did not match their experimental and control groups, even not on individual characteristics of the patients. Moreover, they gave an incomplete picture of the studied groups (see Table 1).

Concerning the *pathogenic nature* of the model, Vandereycken (1980) and Yager (1981,1982) postulate that the typical family organization might be a reaction to a particular stress-situation as well as a causal element for the psychosomatic disease. According to Yager (1982), prospective research on a highly vulnerable but as yet unaffected population is required to arrange this cause-consequence controversy.

Research Method

With regard to the investigated *subjects,* the various experimental and control groups are too small (see Table 1) and even not representative. For instance, the anorexia nervosa sample comprises only young patients with a short illness history of food refusal or restriction, and no other symptoms such as bulimia, vomiting or purging. Vandereycken and Pierloot (1983) showed, however, that characteristics such as age, duration of illness and anorexic symptomatology do have prognostic significance. Moreover, there is considerable evidence to support the idea that differences in anorexic symptomatology are related to different family interaction styles (see Chapter 3). In general, restricting anorexics do have a more favorable family environment. So, the 86 percent success rate of Minuchin's family therapy could, at least partially, be explained by his sample selection, especially with regard to the anorexia nervosa families.

Concerning the research *procedure,* Minuchin et al. (1978) used the behavioral observation method, based on semi-structured interaction tasks. Members of his own clinical team scored the behavioral data. Thus, their initial formulations may have colored what they subsequently saw in families. The results were not controlled by independent observers who were blind to the hypotheses and diagnostic status of the families. Thus, the reliability of the behavioral observation data has not been tested (Yager, 1981, 1982). The observation by clinician researchers is also limited by neglecting the perception of the family members themselves with regard to their family interaction.

Investigated Family Concepts

We question Minuchin's conceptualization with regard to two major issues. Firstly, we criticize the overemphasis of pathological extremes (see also Wood & Talmon, 1983) of the interactional features, and, hence, the lack of attention to situational and temporal variability of family interaction. We prefer to use dimensional instead of categorical terms to characterize the interactional features. We had difficulties in grasping the essence of this concept, especially with regard to overprotectiveness. In our view, this might be a superfluous concept because of its considerable overlap with lack of conflict resolution and enmeshment. Minuchin et al. (1978) state that the four characteristics have to be considered as one clinical picture: "No one of these characteristics alone seemed sufficient to spark and reinforce psychosomatic symptoms" (p. 30). Nevertheless, if one distinguishes four characteristics, the meaning of each of them has to be — at least partially — different from the others. This overlap in meanings of Minuchin's definitions was our second criticism, concerning conceptualization.

Since Minuchin's investigation has been criticized from a methodological point of view, we designed a partially new model of interactional research in families with an anorexia and bulimia nervosa patient. Our study is focused on the operationalization as well as on the verification of Minuchin's four interactional characteristics. Thus, we partially redefined the characteristics; the content as well as the term have been adapted after an in-depth discussion on the use of each and similar interaction features by different authors (Kog et al., 1985).

Dimension A, *the intensity of intrafamilial boundaries* (relabeling of "enmeshment"), has been defined as a continuum according to the degree to which family members behave, think and feel conformably (enmeshment pole) or differently from each other (disengagement pole). This concept reveals something about the nature of the family interaction, not about its quality. It is comparable to the family typology of Reiss (1971a, 1971b, 1981), who differentiates three types of families. The "environment-sensitive families" (comparable to the middle position of our dimension) function according to the paradigm that the problems are "out there:" problems have no personal relevance, they have to be observed and studied accurately in order to solve them. "Interpersonal distance-sensitive families" (comparable to families with a high intensity of intrafamilial boundaries) consider problems as "something personal:" problem-solving is seen as an evidence of someone's independence in the family. Finally, "consensus-sensitive families" (comparable to families with a low intensity of intrafamilial boundaries) consider problems as "in here:" the solution is viewed as a means to reach consensus in the family.

Dimension B, *the degree of the family's adaptability* (relabeling of "rigidity"), has been defined as a process variable: the evolution of the family in its stability and change on different system levels. The family is characterized by a "coherence" (Dell, 1982) with minor fluctuations or greater changes in reaction to forces from within or from outside the family system. So, we endorse "the evolutionary paradigm" (Hoffman, 1981) in systems theory.

We hypothesized that dimension C, *the degree of avoidance/recognition of intrafamilial tension* (relabeling of "overprotectiveness,") might be a superfluous dimension because of its considerable overlap with dimension A and D. However, in order to test this hypothesis in our own study, we had to operationalize this concept. We focused on the acceptance versus avoidance of intrafamilial tension, because we judged this aspect as most specific and thus most different from "enmeshment" and "lack of conflict resolution."

Finally, dimension D, *the family's way of handling conflicts,* finally, refers to the family's way of solving problems with regard to intrafamilial conflicts (predominantly between parents and children). As to the degree of conflict, this concept, once again, has to be considered in the dimensional sense with conflict avoidance at one end and conflict escalation at the other. As to the modality of conflict resolution, parents and children can take different positions which will be discussed later on.

We used these dimensional definitions as a basis for our operationalizations. The preliminary results of a pilot study of ten families with an anorexia or bulimia nervosa patient (Kog et al., 1985a) suggest some support for our conceptualization of family functioning, especially with regard to the dimensional nature of the interaction concepts. For each of the operational definitions, there seemed to be sufficient variability to conclude that anorexia/bulimia nervosa families can take variable positions on these dimensions. This means that, unlike Minuchin et al. (1975, 1978), we did not find a specific or consistent interaction pattern or family profile.

We presumed that the conclusions of Minuchin and colleagues are biased by their focus on the extreme positions on the dimensions as well as by their use of a selected sample of anorexic families. We, on the contrary, studied intact as well as broken families from different social classes and with a child belonging to various symptomatic subgroups. Thus, we studied a *heterogeneous* sample of families, but nevertheless all of them had a child with an eating disorder. A representative sample of these eating disorders was investigated in our pilot study in order to test whether these families scored sufficiently differently on the dimensions because a concept-validation requires a sufficient degree of variability. The eating disorder families indeed took variable positions on the dimensions, so we confined ourselves to this clinical sample. Our main purpose was to develop a clear conceptual framework within which empirical operationalizations are directly linked to the interactional dimensions. We believe that this will be a better basis for further comparative and longitudinal research because, in the past, too much energy has been invested in simply comparing various families which were classified according to general or theoretical ideas without sufficient empirical support. Interactional dimensions have to be translated in clear and neutral behavioral operationalizations in order to generate a valuable and reliable family classification based on crucial interactional dimensions.

CONCEPT-VALIDATION OF THE PSYCHOSOMATIC FAMILY MODEL

Subjects

We investigated the families of 55 female eating disorder patients. The entire family of each patient treated in the Anorexia Nervosa Unit of the University Psychiatric Center St. Jozef (Kortenberg, Belgium) between March 1983 and October 1984 was asked to participate if the patient still lived at home at the beginning of the therapy (one family did not want to participate because of the long traveling distance). The results of two families were incomplete: one family dropped out during the study because of an escalation of conflicts and another family was not able to fill out the questionnaire. So, the final data were drawn from 53 Flemish families. The general characteristics of these families are comparable to other samples of eating disorder families (Kog & Vandereycken, 1985).

Intact versus broken home: in 45 cases (85%) the parents were still living together, while 15% of the cases showed a broken home situation (in three cases the parents were divorced and in five families one parent was deceased; in seven of the cases the father was the absent parent).

Social class (according to father's occupation): 23% belonged to the lower social class; 32% to the lower-middle, 19% to the upper-middle, and 26% to the upper social class.

Number of children: in 2 cases the patient was the only child, 15 families had two children, 16 families had three children, 13 families had four children, and 7 families had five or more children.

Family life cycle: 19% were situated in the pubertal or young adolescent phase (the middle child being between 12 and 15 years of age), 32% in the middle adolescent phase (16 to 18 years), and 49% in the late adolescent or launching phase (19 years and older).

Patients' age averaged 19 years, ranging from 14 to 34 years.

Patients' duration of illness varied between 6 months and 5 years (average of 2.2 years).

Patients' diagnosis according to DSM-III (American Psychiatric Association, 1980): 74% met the criteria for anorexia nervosa, 57 % belonging to the subgroup of "pure" dieters and 17% to the binge eaters/vomiters/purgers (see Vandereycken & Pierloot, 1983); 17% showed the bulimia syndrome, referred to as bulimia nervosa (Russell, 1979); 9% had an atypical eating disorder (which means that they did not fulfill all criteria of the previous categories).

Treatment format: 23% of the patients were only in outpatient therapy while 77% were treated in a structured inpatient program (see Vandereycken, 1985).

Procedure

The family interaction concepts are validated with a multitrait-multimethod approach (Campbell & Fiske, 1959). Two behavioral methods (behavioral process or direct observation and behavioral product measures) and one self-report method are used to operationalize each concept. Behavioral data are based on a range of semi-structured tasks that differ with regard to the subsystem that is engaged (individual family members, parents/children, and entire family) and the nature of the induced interaction (decision making, conflict resolution and structure-free situation). The final result of each interaction task (the behavioral product measure) as well as the interaction process (on the basis of videotaped observation) are studied. Immediately following completion of the interaction tasks, each family member is asked to fill out the Leuven Family Questionnaire. This two-hour-long session occurs before the beginning of the outpatient treatment or within the first 10 days after hospitalization. This research procedure is the end product of a process of trial and error in the course of a pilot study of 10 families with an anorexia or bulimia nervosa patient (Kog et al., 1985a). This procedure appeared to be a clear, practical and fruitful approach for studying family interaction, and is, as such, ready and easily applicable for use on a larger scale. We will now briefly describe the different phases of our standardized research procedure.

Introduction: the investigator (first author) explains the purpose of the family meeting and also the use of the video-recording (confidentiality of all information is guaranteed). She then announces that she has to prepare a few things before the first task can be started and moves to the adjacent observation room that is linked with the research room by means of a one-way mirror (the investigator will always leave the research room after having explained a task). The interaction during this three-minutes-long wait is videotaped in order to observe the family's first reaction to the research setting. This observation period is inspired by the investigation of Ketelaar-Van Ierssel (1982).

Interest task: this task comprises an individual and an interactional component. First, the *individual component.* The investigator gives each family member a 12-item questionnaire (see Appendix 1) concerning different aspects of the adolescent phase of the family life cycle. Each question is followed by 7 response possibilities. Every family member has to individually choose two answers that he/she likes the most and two answers that he/she likes the least. Members are told not to discuss or to compare each other's answers. This part lasts approximately 20 minutes. For the *interactional component,* the family is given the same questionnaire now only listing the first 6 items. The task has changed such that each family member has to choose only 1 of the 7 response alternatives and must specify with whom he/she prefers to engage in the activity described. Therefore, a deliberation within the family is needed. There are many possible outcomes of this deliberation: each family member may choose different possibilities, or some family members may choose the same possibilities and others do not, or the whole family may prefer to do something together. Again, the final answers have to be filled in on the questionnaire. This decision-making task, that may last at most 20 minutes, is an adaptation of the "Unrevealed Difference Technique," developed by Ferreira and Winter (1965).

Family criticism task: this task also comprises an individual and an interactional component. During the *individual component,* each family member is given three cards. On each card they have to write one thing they do not like in the way the family interacts at home. This must be clearly formulated, because these issues will be discussed later on. When this is completed (10 minutes), the *interactional component* starts. First, the family members have to read each criticism out loud. Then, they have to deliberate which criticism is most important for the family at that moment. Afterwards, the remaining criticisms have to be ordered from the most to the least important. This second component of the task lasts at most 20 minutes. The idea of formulating family criticisms is based on the "Blame Technique," originally described by Watzlawick et al. (1970).

Break: the break, as used by Ketelaar-Van Ierssel (1982), lasts 10 minutes, during which time the family is given soft drinks and biscuits. They are asked to stay in the room. The videotape of this break gives an impression of the family interaction in a structure-free situation wherein food is available.

Disagreement task: this is a conflict management task to be carried out between the subsystems "parents" and "children," separated in the room. The *preparing phase* of this task is carried out by each of the subsystems on their own. Each subsystem has to choose one subject (problem) on which they disagree with the other subsystem and write it down on a card. They have to put the card on the table, so that the other subsystem can read the problem without discussing it. Then, each subsystem has to write down on a separate list their proposal for resolution of their own problem and of the problem formulated by the other subsytem (see Appendix 2). Once this is done, the *negotiation phase* can start. First, the parents explain the problem they have chosen, the children say what they think about it, and finally parents and children try to achieve resolution. The parents write this agreement on their card. Afterwards, the children explain their problem and a similar negotiation follows. The preparation and negotiation phases must be completed in 30 minutes.

Leuven Family Questionnaire: finally, each family member has to fill out a questionnaire comprising 106 items concerning family life. For each of the items, they have to score on a 6-point scale if this statement is definitely not true, not true, rarely true, true some of the time, true most of the time or true all of the time, for their family. The items are operationalizations of the two poles of each of the four dimensions (see Appendix 3).

Data Analysis

As mentioned above, each of the four interactional dimensions is operationalized by means of two behavioral methods (a direct observation and a behavioral product method) and a self-report method. We will now discuss the four operationalizations in the three methods.

Behavioral Product Method

Each of the four interaction dimensions is operationalized in one product measure, i.e., the written result of one of the interaction tasks.

In order to measure *the intensity of intrafamilial boundaries* (dimension A), we rely upon the results of the individual component of the interest task. The questionnaires of all possible dyads in the family are compared with respect to *spontaneous agreements:* i.e., similarity in choices without consulting together. Inspired by Ferreira and Winter (1965), we use the following scoring system for each of the 12 items:

1. Conformity in choices is scored positively, i.e., $+1$ point for each response alternative similarly chosen by each member of the dyad. Thus the maximum conforming score for a single item is $+4$.
2. Difference in choices is scored negatively, i.e. -1 point if the members of a dyad disagree about a response alternative. As above this yields a maximum difference score of -4 for any individual item.

The scores for the 12 items are added and may thus theoretically vary between -48 and $+48$ for each dyad. We apply the following formulas to this spontaneous agreement (SA)-measure:

1. *On the system level:*

$$\frac{\text{addition of all SA-scores}}{\text{total of all possible dyads in the family}}$$

The result is the average intensity of boundaries within the family. This measure can be compared between families of different size, regardless of the number of possible dyads.

2. *On the generational level:*

$$SA_{\text{parents}} - \text{highest } SA_{\text{parent/child}}$$

If this measure is positive, there are firm generational boundaries. The SA between the parents (generational SA) is higher than the SA between one parent and one child (transgenerational). A negative result, on the contrary, reflects cross-generational intrusion (higher transgenerational than generational SA).

3. *On the individual level:*
   (a) highest SA score
   (b) lowest SA score
   (c) difference between score (a) and (b)

The difference-score (c) reflects the degree of intrafamilial differences with respect to boundaries.

We have reinterpreted Minuchin's concept of "rigidity" according to *the degree of the family's adaptability* (dimension B). This process variable may be measured either in the same situation over a longer time period (e.g., during the course of family therapy) or in different situations at one given moment. The latter is the case in the present investigation where we measure the degree of the family's adaptability as reflected in the outcome (written information) of the interactional part of the interest-task. We determine the organization for each of the six situations by studying the pattern of "who prefers to do what with whom." For intact families with at least two children, we differentiate 6 organization patterns that we consider important according to family interaction theory: (1) the whole family; (2) each family member separately (alone or with people outside the nuclear family); (3) parents together and children separately or together; (4) parents separately and children partly together or altogether; (5) one parent with one or more children and the other parent alone or with other children; and (6) both parents with one or more children but not all of them. For intact families with only one child, organization pattern 1 and 6 are identical, so there are but five organization patterns available. For broken families only organization pattern 1, 2, 4 (one parent separately and the children partly together or altogether) and 6 (one parent with one or more children but not all of them) are available. Families with one parent and one child only have two patterns available: they carry out the activity together or separately.

After having determined the organization pattern for each situation, we examine to what extent the family organizes itself identically or differently in the six situations. Each of the six situations is compared with each other (a total of 15 comparisons): one point is scored when the organization of the family is totally identical and zero is scored when the organization is different. However, the constancy by chance is different for the different types of families because the number of available organization patterns differs. Therefore, we applied a correction for the constancy by chance, that is based on the formula of correction for guessing. This correction depends upon the number of available organization patterns. The degree of organizational constancy is expressed in a percentage, according to the following formula:

$$[N_c - N_v/p-1] \times 100/15$$

N_c = number of organizational constancies (min. = 0; max. = 15)
N_v = number of organizational variabilities (min. = 0; max. = 15)
p = number of available patterns (6, 5, 4, or 2 according to the type of family)

Hence, families may score from 0 (extreme organizational variability) to 100 (extreme organizational constancy). Some families may score negatively (min. = -12) because of a slight overcorrection in certain types of families, but these negative scores are transformed to 0. The position of a family on this continuum is comparable between different types of families.

In our view "overprotectiveness" represents a process variable which involves *the degree of avoidance/recognition of intrafamilial tension* (dimension C). Avoidance or recognition of intrafamilial tension is based upon the results of the family criticism task. In this measure, we do not take into account the order of the criticisms, nor who wrote it. We only categorize the written criticisms, on the basis of their content, into two classes: "recognition" or "avoidance" of intrafamilial tension. The class of "avoidance of criticism" is further subdivided into 6 modalities, with a different score. Criticisms may be avoided by:
1.   denial, were there is no criticism (score = -3);
2.   primary projection, in which someone outside the nuclear family is criticized (score = -2);
3.   self-criticism, in which a family member criticizes oneself (score = -2);
4.   detouring, in which the illness is mentioned (score = -2);
5.   neutralization, where the conflict is ascribed to some impersonal cause (score = -2);
6.   disqualification, in which the criticism is situated in the past or is retracted (score = -1).
The class of "recognition of criticism" is further subdivided into 7 modalities:

1. personal criticism, i.e., one particular person is blamed for interpersonal problems (score = +3);
2. guilt-induction, where an unidentified person or persons is/are blamed for some personal sorrow (score = +3);
3. concrete interactional criticism, which makes reference to at least 2 persons, without blaming a particular one (score = +2);
4. vague interactional criticism; the family interaction in general is criticized (score = +1);
5. minimization: an interactional criticism is formulated, but accompanied by "sometimes," "a little," "may be" (score = +1);
6. wish; this means that no criticism but a wish for a better interaction is expressed (score = +1);
7. organizational criticism, i.e., home rules or habits are considered the cause of tensions in the family (score = +1).

After this categorization, we add all the scores and divide this sum by the number of criticisms (9 if there are 3 family members, 12 if there are 4 family members). This avoidance/recognition ratio (min. = -3, max. = +3) is comparable between families of different size.

"Lack of conflict resolution," as a final characteristic, has been redefined according to *the family's way of handling conflicts,* i.e., the degree and modality of problem-solving with regard to intrafamilial conflicts. This variable is measured using the results of the negotiation phase of the disagreement task between parents and children. We determine the modality of conflict resolution by comparing the starting position of each subgroup (on the separate list) and the solution (on the card) for the two problems. There are 5 possibilities for each of the problems:

1. No conflict (score = 1): no problem is formulated or discussed;
2. Spontaneous agreement (score = 2): the two subgroups have the same proposal for resolution of the problem;
3. Compromise (score = 3): the two subgroups have a different proposal for resolution but they agree upon a compromise solution;
4. Approval/conviction (score = 4): the two subgroups have a different proposal for resolution; the final solution approves the proposal for resolution of one subgroup;
5. Conflict escalation (score = 5): the discussion ends without reaching a solution.

The total degree of conflict equals the sum of the scores of the two problems (min. = 2, max. = 10).

Behavioral Process Method

Because non-verbal interchanges and spatial aspects are so important in structural family theory, we chose to study the interaction directly on the videotape without typing out the verbal transcript. Consequently, we were only able to study more global interactions because the camera had to be fixed in a standardized position in which large as well as small families could be videotaped integrally. Because global ratings over a longer period are not reliable (Harris & Lahey, 1982), we restricted the observation period and formulated the behavioral referents of the interaction characteristics as concretely as possible, adding examples that we extracted from the preliminary investigation of 10 families. Each interaction task was observed during a specific time period (minimum of 3 minutes, maximum of 7 minutes) during which 4 to 8 behavioral interaction categories had to be studied. The behavioral categories were operationalizations of the 4 interactional dimensions mentioned above. Two raters scored each videotape independently; they watched the tape during the specified interval and scored immediately after each time period on a three-point scale. For example, during the first five minutes of the interactional part of the interest task, one example of the behavioral categories that had to be scored was "the evolution of distance between the family members." The raters had to score "1" when the distance did not narrow, "2" when family members reduced distance by means of eye contact or body gesture, "3" when family members moved their seats toward one another or touched each other.

We did a pre-training on the material of the pilot study and frequently checked the agreement between the two raters, following the suggestions of Harris and Lahey (1982). Nevertheless, some interaction categories seemed to abstract to reach a reasonable degree of interscorer agreement. The behavioral category "guidance" (Is the conversation structured? Are decisions made?) appeared to be extremely difficult to score ("1" there is no guidance; "2" there is guidance to some degree; "3" there is a high degree of guidance). The interrater reliability of this category was 0.512 (Pearson-correlation) and the interrater agreement was 0.278 (kappa-coefficient). Other interaction categories were satisfactorily reliable (e.g., Are there critical remarks with regard to the task, by means of verbal or nonverbal criticisms?: "1" = no; "2" = once; and "3" = more than once; interrater reliability = 0.722; interrater agreement = 0.567). The overall average interrater agreement was 0.31 and the average interrater reliability 0.50.

The interrater reliability is higher than the interrater agreement most of the time, because the first measure does not take into account the "between-raters" variance but only the consistency of the various raters over the subjects (the raters can differ absolutely). The interrater reliability is the relevant measure of the reliability of the scores in the studied sample, such as in this concept-validation study. The interrater agreement, which takes into account the between-raters variance, is the relevant measure when the scores will be generalized to other samples (Tinsley & Weiss, 1975).

The interrater reliability — which is important in our research project — is also reflected in the measure of internal consistency of those behavioral categories that were operationalizations of the same interactional dimension. We used the

Gulliksen item analysis program to select the most reliable categories for each dimension (Verhelst & Vander Steene, 1972). For dimension A, ten behavioral categories were selected out of 28, with an internal consistency of coefficient alpha = 0.73. The behavioral category "Do the parents talk with each other?" (during the preparation phase of the third task, in which the parents had to deliberate together) was the best measure of this dimension. Seventeen behavioral categories out of 27 were selected for dimension B, but nevertheless this scale remains relatively heterogeneous (coefficient alpha = 0.50). This latter dimension is measured by means of the comparison between the results of the same interaction categories, scored during two different tasks. The comparison between "the degree of attention seeking behavior" during the individual component of the interest- and criticism-task was the best measure of this dimension. For dimension C, 10 out of 19 behavioral categories were selected, with an internal consistency of 0.67. The interaction category: "Does one talk about the eating problem in the family?" (during the individual part of the interest- task) was the best operationalization of this dimension. Finally, we selected 9 out of 21 behavioral categories for dimension D, with an internal consistency of 0.71. The category "Is there a tense atmosphere in the family?" (during a free moment after the criticism task) was the best measure of this dimension.

Because the direct observation method has disadvantages that prevent its use in clinical practice (time-consuming, check of interrater reliability), we compared these data with the previously discussed behavioral product measures that operationalize the same four interactional dimensions and are more easy to use in clinical practice.

Self-Report Method

The *Leuven Family Questionnaire* is decribed in detail elsewhere (Kog et al., 1985b; see also Chapter 6). The original self-report questionnaire comprised 106 items, describing the various components that were associated with the four interaction features in the literature (Kog et al., 1985). We operationalized the two poles of each subcomponent with several items. The internal consistency of the items that had to measure the same interaction feature was, however, low. Thus we first selected the items with the lowest item-test correlation until we reached the maximum possible homogeneity, by means of the Gulliksen item analysis method (Verhelst & Vander Steene, 1972). Seven out of 13 items were selected for dimension A. The internal consistency of this final scale was 0.80. The item "We feel very close to each other" was the best representation of this dimension. Ten out of 24 items were selected for dimension B (coefficient alfa = 0.64), best represented by the item "Coalitions are often formed between the same persons in our family." Fifteen out of 28 items were selected for dimension C, with an internal consistency of 0.77. The item "I feel more comfortable within our family than outside of it" was the best representation of this scale.

Finally, 12 out of 24 items are selected for dimension D, with an internal consistency of 0.85. The item "Parents and children are unable to reach an agreement on certain issues" was the best measure of this dimension.

Multitrait-Multimethod Analysis: Hypotheses

We consider the three methods as congruent with a systemic view of the family and thus yielding transactional data. The nature of the data are, however, quite different. The greatest divergence is expected between each of the two behavioral methods on the one hand and the self-report method on the other because the research context is totally different. The self-report method is based on the insider's view; the evaluation of system functioning to which the evaluator (each family member) takes part. The two behavioral methods are based on the evaluation of the same system functioning by an outsider (the researcher-observer). The two behavioral methods are similar with regard to this research context but differ in the technique to analyze the information.

According to Campbell and Fiske (1959), the convergent as well as the discriminant validity of the operationalizations can be determined by an investigation of the correlations in the multitrait-multimethod matrix. There has to be a significant correlation between different measures of the same dimension (*convergent validity*). But these latter correlations also have to be higher than the correlations between measures of different dimensions, even if the same method was used (*discriminant validity*).

We do expect convergent as well as discriminant validity for at least the two behavioral operationalizations of dimension A, B and D. It seems to us that dimension C is too little specific in meaning, so that its operationalizations will correlate as highly with operationalizations of other dimensions as with each other. Thus, we do not expect convergent nor discriminant validity for the operationalizations of dimension C. As to the methods, we expect higher correlations between the two behavioral measures than between the behavioral measures and the self-report measure for every dimension. However, these inter-method correlations have to be higher when measuring the same dimensions as opposed to different dimensions.

Results

Multitrait-Multimethod Matrix

We tested the convergent and discriminant validity of the operationalizations on the basis of the intercorrelation matrix of the results of the four interaction features, measured with three different methods (see Table 2).

Qualitative Analysis of the Multitrait-Multimethod Matrix

We then tested the convergent and discriminant validity of the operationalizations by means of the heuristic guidelines of Campbell and Fiske (1959).

Table 2. Multitrait-Multimethod Matrix

Operationalizations§		Method 1 Behavioral product method				Method 2 Behavioral process method				Method 3 Self-report method			
		Bound.	Adapt.	A/R T.†	Confl.†	Bound.	Adapt.†	A/R T.	Confl.†	Bound.	Adapt.	A/R T.	Confl.
Method 1	Bound.	X											
	Adapt.	0.198	X										
	A/R T.	0.191	-0.085	X									
	Confl.	0.243	0.012	0.243	X								
Method 2	Bound.	0.361**	-0.058	0.126	0.181	X							
	Adapt.	0.286*	0.354**	0.212	-0.096	0.042	X						
	A/R T.	-0.050	-0.320*	0.182	0.233	0.300*	-0.101	X					
	Confl.	0.255	0.063	-0.078	0.154	-0.119	0.257	-0.019	X				
Method 3	Bound.	0.157	0.046	0.198	0.233	0.071	-0.016	-0.084	0.326*	X			
	Adapt.	-0.109	-0.065**	-0.399**	-0.246	0.068	0.169	-0.109	-0.282*	-0.432**	X		
	A/R T.	-0.001	0.090	0.210	-0.130	-0.112	-0.047	0.004	0.300*	0.790***	-0.373**	X	
	Confl.	0.218	0.125	0.405***	0.446***	0.117	0.031	0.030	0.433***	0.675***	-0.643***	-0.688***	X

°The numbers in bold type refer to the correlations in the validity diagonals. The heterotrait-monomethod triangles are marked by a solid line. The heterotrait-heteromethod triangles are marked by a broken line.

§Bound. – intensity of intrafamilial boundaries; Adapt. – degree of the family's adaptability; A/R T. – degree of avoidance/recognition of intrafamilial tension; Confl. – the family's way of handling conflicts.

†We changed the sign of the intercorrelations with this measure because a low score on this measure referred to the pole of the dimension that Minuchin stressed. The intercorrelations with measures that operationalized the dimension in the same direction have not been changed.

*p < .005   **p < 0.01   ***p < 0.001

Firstly, the correlations in the validity diagonals (indicated in bold type in Table 2) have to be sufficiently high (convergent validity). This is partially so for the operationalizations of dimensions A, B and D. The correlation between the two behavioral operationalizations of dimension A and B, and the correlation between the behavioral product measure and the self-report measure and, finally, the correlation between the behavioral process measure and the self-report measure of dimension D are significant. Not one of the operationalizations of dimension C correlates sufficiently with another operationalization of this same dimension. Thus, the measures of dimension C do not show convergent validity.

Secondly, the correlations in the validity diagonals have to be higher than the correlations in the heterotrait-heteromethod triangles (marked in dotted line in Table 2). This is one of the criteria for discriminant validity. Dimension A and B, measured with the two behavioral methods and dimension D, measured with the self-report method and each of the two behavioral methods, fulfill this requirement.

Thirdly, the correlations in the validity diagonals have to be higher than the correlations in the heterotrait-monomethod triangles (marked in full line in Table 2). This is the second demand for discriminant validity. Within the behavioral product method, this requirement is fulfilled for the operationalizations of dimension A, B and D: each of these operationalizations correlates higher with another operationalization of the same dimension than with the same-method-operationalizations of other dimensions. This is not so for the operationalization of dimension C, which shows a bad discriminant validity for the behavioral product measure of dimension C. Within the behavioral process method, all of the operationalizations fulfill this requirement. Finally, not a single operationalization with the self-report method fulfills this requirement. Even the self-report measure of dimension D, that correlates significantly with the two behavioral measures of this dimension and thus shows convergent validity, correlates higher with the three other dimensions, measured by the same method. Thus, there is more method-variance than trait-variance in the operationalizations with the self-report method.

Fourthly, the pattern of intercorrelations between the operationalized dimensions has to be similar in the monomethod and heteromethod triangles. This last demand for discriminant validity is only partially fulfilled. Even for the two behavioral methods, the pattern of intercorrelations is different, especially for the intercorrelations with the operationalizations of dimension C.

We conclude that convergent and partially discriminant validity has been proven for dimension A, B and D. However, this convergent and discriminant validity does not apply to all operationalizations of the dimensions. The two behavioral methods fit best with the model. The self-report method seems to measure other dimensions than those that are tested here, except the conflict measure that shows convergent validity.

Explorative Factor Analysis of the Self-Report Method

On the basis of the previous results, we hypothesized that a family member might evaluate his or her own family system functioning with different concepts than an outsider. That's why we carried out an explorative factor analysis on the 106 original items of the family questionnaire.

The first factor measures all kinds of *conflict* behavior, e.g., quarrelling, blaming, coalitions, violence, and interpersonal tension without open conflict. The second factor measures the amount of sharing of contact, personal body space, emotional space, information and conversation. It is most comparable to the concept of "proximity," that Wood and Talmon (1983) consider as just one component of the boundary concept. We prefer to call this scale *cohesion* because this is a more generally used term for emotional togetherness and concern in the family. The third factor is most comparable to the other component that Wood and Talmon (1983) differentiate in the broad concept of boundaries. It refers to the boundary between generations in the family and the roles that accompany this generational differentiation; nurturance, control, alliances and coalitions. While our items predominantly refer to rather negative aspects — indicating a lack of nurturance and control and cross-generational alliances and coalitions — and do not refer exclusively to the generational differentiation but to the general functions of "a family" as described above, we call this scale *disorganization*. Thus, the final "Leuven Family Questionnaire" (see Appendix 3) comprises three scales: conflict (30 items), cohesion (21 items) and disorganization (22 items).

Cluster Analysis of the Behaviorally Measured Dimensions

In order to test Minuchin's psychosomatic family model, we investigated if we could distinguish different types of families on the basis of their response pattern with regard to the three validated concepts (the intensity of intra-familial boundaries, the degree of the family's adaptability, and the family's way of handling conflicts) measured with the behavioral product method because this latter method showed reliability as well as validity. For this purpose, we used a non-hierarchical cluster analysis (Rubin & Friedman, 1967), resulting up in seven types of families. Cluster one comprises three families with a clear interaction profile. They show loose intra-familial boundaries, a low degree of adaptability and an absence of conflict in the family. We called this cluster "the *enmeshed* family." Cluster two, which is called "the *unpredictable* family," is characterized by a high degree of conflict and adaptability. Seven families show this interaction profile. Cluster three is the largest cluster. It comprises thirteen families. We defined it as "the *pseudo-happy* family" because these families show the least conflict but also rather fixed boundaries. Thus there is absolutely no conflict in these families, but neither is there cohesion. Cluster four consists of ten families, which show very fixed boundaries and a rather high degree of adaptability. We defined this type as "the *uncohesive* family." Cluster five is grouping ten families. Their interaction pattern is difficult to interpret. They show a medium degree of conflict and intrafamilial boundaries, and a rather high degree of adaptability. We called this cluster "the *ambivalent* family" because dependency (cf. boundaries) and independency (cf. conflict) are present in a less-structured way (cf. adaptability). Cluster six consists of three families, which we defined as "the *conflicted* family" because they show the highest degree of conflict, a rather low degree of adaptability and loose boundaries. They seem to be conflictually attached to each other. Finally, cluster seven, finally, comprises 7 families, which show a rather high degree of adaptability, a low degree of conflict, and clear boundaries. We called this cluster "the *socially-desirable* family" because they seem to fulfill the social norms for a "good family."

The clusters "enmeshed family" and "conflicted family" (quarrelling without reaching a solution) approach Minuchin's psychosomatic family model. The dimensional redefinition generated, however, important nuances of Minuchin's extreme family model, such as the "unpredictable family," the "ambivalent family" and the "pseudo-happy family." In these latter types, at least one variable is less extreme or even leans toward the other pole of the dimension. The two remaining types; the "socially-desirable family" and the "uncohesive family," do not even resemble Minuchin's typology.

CONCLUSION

This concept-validation study lent considerable support for our hypothesis that "overprotectiveness" (redefined and operationalized as "the degree of avoidance/recognition of intrafamilial tension") was a superfluous dimension, because the three methodological operationalizations failed to show convergent as well as discriminant validity.

Our hypothesis that the two behavioral methods would correlate higher with each other than with the self-report method is sustained by most of the data, with one important exception. The two behavioral measures for "the intensity of intrafamilial boundaries" and "the degree of the family's adaptability" showed convergent as well as discriminant validity. Curiously, however, both behavioral measures for "the family's way of handling conflicts" correlated significantly with the self-report measure for this dimension but did not correlate significantly with each other. Thus, the insider/outsider contrast, or self-report/behavioral method contrast seems to explain some of the correlations between the operationalizations, but not all of them. Family members appear to use the same conceptual scheme as an outsider-observer with regard to the evaluation of conflict. The insiders' evaluation is a global experience of negativity, referring to both the occurrence of quarrels in the family (e.g., "In our family opinions regularly differ") and the lack of conflict resolution (e.g., "Parents and children are unable to reach an agreement on certain issues"). The existence of conflict, however, does not have to be related to a lack of conflict resolution in the family. This may be the reason why the behavioral product measure (which focuses on the method of conflict resolution) and the behavioral process measure (which focuses on the existance of conflict in the family) do correlate significantly with the self-report measure (which measures both aspects), but not significantly with each other.

The insider-perspective is a more global evaluative judgment of family interaction, not only for the evaluation of conflict, but also for the evaluation of other dimensions. The factor analysis of the self-report method revealed three dimensions: conflict, cohesion and disorganization. The behavioral methods measure more specific dimensions. The dimension "intensity of intrafamilial boundaries" refers to the degree of differentiation of subsystems in the family in order to carry out their functions. The dimension "degree of the family's adaptability" refers to the degree of variability in coalitions, guidance, affective atmosphere and habits. With regard to the third dimension, "the family's way of handling conflicts," we hypothesize that it comprises two separate dimensions "the degree of conflict-behavior" (e.g., quarrelling, coalition formation) and "the degree of conflict resolution" (e.g., negotiation and reaching an agreement). This hypothesis has to be further tested by means of at least two behavioral operationalizations of these two aspects.

This concept-validation study is but a start of the empirical test of important structural family dimensions. Many questions remain open. It would be interesting to reinvestigate the correlations between the factor analyticly derived self-report scales and the behavioral measures, and between separate measures for conflict-behavior and conflict resolution in order to test some of the hypotheses stated above. Another perspective for future research is the differentiation between a behavioral and an experiential outsider-method (e.g., a global evaluation by the therapist) and between a behavioral (e.g., self-monitoring) and an experiential insider-method (Olson, 1981), in order to study to what extent the frame of reference (insider versus outsider) and the type of information (observation versus experiential evaluation) explain the correlations between operationalizations of the same dimensions.

Finally, we investigated Minuchin's typology of anorexic families applied to our large and more differentiated sample of eating disorders. We distinguished seven types of families in our sample, some of which approach Minuchin's psychosomatic family model, others however being less extreme and even opposite types of family interaction. The selection of Minuchin's sample of anorexic families does not seem to offer an explanation for his more coherent family characterization because we found that families with young as well as old patients and families with restricting as well as other types of anorexics and bulimics were spread over the various family types. In other words, the type of eating disorder does not seem to be clearly connected to a particular type of family functioning as analyzed in our study. Thus, we hypothesize that Minuchin's focus on more extreme positions on the interaction dimensions resulted in a selective attention for behaviors that refer to these extreme positions. In our view, it is important to stress even small differences in family interaction. Less extreme positions on the dimensions are very important in the assessment of family interaction because the abilities of the family are important data in family therapy. Before we can generalize this family typology, we have to investigate a larger and still more differentiated sample of families, especially "normal" families without overt pathology or an individual symptom bearer.

REFERENCES*

American Psychiatric Association (1980) *Diagnostic and Statistical Manual of Mental Disorders (DSM-III)*. Washington, D.C.: American Psychiatric Association.

Blakar, R.M. (1979), *Studies of Familial Communication and Psychopathology. A Social-Developmental Approach to Deviant Behavior*. Oslo: Universitetsforlaget.

Campbell, D.T. & Fiske, D.W. (1959), Convergent and discriminant validation by the multitrait-multimethod matrix. *Psychological Bulletin*, 56:81-105.

Dell, P. (1982), Beyond homeostasis: Toward a theory of coherence. *Family Process*, 21:21-41.

Ferreira, A.J. & Winter, W. (1965), Family interaction and decision making. *Archives of General Psychiatry*, 13:214-223.

Harris, F. & Lahey, B. (1982), Recording system bias in direct observational methodology. A review and critical analysis of factors causing inaccurate coding behavior. *Clinical Psychology Review*, 2:539-556.

Hoffman, L. (1981), *Foundations of Family Therapy: A Conceptual Framework for Systems Change*. New York: Basic Books.

Jacob, T. (1975), Family interaction in disturbed and normal families: A methodological and substantive review. *Psychological Bulletin*, 82:33-65.

Ketelaar-Van Ierssel, A. (1982), *Afgrenzingsprocessen in Gezinnen. Een Vergelijkend Onderzoek tussen Gezinnen met Kinderen met Gedragsproblemen en Zogenaamde Normale Gezinnen* (Boundary Processes in Families. A Comparative Study of Families with Children with Behavioral Problems and Socalled "Normal" Families). Lisse: Swets & Zeitlinger.

Kog, E., Vandereycken, W. & Vertommen, H. (1985), The psychosomatic family model. A critical analysis of family interaction concepts. *Journal of Family Therapy*, 7:31-44.

Olson, D.H. (1981), Family typologies: Bridging family research and family therapy. In: Filsinger, E.E. & Lewis, R.A. (Eds.), *Assessing Marriage. New Behavioral Approaches*. Beverly Hills-London: Sage Publications.

Reiss, D. (1971a), Varieties of consensual experience. I. A theory for relating family interaction to individual thinking. *Family Process*, 10:1-28.

Reiss, D. (1971b), Varieties of consensual experience. II. Dimensions of a family's experience of its environment. *Family Process*, 10:28-35.

Reiss, D. (1981), *The Family's Construction of Reality*. Cambridge-Massachusetts: Harvard University Press.

Rubin, J. & Friedman, H. (1967), *A Cluster Analysis and Taxonomy System for Grouping and Classifying Data*. New York: IBM Corporation.

Russell, G. (1979), Bulimia nervosa: An ominous variant of anorexia nervosa. *Psychological Medicine*, 9:429-448.

Tinsley, H. & Weiss, D. (1975), Interrater reliability and agreement of subjective judgments. *Journal of Counseling Psychology*, 22:358-376.

---

* This list contains only secondary literature, whereas the other references are mentioned in the final section of this book: "Bibliography on Family Aspects of Eating Disorders."

Vandereycken, W. (1985), Inpatient treatment of anorexia nervosa: Some research-guided changes. *Journal of Psychiatric Research,* 19:413-422.

Vandereycken, W. & Meermann, R. (1984), *Anorexia Nervosa. A Clinicians' Guide to Treatment.* Berlin-New York: Walter de Gruyter.

Vandereycken, W. & Pierloot, R. (1983), Drop-out during in-patient treatment of anorexia nervosa: A clinical study of 133 patients. *British Journal of Medical Psychology,* 56:145-156.

Verhelst, N. & Vander Steene, G. (1972), A Gulliksen item analysis program. *Behavioral Science,* 17:491-493.

Watzlawick, P., Beavin, J., Sikorski, L. & Mecia, B. (1970), Protection and scapegoating in pathological families. *Family Process,* 9:27-39.

Wood, B. & Talmon, M. (1983), Family boundaries in transition: A search for alternatives. *Family Process,* 22:347-357.

APPENDIX 1: INTEREST TASK – INDIVIDUAL COMPONENT

1. *What do you like to do the most and the least in leisure time?*
   doing sports/doing carpentering/visiting friends/watching T.V. at home/engaging in corporate life/going to the movies/reading

2. *Which type of movie do you like the most and the least?*
   science fiction/historical film/psychological film/thriller/cartoon/comedy/western

3. *Where do you like to dine out the most and the least?*
   hamburger house/fish restaurant/vegetarian restaurant/sandwich bar/chinese restaurant/gastronomic restaurant/self-service

4. *In what do you like to engage yourself the most and the least?*
   nature/Third World/your neighborhood/sports/theatre/encounter-group/hobby club

5. *In which way do you like to travel or spend your holiday the most and the least?*
   with a house trailer/in a tent/in a bungalow/in a hotel/in an apartment/a cruise/to hitchhike with a rucksack

6. *Which type of work do you like the most and the least?*
   housework/lace-work/to trade/to take care of patients/research activities/to give guidance to

7. *Which dish do you like to eat the most and the least?*
   Jacob's shell/steak/tonguelet/rabbit/asparagushamrol/lamb/turkey

8. *Which values do you find most and least important?*
   liberty/honesty/egality/friendliness/forgiveness/responsibility/will-power

9. *Which color do you like the most and the least?*
   blue/yellow/green/red/white/black/brown

10. *Which kind of profession do you like the most and the least?*
    craftsman/self-employed/teacher/sportsman/researcher/medical assistant/artist

11. *Which animal do you like the most and the least?*
    dog/hot-water fish/cat/rabbit/monkey/lamb/canary-bird

12. *In what type of residence do you like to live the most and the least?*
    apartment/gentlemen's house/country house/farm/community/welfare
    house/an isolated house

APPENDIX 2: DISAGREEMENT TASK — PREPARING PHASE

PARENTS

I. Concerning the problem of the parents:

1. *To whom applies this problem especially?* (mark which alternative applies
   to your problem)
   — to all children
   — especially to certain children
   — to one of the children
2. *Who is involved in this problem?* (mark which alternative applies to your
   problem)
   — both parents are equally involved in this problem
   — especially father is involved in this problem
   — especially mother is involved in this problem
3. *Your proposal for resolution of this problem:* (write this down in a few
   words)

II. Concerning the problem of the children:

1. *Your proposal for resolution of the problem of the children:* (write this down
   in a few words)
2. *Who shares the proposal for resolution of the problem?* (mark which alternative applies to this problem)
   — both parents
   — especially father
   — especially mother

CHILDREN

I. Concerning the problem of the children:

1. *To whom applies this problem especially?* (mark which alternative applies
   to your problem)
   — to both parents
   — especially to mother

— especially to father
2. *Who is involved in this problem?* (mark which alternative applies to your problem)
    — all children are equally involved in this problem
    — especially some children are involved in this problem
    — especially one of the children is involved in this problem
3. *Your proposal for resolution of this problem:* (write this down in a few words)

II. Concerning the problem of the parents:

1. *Your proposal for resolution of the problem of the parents:* (write this down in a few words)
2. *Who shares the proposal for resolution of the problem?* (mark which alternative applies to this problem)
    — all of the children
    — especially some of the children
    — especially one of the children

APPENDIX 3: LEUVEN FAMILY QUESTIONNAIRE*

1. Questionnaire**

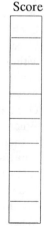

Score

1. It is very clear who likes or dislikes each other in our family.
2. Family members are completely involved in each other's lives.
3. In our family, everybody has to solve his own problems.
4. If in our family something has to be decided, each parent has his supporters among the children.
5. We defend our family, regardless of what has happened.
6. The parents let the children live their own lives without interfering a lot.
7. Some physical complaints reoccur again and again in our family.
8. I do not know any family that is closer than ours.

---

*　The six response possibilities (definitely not true, not true, rarely true, true some of the time, true most of the time, true all of the time) are scored 1 to 6 or the reverse for the negatively keyed items (*). Thus, the result for the conflict scale is minimally 30 and maximally 180; the result for the cohesion scale is minimally 21 and maximally 126; the result for the disorganization scale is minimally 22 and maximally 132.

**　If the parents in your family are divorced or if one of the parents has deceased, you do not have to answer the questions which are marked with "*"

9.   It seems there is no room to be alone in our house.
10. The same family members usually take sides with each other.
11. We weigh our words carefully while discussing, because we are all very sensitive.
12. In our family, there is no regularity.
13. We easily blame other family members.
14. I feel more comfortable within our family than outside of it.
15. In our family decisions are made without consultations.
16. Parents and children regularly quarrel with each other.
17. We easily take the blame.
18. We feel more comfortable with friends than at home.
19. Each family member wants to have his own say, so we usually cannot reach a decision.
20. I feel guilty when I go my own way.
21. We do not feel friendship for each other.
22. We talk a lot about our conflicts but do not reach an agreement.
23. I feel responsible for the other family members.
24.* When the parents quarrel, they both try to get the children on their side.
25. In our family, opionions regularly differ.
26. When we are having a pleasant time, we do not keep track of time.
27. Each of us lives his own life.
28. Physical complaints are merely an expression of all tensions within our family.
29. Without the support of the family, it would be difficult to undertake anything.
30.* Our parents do not agree on the education of the children.
31.* When the parents quarrel, the children take sides with one of them.
32. Our family is so well-organized that everything goes smoothly (e.g., fixed meal-times, fixed weekend activities and week menu).
33. We do not have meals together.
34. When we are angry with each other, there can be great turmoil.
35.* The parents always side with each other and so do the children.
36. We do not feel responsible for the other family members.
37. Family members have conflicts that cannot be talked out.
38. Our family hates quarrelling and shouting.

39. We feel little love for each other.
40. Most of the time, we have to agree with those who criticize our family.
41. In a discussion, parents and children are able to reach an agreement.
42. We do not know whether we can count on each other.
43. The least cause can greatly upset our family.
44. We comfort each other when one of us is in trouble.
45.* The parents decide together without consulting the children.
46. In family interactions, we always return to the same habits.
47. We hate tensions and quarreling in our family.
48. We do not appreciate the advice and support that are given by the family.
49. Tensions between family members are inevitable.
50. We spend the evenings together.
51. We bottle up all tensions.
52.* Certain children always support one particular parent.
53. We always agree on major issues.
54. Family members decide on the basis of their own judgments.
55. A discussion easily results in reproaches.
56. Family ties are more important to us than friendships.
57. Family members do not cling together.
58. The same persons always decide for the whole family.
59. We try to avoid quarrelling at all costs.
60. We easily take out our problems on the family, even if they have nothing to do with the family.
61. The parents worry a lot about the children.
62. A tense atmosphere sometimes lasts several days.
63. Some members of our family interfere with one another.
64. Parents and children are unable to reach an agreement on certain issues.
65. The atmosphere in our house can change from one moment to the next.
66. When the children quarrel, each of them tries to get the parents on his side.
67. We easily take out tensions on our family.
68. Major conflicts exist in our family.
69. There is a lot of friendship in our family.
70. Our parents always agree.
71. Before we make a decision, we ask for the approval of the other family members.

72. Conflicts do not occur in our family.
73. We feel very close to each other.

2. Scoring system (see footnote, page 103)

Conflict scale:
   item 1, 4, 7, 10, 13, 16, 19, 22, 25, 28, 31, 34, 37, 40, 43, 46, 49, 52, 55, 58, 60, 62, 63, 64, 65, 66, 67, 68, 70*, 72*

Cohesion scale:
   item 2, 5, 8, 11, 14, 17, 20, 23, 26, 29, 32, 35, 38, 41, 44, 47, 50, 53, 56, 59, 61

Disorganization scale:
   item 3, 6, 9, 12, 15, 18, 21, 24, 27, 30, 33, 36, 39, 42, 45, 48, 51, 54, 57, 69*, 71*, 73*
   * Negative load.

Chapter 6

Self-Report Study of Family Interaction in Eating Disorder Families Compared to Normals

Elly Kog, Hans Vertommen and Walter Vandereycken

In our concept-validation study of the psychosomatic family model (see Chapter 5), we used two behavioral methods and one self-report method. In this chapter, we will confine ourselves to the discussion of the results of the self-report method, which is based on the Leuven Family Questionnaire. We will briefly mention the construction of this questionnaire and then discuss some results of a comparative study between eating disorder families and normal families, and of intrafamilial comparisons in both types of families.

SUBJECTS

This family questionnaire was used to study the perception of family interaction in a clinical and a normal sample. The clinical sample was a randomly selected group of 53 families with an eating disorder patient (anorexia nervosa and bulimia) treated at the University Psychiatric Center St. Jozef in Kortenberg (Belgium). We chose this syndrome because anorexia nervosa families would be characterized most significantly by the psychosomatic family model, according to its authors (Minuchin et al., 1978). The normal sample was a group of 220 nonpatient control families (representative of the Flemish population) who were contacted with the help of first year psychology students. Each student had to research a family of a certain social class (determined by father's occupation), family size and status of the family life cycle (determined by the middle child). All family members still living at home but older than 12 years of age were asked to fill out the questionnaire.

The eating disorder group comprised somewhat more (15%) divorced or deceased parents than the normal group (5%). There were more families of higher social status in the eating disorder sample. The greatest differences are within the most extreme social classes: There were more working-class families in the normal sample and more higher employees and employers in the eating disorder sample. Families of both samples were within the pubertal (12-15), adolescent (16-18) or launching (19+) stage of the family life cycle, according to the age of the middle child (see Chapter 5, "subjects"). Eating disorder families were found to be predominantly in the older stages and normal families were approximately equally distributed over the three stages. In the eating disorder sample, we differentiated four subgroups according to the clinical symptomatology of the patient. In the anorexia nervosa syndrome, defined according to DSM-III (American Psychiatric Association, 1980), we further differentiated restricting and bulimic anorexics. The normal-weight bulimics fulfill the requirements for bulimia in DSM-III, except that a previous history of weight loss is not considered a negative criterion for the diagnosis. The atypical cases are patients with weight or eating problems who do not fulfill the DSM-III criteria for anorexia nervosa or bulimia.

PROCEDURE

Each family member still living at home was asked to fill out a list of 106 items on a six-point scale. The original questionnaire comprised items describing the various components that Minuchin and coworkers associated with the four psychosomatic family features. But we soon found that neither the patient families nor the control families perceived their family in the concepts Minuchin described. The congruence analysis of the first four empirical factors of a factor analysis and Minuchin's four hypothetical characteristics yielded coefficients no higher than 0.55 for both groups. That is why we abandoned the hypothetical structure inspired by Minuchin's concepts and used an explorative factor analysis in order to determine the latent structure of the questionnaire (see Kog et al., 1985b). On the basis of an orthogonal factor analysis — using the normalized varimax criterion — and a subsequent item analysis, the Leuven Family Questionnaire was subdivided into three scales (see Table 1).

The *conflict* scale measures open conflict — such as quarrelling, blaming, coalitions and violence — as well as interpersonal tension without open conflict. This scale is most comparable to Minuchin's characteristic of "lack of conflict resolution," because both of them comprise these two conflict patterns. The item "family members have conflicts that cannot be talked out" is the best representation of this scale.

The *cohesion* scale measures the amount of sharing of contact time, personal body space, emotional space, information, conversation and decision space of each person in the family. This scale is most comparable to the concept "proximity" that Wood and Talmon (1983) regard as just one component of the boundary concept. This scale also refers to the concern for each other's welfare

Nr.	Scale	Nr.	Subscale	Definition	N items
1	Conflict	1	Tensions	Unresolvable disagreements create a tense atmosphere in the family	23
		2	Coalitions	The family is subdivided in groups which disagree	7
2	Cohesion	3	Sense of security	The family is perceived as a secure nest; one adds and supports each other against the threatening outside world	13
		4	Conflict Avoidance	Family members avoid divergences of opinion and personal views	8
3	Disorganization	5	Separation	Each person in the family lives his own life; affective involvement is lacking	11
		6	Lack of Organization	There is no leadership in the family and no regularity in family life	11

in the family, that Minuchin called "overprotectiveness." We prefer to call this scale "cohesion" because this is a more generally used term. The item "we comfort each other when one of us is in trouble" has the highest item-test correlation.

The *disorganization* scale is most comparable to the other component that Wood and Talmon (1983) differentiate in the broad concept of boundaries. It refers to the boundary between generations in the family and the roles that accompany this generational differentiation: nurturance, control, alliances and coalitions. While our items predominantly refer to rather negative aspects, indicating a lack of nurturance and control, loose alliances and cross-generational coalitions, we call this scale "disorganization." This scale is best represented by means of the item "we do not know whether we can count on each other."

So, the final Leuven Family Questionnaire consists of 73 items: 30 items for the conflict scale, 21 items for the cohesion scale and 22 items for the disorganization scale (see Appendix 3, Chapter 5).

RESULTS

We did a series of intergroup comparisons between the results of the 53 eating disorder families and the 220 normal control families, on the three scales (intergroup comparisons). Moreover, we compared the results of father, mother, and eating disorder child in the patient sample and the results of father, mother and oldest child in the nonpatient sample (intrafamilial comparisons).

Table 2: Clinical subtypes versus normals*

	Conflict		Cohesion		Disorganization	
	X	SD	X	SD	X	SD
A. Normals (N- 837)	90.17	22.97	86.41	13.20	51.67	14.81
B. Restricting anorexics (N = 134)	99.49‡	23.88	87.76	13.71	55.85‡	16.61
C. Bulimic anorexics (N = 40)	106.49‡	20.36	83.20	15.09	62.02‡	14.24
D. Normal-weight bulimics (N = 38)	106.10‡	14.21	86.03	12.52	60.17‡	11.45
E. Atypical cases (N = 23)	113.57‡	15.48	80.48†	11.85	67.26‡	13.22

*Average scores of all members of each of the eating disorder subtypes versus average scores of all members of normal families.
‡ = p < 0.01
† = p < 0.05 (two-tailed t-tests: levels of significance of the comparisons between group B versus group A, group C versus group A, group D versus group A, and group E versus group A)

Intergroup Comparisons

Totals. When we compare the average scores of all family members of the eating disorder families (235 subjects) with the average scores of all family members of the normal families (837 subjects), the patient families report significantly more conflict (p < 0.01) and more disorganization (p < 0.01), but do not differ from nonpatient families with regard to perceived cohesion in the family.

Clinical subtypes. When we compare the average scores of all family members of the various eating disorder subgroups with the average scores of all family members of the normal group (see Table 2), all eating disorder subgroups report significantly more conflict and more disorganization. However, restricting anorexics show a response pattern which is most similar to that of the normal control families. Bulimic anorexics and normal-weight bulimics show a mutually comparable, more differing response pattern. These three subgroups do not differ significantly from the normal sample on cohesion but the atypical cases report significantly less cohesion too. Moreover, this latter subgroup scores most extremely on conflict and disorganization.

Then, we matched the eating disorder sample and the normal sample each time on one variable and checked if the differences between groups were still significant. First, we matched groups for *social class.* The same differences were again evident: all eating disorder subgroups scored more conflict and more disorganization than their normal counterpart, but the higher the social class, the

Table 3: Eating disorder families versus normal families, situated in the same phase of the family life cycle

| | Conflict | | | | Cohesion | | | | Disorganization | | | |
| | Eating Disorders | | Normal Controls | | Eating Disorders | | Normal Controls | | Eating Disorders | | Normal Controls | |
	X	SD	X	SD	X	SD	X	SD	X	SD	X	SD
Pubertal Phase (44/218)*	104.74	21.90‡	87.90	23.27	85.97	15.42§	90.49	14.37	59.26	16.50‡	50.21	15.39
Adolescent Phase (82/323)	101.01	22.81‡	90.57	22.73	84.59	13.35**	85.16	12.75	54.72	14.65†	51.28	14.50
Launching Phase (109/296)	104.09	21.42‡	91.30	23.06	87.2 6	13.79§	84.51	11.95	62.91	15.51‡	53.51	14.66

*Between brackets: number of subjects in eating disorder group/normal control group.

‡ = p < 0.01
† = p < 0.05
§ = p < 0.10
** = nonsignificant (two-tailed t-tests)

smaller the differences between groups. Differences were no longer significant for the upper social class families. So, when one compares eating disorder families with normal families on their perception of family interaction, it is important to control for social class.

Secondly, we compared patient and nonpatient families, situated in the same *phase of the family life cycle* (see Table 3). In the three phases, patient families reported significantly more conflict and more disorganization, but patient families in the pubertal and in the launching phase reported respectively less cohesion and more cohesion than their normal counterparts. This is an interesting finding that can be further explored by means of an internal comparison among families in different phases of the family life cycle in the eating disorder and the normal sample (see also Table 3). Normal families report more conflict, less cohesion and more disorganization in the older phases, with the greatest difference between the pubertal and the adolescent phase. This is what one would expect in the evolution of family life: during adolescence, children develop their own opinions which can differ from those of the parents. In the patient families, however, the pattern is totally different. The evaluation of family interaction in this group is most favorable in the adolescent phase: patient families report the least conflict and disorganization in this phase. Patient families in the launching phase report more conflict and more disorganization, which is comparable to the evolution in normal families, but also more cohesion, and this is the opposite of normal families.

We were wondering if these differences would apply in the same degree to all family members. We compared the results of the *fathers, mothers and patients* of eating disorder families with these of the fathers, mothers and eldest children of normal families, first for the total group and then separately for the families in the same phase of the family life cycle (see Table 4). We ascertained that fathers, mothers and patients report significantly more conflict and disorganization than their normal counterparts. The three of them also note more cohesion but not significantly so. In general, patients and their mothers differ more from their normal controls than do patient fathers. When we studied the results for the different phases, curiously the patient fathers only reported significantly more cohesion in the launching phase, compared with the normal fathers.

For the mothers, the differences were more pronounced. Compared to their normal counterparts, mothers of eating disorder families in the adolescent phase reported significantly more conflict and less disorganization, while mothers in the launching phase reported significantly more conflict, cohesion and disorganization. This latter phase seems to be very problematic for the patient mothers: they report a great deal more conflict and more disorganization but also somewhat more cohesion than the patient mothers in the adolescent phase. Normal control mothers in the launching phase report somewhat more conflict and disorganization but also less cohesion than control mothers in the adolescent phase.

Table 4: Fathers, mothers and patients of eating disorder families versus fathers, mothers and oldest children of normal families, situated in the same phase of the family life cycle

	Conflict				Cohesion				Disorganization			
	Eating Disorders		Normal Controls		Eating Disorders		Normal Controls		Eating Disorders		Normal Controls	
	X	SD	X	SD	X	SD	X	SD	X	SD	X	SD
Fathers:												
Total (46/208)*	93.32	21.00‡	84.50	22.16	93.21	13.72**	89.81	12.22	55.49	15.67†	50.25	15.40
Pubertal phase (10/62)	92.56	17.48**	84.95	21.72	95.00	18.57**	92.54	13.83	54.00	16.80**	49.77	14.97
Adolescent phase (16/75)	91.69	21.64**	83.67	22.13	89.31	14.53**	89.48	11.59	51.50	13.58**	48.97	14.05
Launching phase (20/71)	92.55	20.16**	84.89	22.97	95.95	10.46§	87.44	10.62	58.50	15.57†	52.11	17.16
Mothers:												
Total (52/210)	102.12	21.73‡	85.51	21.78	95.05	11.14**	92.28	11.91	58.35	14.28‡	48.83	13.73
Pubertal phase (10/65)	96.67	16.56**	85.48	23.98	93.78	8.89**	93.97	14.53	54.44	13.24**	47.55	14.27
Adolescent phase(19/77)	97.79	22.79‡	84.35	20.09	94.11	13.10**	92.49	10.28	53.89	11.39†	46.92	12.93
Launching phase (23/68)	106.05	21.94‡	86.49	21.67	96.32	10.93†	90.26	10.72	63.45	15.75‡	52.16	13.78
Patients/Oldest Children												
Total (53/200)	111.38	22.07‡	94.48	23.01	81.96	12.23**	80.44	13.72	60.25	18.31†	55.16	16.01
Pubertal phase (10/61)	123.89	26.46‡	93.43	23.81	75.33	11.82§	84.58	15.40	68.56	21.61†	54.23	17.57
Adolescent phase (20/78)	106.35	20.15§	96.38	22.05	83.20	11.77§	78.04	11.75	53.15	16.14**	55.55	15.74
Launching phase (23/61)	108.68	19.55‡	93.10	23.86	84.41	12.08**	79.03	13.36	61.23	14.81**	55.77	14.97

*Between brackets: number of subjects in eating disorder group/normal control group.

‡ = p < 0.01

† = p < 0.05

§ = p < 0.10

** = nonsignificant (two-tailed t-tests)

Table 5: Intrafamilial comparisons in eating disorder families

	Conflict			Cohesion			Disorganization		
	12-15§	16-18	19+	12-15	16-18	19+	12-15	16-18	19+
Father-Mother	93-96‡	92-102**	93-106***	95-94	89-92	96-96	54-54	52-56	59-63
Father-Patient		93-124***	92-109***	93-107**	95-75**	89-83**	96-84***	54-69*	52-53	59-60
Mother-Patient		96-124***	102-109**	106-107	94-75***	92-83**	96-84***	54-69*	56-53	63-60

§12-15 = pubertal group; 16-18 = adolescent group; 19+ = launching group
‡All numbers (average scores) are rounded off
*** = p < 0.01; ** = p < 0.05; * = p < 0.10 (two-tailed paired t-tests)

Finally, the patients differed most from the eldest children of normal families when they were in the pubertal phase: they reported much more conflict, more disorganization and less cohesion. Patients of families in the adolescent phase still reported significantly more conflict and more cohesion, whereas those in the launching phase only noted significantly more conflict.

Intra-Familial Comparisons

We compared the results of father, mother and child of the same family and afterwards tested the average differences among these three family members in the same phase of the family life cycle. We carried this out separately for eating disorder families (see Table 5) and normal families (see Table 6).

The *parents* of eating disorder families (see Table 5) differed significantly with regard to the perception of conflict in the adolescent and launching group; the mother reported more conflict than her husband in these phases. The parents of normal families (see Table 6) differed significantly in their perception of cohesion in the adolescent and launching group. Mothers report more cohesion than their husbands in these stages, but the difference is minimal (because of the large group – 410 normal parents – small differences are significant). So, we may conclude that normal parents are more similar in their perception of family interaction than parents of eating disorder families, especially in the older groups.

The *children* in the patient as well as in the normal families (see Tables 5 and 6) report significantly more conflict and less cohesion than both of their parents, in the three age groups. The control children also report more disorganization than both parents in the three age groups. The patients only report significantly more disorganization in the pubertal group. So, the control child differs somewhat more from both parents on the disorganization scale. When we checked

Table 6: Intrafamilial comparisons in normal families

	Conflict			Cohesion			Disorganization		
	§12-15	16-18	19+	12-15	16-18	19+	12-15	16-18	19+
Father-Mother	86-85‡	84-85	87-87	93-94	89-92**	87-90**	50-47	49-47	53-52
Father-Child	86-94*	84-97*	87-93*	93-85*	89-78*	87-79*	50-55**	49-55*	53-55***
Mother-Child	85-94*	85-97*	87-93**	94-85*	92-78*	90-79*	47-55**	47-55*	52-55**

§12-15 = pubertal group; 16-18 = adolescent group; 19+ = launching group
‡ all numbers (average scores) are rounded off
* = $p < 0.01$
** = $p < 0.05$
*** = $p < 0.10$ (two-tailed paired t-tests)

the differences among subgroups in the eating disorder sample, we ascertained that the patient differs most from both parents in the pubertal group and least in the launching group. The control child, on the other hand, differs most from both parents in the adolescent group. So, the same pattern as discussed before, is emerging. The child of a normal family develops his/her own opinions in the adolescent phase, while the patient child diverges most in the pubertal phase. In the launching phase a peculiar pattern is shown. The difference on the conflict scale between mother and patient is no longer significant because the former reports more and the latter less conflict, compared with younger groups. Father reports a similar degree of conflict in the three groups. Consequently, the difference between the patient parents becomes significant in the adolescent and launching group.

CONCLUSION

To summarize, eating disorder families report more conflict and disorganization but do not report significantly more cohesion than normal families. So, the tightly-knit family structure clinicians appear to observe in eating disorder families (e.g., Crisp et al., 1980; Minuchin et al., 1978)) is not reported by family members themselves. This interpretation, however, has to be shaded according to clinical subtypes of eating disorders and according to the stage of the family life cycle.

With regard to *clinical subtypes,* restricting anorexics scored most similarly to normal families. Bulimic anorexics report more conflict and disorganization and lower levels on cohesion, compared with their restricting counterparts. Similar results are obtained by Strober (1981), using the "Family Environment Scale." Bulimic anorexics and normal-weight bulimics showed a quite comparable response pattern and differed both from the restricting group. Garner et al. (1985) suggest, on the basis of similar findings with the "Family Assessment Measure" (and psychometric tests), that the presence or absence of bulimia might be a more significant subdividing criterion than the presence or absence of weight loss.

With regard to the *phase of the family life cycle,* eating disorder families in the pubertal phase also differ from normal families in their perception of cohesion, but they report less cohesion than their normal counterparts. On the other hand, eating disorder families in the launching phase, report more cohesion than normal families in the same phase. In the adolescent phase, both groups do not differ significantly in their perception of cohesion in the family. On the basis of these results, we hypothesize that eating disorder patients of different age groups might be confronted with different problematic family issues: (1) eating disorder families in the pubertal phase overreact negatively; (2) the normal family dissociation in the adolescent phase does not take place in eating disorder families; and (3) family members get conflictually attached to the nuclear family in the launching phase.

We were wondering if these differences between phases would apply to the same degree to all *family members.* We ascertained that the patient and the mother in particular showed different results when compared with their normal counterparts. Patients of families in the pubertal phase seem to overreact in their negativity toward their family, but this reaction is congruent: they report more conflict, less cohesion and more disorganization than the oldest children of normal families. Patients of families in the adolescent phase seem to underreact: the normal disengagement does not take place because they report significantly more cohesion in this phase. Patients of families in the launching phase seem to be attached to their families in a conflictual way: they report significantly more conflict and more disorganization but also more cohesion. The same applies to the mother in this latter phase. Dally (1977) reported a higher incidence of family discord in the 11-14 years group, compared with the 15-18 years group and the 19 and older group. This information was obtained from the child. Thus, our finding with regard to conflict partially confirms Dally's because the patient reports more conflict in the pubertal group than in the adolescent and launching group. But at the same time we ascertain that such general statements are not justified because, if the information had been based on the view of the mother, Dally would have obtained reverse results when taking into account our finding that the mother reports the highest level of conflict in the launching phase.

Finally, we compared the results of *father, mother and child of the same family.* The patient child differs most from both parents on the three scales in the pubertal group and the normal child in the adolescent group. In the launching phase the patient approaches the mother's opinion. The parents of eating disorder families differ more in these older phases. So, we conclude that there is a clearer differentiation in the perception of family interaction between parents and child in normal families and this is most pronounced when the child is in the adolescent and launching phase of the family life cycle. Garfinkel et al. (1983), who investigated anorexia nervosa families in the adolescent and launching phase, also noted a similar response pattern on the part of the anorexic daughters and their mothers on the self-reporting "Family Assessment Measure." Mother and daughter both mentioned more family problems than the father who did not note any family abnormality. Houben, Pierloot and Vandereycken (see Chapter 8), investigating anorexia nervosa families in these latter phases, also reported a lack of differentiation between the parent-child and the husband-wife relationships. This latter finding seems also applicable to the results of both our intergroup and intrafamilial comparisons. As to the intergroup comparisons, patient families report more cohesion in the launching phase of the family life cycle. When we checked if this applied to the three family members, we found that mother and patient, especially, experience more cohesion but also more conflict and more disorganization than their normal counterparts. It seems as if mother and patient are conflictually attached to the family in the older phases. The intrafamilial comparisons indeed show that mother and patient approach each other in the perception of conflict in these phases and both of them experience more disorganization and more cohesion as well. The normal separation between patient and parents seems to be replaced by a distance between the parents and an approach between mother and patient. However, this family pattern is experienced as problematic, especially by mother and child.

REFERENCES*

American Psychiatric Association (1980), *Diagnostic and Statistical Manual of Mental disorders.* *3rd ed.* Washington D.C.: American Psychiatric Association.

Crisp, A.H., Hsu, L., Harding, B. & Hartshorn, J. (1980), Clinical features of anorexia nervosa: A study of a consecutive series of 102 female patients. *Journal of Psychosomatic Research,* 24:179-191.

Dally, P. (1977), Anorexia nervosa: Do we need a scapegoat? *Proceedings of the Royal Society of Medicine,* 70:470-474.

Garner, D., Garfinkel, P. & O'Shaugnessy, M. (1985), The validity of the distinction between bulimia with and without anorexia nervosa. *American Journal of Psychiatry,* 142:5 81-587.

Strober, M. (1981), The significance of bulimia in juvenile anorexia nervosa: An exploration of possible etiologic factors. *International Journal of Eating Disorders,* 1(1):28-43.

Wood, B. & Talmon, M. (1983), Family boundaries in transition: A search for alternatives. *Family Process,* 22:347-357.

---

* This list contains only secondary literature, whereas the other references are mentioned in the final section of this book: "Bibliography on Family Aspects of Eating Disorders."

Chapter 7

An Explorative Study on Parenting in Eating Disorder Families

Claire Perednia and Walter Vandereycken

INTRODUCTION

This chapter attempts to assess the parenting style in families with an anorexic or a bulimic patient. Our motivation is mainly pragmatic. We wanted to make an exploratory study that yields useful data for our everyday clinical practice with these families. This is very important since our treatment is based upon a family-oriented approach. It is often our experience that the parents of our hospitalized patients have a great need for counseling and guidance. On the one hand they feel responsible for what happened ("we have failed as parents") and, on the other hand, they are afraid of the future ("what can or should we do when the problems eventually recur?"). Our treatment appears to be more successful when the family (especially the parental dyad) is involved in the treatment. But while practically all of the parents are expecting some guidance, not every case requires family therapy.

In the literature on families of eating disorder patients, the educational role of the parents and their parenting style have been almost completely neglected. No systematic attention has been paid to this aspect. The very first family investigations — also in anorexia nervosa — overemphasized the mother-child interactions, reflecting the myth that "parenting means mothering." In later publications the "absent father" came into the picture. But soon the importance of the whole family was stressed by the systems theory approach, considering the parents as a subsystem. The interaction, however, between the parental subsystem and the children was usually analyzed in terms of communication, problem-solving, boundary setting etc., while the more specific educational role of the parents was overlooked. Though each family starts from the desire of two partners to become parents — an important shift in the family life cycle — systems theorists were usually not interested in "parenting," in the educational influence of *both* parents.

Although a theoretical model of effective parenting is lacking (see e.g., Belsky & Vondra, 1985), reviews in the area of child-rearing suggest that parenting consists of two principal dimensions (Arrindell & van den Ende, 1984): the *parental affection or care* (warmth versus hostility), and the *parental control* (permissiveness versus restrictiveness). When looking at the literature, one recognizes these two dimensions under various names used by different authors.

Anderson (1981), for instance, stresses the reciprocal developmental influence in parent-child relations. But it is also a fact that the relations are asymmetric. The adult caregivers (generally the parents) carry an important responsibility by the continuous choices they make and by the resulting influence on the development of the children. "There is little question that parents influence children's development in important ways. However, the nature of that influence is determined by the particular configuration of variables in a given family, which includes the range of parents, child and sibling characteristics as well as characteristics of the community and cultural settings in which they reside. Indeed, *the combination of parental warmth, reasonable control,* and *high expectations* has emerged repeatedly in descriptions of families of well functioning children, and such children seem to elicit more of the same from others" (Anderson, 1981, p. 41; italics added).

Bowlby (1977) suggests a strong causal relation between an individual's experiences with his parents and his later capacity to make affectional bonds, with deficiencies manifesting themselves in psychopathology. He also emphasizes the importance of the way in which parents perform their role. "The main variable to which I draw attention is the extent to which a child's parents (a) *provide him with a secure base,* and (b) *encourage him to explore from it...*, the extent to which parents recognize and respect a child's desire for a secure base and his need of it, and shape their behaviour accordingly.... Complementary in importance to a parent's respect for a child's attachment desires is respect for his desire to explore and gradually to extend his relationships both with peers and with other adults" (Bowlby, 1977, p. 206; italics added).

Important contributions by Maccoby and Martin (1983) and Parker (1983, 1984) also distinguish similar dimensions in style and practice of parenting. According to the former, security/responsivity versus demand/control are the major dimensions of parenting. In the first dimension (*security*) the concept of responsivity takes a central position as to the needs of the child and the signals it sends out, i.e., the mutual understanding of the interactions between child and parent(s). The second dimension (*controlling behavior*) refers to the demands the parents make on the child. On the basis of these dimensions four "educational styles" may be distinguished (Maccoby & Martin, 1983):

a.   An *authoritarian-autocratic style:* The parents show little responsivity and make a lot of demands on the children in whom usually little initiative, spontaneity and social competency can be observed.

b. A *spoiling-much allowing style:* The parents show a great responsivity but little demanding; the children show often impulsive and aggressive behavior, little independence and it is difficult for them to take responsibility.

c. An *indifferent and uninteressed style:* The parents show little responsivity and few demands; the child lives at a great distance from his parents and the risk for antisocial and delinquent behavior is high.

d. An *authoritative and interactional style:* The parents are responsive and demanding; the children show more independent behavior, self-confidence and social responsibility.

Parker (1983, 1984) is especially interested in *parental overprotection* as a style by which parents fail to give warmth, affection and closeness to their child, and, at the same time, fail to allow the child enough space for exploring the environment and thus gaining life experience. According to Parker, this parental overprotection is a nonspecific risk factor in the psychosocial development of the child. Once again, this author finds two dimensions in factor analytical studies of parental characteristics; a *care* and a *protection* dimension. By means of a self-reporting questionnaire he developed (the "Parental Bond Instrument"), Parker defines four parenting styles which, to some extent, correspond with the educational styles mentioned above:

a. *Optimal parenting,* characterized by high care and low protection (cf. authoritative-interactional).

b. *Neglectful parenting,* with low care and low protection (cf. indifferent uninterested).

c. *Affectionate constraint* with high care and high protection; this parental style has also been described as "indulging," in contrast to "controlling" overprotection (cf. spoiling-much allowing).

d. *Affectionless control* with low care and high protection (cf. authoritarian-autocratic).

We hypothesize that with regard to eating disorders, the dimension of parental control/protection is a very important one. According to Vandereycken and Meermann (1984), one feature is common to all these families: the lack of adequate joint authority of the parents. This means that the parents have problems finding a balance between an adequate (i.e., rational and flexible) control and the amount of age-appropriate autonomy they give to their child. Indeed, we saw very contrasting families, some with parents being very controlling and overprotective, and others with a serious lack of control, being almost chaotic. This brings us to another important observation: that the parents generally fail to reach a basic agreement about child-rearing issues.

In order to systematically examine these clinical observations as well as the aforementioned theoretical propositions, we designed an exploratory study on the parenting style in families of anorexic and bulimic patients who came to our unit for inpatient treatment. Because of the lack of a model for effective parenting—which might provide guidelines for the assessment of child rearing-behavior — the questionnaires (EMBU, PBI) we used investigated the underlying dimensional structure of parental rearing behavior as perceived by recipients (Arrindell & van den Ende, 1984).

This parenting style is influenced by several factors that we attempted to explore by an interview and self-reporting questionnaires:
- the psychological well-being of the parents as individuals (interview plus SCL-90),
- the parents' marital relationship (interview plus MMQ),
- the child-rearing experiences in the parents' families of origin; how one experienced one's own education may influence the way one is rearing own children (interview plus EMBU and PBI); this might reveal some information about transgenerational issues.

With regard to this last topic, we were also interested to know how the patient herself experienced the way she was raised by her parents before onset of the eating disorder.

METHOD

Procedure

The study was done with anorexic or bulimic patients who had been hospitalized in our unit and who were still living with their families. We utilized a self-designed standardized interview and a number of questionnaires, which we will describe further on. After the intake interview, the research assistant (who was not directly involved in the treatment program) invited the parents — by telephone or by letter — and informed them about the intention of the study, the course and duration (2 to 3 hours), and finally asked for their consent. On the day of the interview, the hospitalized patient was also given two questionnaires (EMBU and PBI) to fill in. To avoid contamination of answers between the parents during the study, the interview as well as the questionnaires were administered separately and they had no contact with each other during the investigation. The parents themselves decided who would be the first to be interviewed. When the study was terminated, the parents had the opportunity to visit their daughter who had already filled in her questionnaires. The standardized interview we used for the parents was self-designed and is reprinted in the Appendix. It consisted of three major parts: questions about the eating disorder, about child-rearing issues and about the marital relationship.

Questionnaires

We limited ourselves to questionnaires which were known in the international literature and which, at the same time, were already tested in a Dutch population (except for the PBI).

EMBU or "Own Memories of Child-Rearing Experience"

The EMBU is an inventory designed by Perris et al. (1980) in order to assess one's memories of parental rearing behavior. It is originally a Swedish inventory, consisting of 14 subscales, each one containing items to be separately scored with respect to one's own father and mother. They describe the degree to which each parent was abusive, depriving, punitive, shaming, rejecting, overprotective, tolerant, affectionate, performance oriented, guilt engendering, stimulating, favoring siblings and favoring the subject. Arrindell et al. (1983c) developed a Dutch version of the EMBU and found, by means of factor analysis, four conceptually clear factors: "rejection," "emotional warmth," "overprotection" and "favoring subject." This Dutch version we used contains 64 items (25 for "rejection," 18 for "emotional warmth," 16 for "overprotection" and 5 for "favoring subject"). The subjects are required to answer all questions concerning the father's behavior first, followed by those having reference to the mother's. Regarding the psychometric qualities of this questionnaire, Arrindell et al. (1983c) write, "that the Dutch EMBU is a highly reliable measure which in many respects resembles the Swedish and the English forms. It thus appears to be an excellent instrument for standardized assessment of the familial environment of upbringing, and in particular for use in the area of mental health research" (p. 175).

The Parental Bonding Instrument or PBI

The PBI was developed by Parker et al. (1979) as a refined self-report measure of parental (paternal and maternal) behaviors and attitudes, as experienced by the child. As already noted in the introduction, Parker defined two major dimensions: "care" and "protection." The questionnaire itself contains 25 items and subjects are asked to score each parent on a 4-point scale as they were remembered in the respondent's first 16 years. The 12 "care" items assess parental warmth, understanding, affection, empathy and closeness, with negatively loaded items assessing indifference and rejection. The 13 "protection" items assess several components of overprotection such as control, intrusion, excessive contact, infantilization and the encouragement of dependency, while negatively loaded items assess the encouragement of independence and autonomy.

The reliability of the PBI has been investigated in clinical as well as in nonclinical groups with a satisfying reliability (Parker, 1983a). There is also support for the validity of the PBI and this, according to this author, there is even a considerable support for the view that the PBI is an acceptable measure of actual as well as of perceived parental characteristics (Parker, 1984). We translated the PBI into Dutch but we do not yet have data on the psychometric qualities of this version. Therefore, we can only compare our data with Parker's normative scores for an Australian population.

The Maudsley Marital Questionnaire (MMQ)

We used this questionnaire to assess how the parents perceive their marital relationship. The MMQ is a self-report inventory designed to assess the degree of favorableness of attitude toward one's own marriage (Crowe, 1978). It is composed of three scales, related to marital, sexual and general life adjustment and with 9-point scales (0-8) appended to each question. The subjects are asked to indicate which alternative best describes the way things have been for them in the past two weeks. Arrindell et al. (1983, a and b) developed a Dutch version of the MMQ and their studies confirm the good reliability and the very satisfying validity of this instrument.

The Symptom Checklist or SCL-90

Arrindell and co-workers (1981, 1986) developed a Dutch version of the well-known Hopkins Symptom Checklist SCL-90 (Derogatis, 1977). This is a self-report symptom inventory, multidimensional in nature and oriented toward the measurement of "psychopathology." It gives a snapshot of the actually experienced (psychological) complaints of the subject. The Dutch version contains nine dimensions: anxiety, agoraphobia, depression, somatization, obsessive-compulsive behavior (insufficiency in thinking and acting), distrust and interpersonal sensitivity, hostility, sleeping problems and psychoneuroticism (i.e., total score). Each item has to be scored on a 5-point scale. Recently, normative scores became available for the Dutch population (Arrindell, 1986).

Subjects

In total, we invited 16 couples to participate (single-parent families and families where the patient was no longer living at home were excluded). Only 15 completed the interview and 14 filled out the complete questionnaires. One couple did not turn up at the appointment because on their way to the hospital they had a fight. Two parents did not fill in the questionnaires because they were French-speaking. First, we describe demographic data of the parents and then we report some demographic and clinical data of the patients. The fathers ranged in age from 39 to 67 years (mean = 52 years) and the mothers from 37 to 63 years (mean = 49 years). The average duration of marriage was 25 years (range 16-38 years) and the average age at which they married was for the fathers, 26.6 years (range 22-49 years), and for the mothers, 24.6 years (range 18-36). For one father this was his second marriage after the death of his first wife. Most of the couples had three children (range 1-6). In the fathers' families of origin the average number of children was 4.3 (range 1-8) and in the mother's 4.8 (1-12). Only one father did not grow up with his two parents (his father died when he was five years old) and only one mother was reared in a single-parent family (her parents divorced when she was three and she was raised by her mother). The mean age at which the fathers left their parents' home was 24.5 years (22-30) versus 23 years (17-36) for the mothers. Most families (50%) were living rather near (in the same town) to their families of origin (the fathers' as well as the mothers'). When rated according to father's occupation, seven families came from the lower social classes, five from the middle class and three from the upper social class. Regarding the diagnosis of the patients (n = 16), the DSM-III criteria were used. Thirteen met the criteria for anorexia nervosa and 3 for bulimia. The mean age at admission was 17.5 years (range 14-25 years).

RESULTS

We will describe successively the results yielded by the interview and by the questionnaires. Finally, some case vignettes will give a more vivid illustration of our findings.

Results of the Interview

We will report successively the answers regarding the eating problems, the child-rearing issues, and the marital relationship of the parents.

1. Questions about the eating disorders
 1a. *Positions of the patient in the family*
 For most parents (67% of the fathers and 53% of the mothers) their eating disordered daughter occupies a special position in the family compared with the other children. The following differences are mentioned:
- fear of contact with other people;
- being more nervous, demanding more attention and being less independent;
- being more quiet, obedient and perfectionist;
- being spoiled and overprotected (for instance, as the first daughter after three sons);
- having more problems at school or at work.

A minority of these parents (13% of the mothers and 7% of the fathers) only noticed a clear difference between the patient and her siblings after the onset of the eating problems. In the majority of the cases (10/15) both parents gave a similar answer.

The vast majority of parents (87%) claim to have no serious problems with the other children. The other parents who do mention problems, refer to psychosomatic complaints (asthma and eczema) and to their own marriage problems.

 1b. *The parents' attitudes toward the eating problems*
 In only one family, *help* for the eating problems was sought by the father. In almost all families (11/15) the mother took the initiative while in the remaining

cases it was a joint decision. In only one third of the families, the parents do agree as to the moment that the existing problems were "officially" recognized (diagnosed) as anorexia nervosa or bulimia. It is remarkable that many parents try to avoid this issue.

When asked about the kind of treatment they considered as necessary, 60% of the parents do agree; 23% thought of a pure medical (somatic) treatment, whereas 50% of the parents considered a psychological or psychiatric treatment (in 10% even considered psychiatric hospitalization) as indicated. Only one parent mentioned a combination of a psychological and a somatic treatment.

The most important *eliciting factors* are mentioned in order of importance are:
- discontent about weight and physical appearance (87%);
- problems at school or work (53%);
- changes due to puberty (47%);
- problems with a boyfriend (27%);
- conflicts between the patient and her parents (23%);
- discord between the parents about child-rearing issues(20%);
- conflicts between the parents (15%);
- conflicts with siblings (15%);
- medical reasons such as an illness or an operation (10%);
- other reasons (like the interference of a grandmother).

Concerning the *interpretation* or conceptualization of the eating problems, both parents adjudge the highest priority to the following statements about the eating disorder:
- it is an obsession or an addiction she is not able to master;
- it is something she did to herself by wanting to lose weight.

The fathers think that the eating problems are surely not:
- a reaction to tensions and problems in the family, or
- a way of getting attention and care from others.

The mothers think that the eating problems are surely not:
- an expression of sexual problems, or
- a lack of character, a weak will.

1c. *The parents' reactions upon the eating problems*

Here, we find a relative similarity between the parents. They react most often with concern and worry (86%), pain and sorrow (84%), patience (54%), support (50%), and comprehension (40%). Mentioned in fewer cases (less than 35%) are helplessness, personal guiltfeelings, authority, distrust and control (more on the part of the mothers), rage and threat of separation.

1d. *Influence of the eating problems on family life*

Most parents—more mothers (80%) than fathers (53%)— experienced that their interaction with the children (i.e., communication, expression of feelings, confidence) suffered the most becuse of the eating problems. About 50% of the parents mention that the eating disorder had some negative influence on the interactions between the children. The anorexia or bulimia was noticed in 56% of the cases to have had no influence at all on the parents' marital relationship. This means that 44% of the parents admit some marital problems as a consequence of the eating disorder! This was more often admitted by the mothers (53%) than by the fathers (33%). The eating problems was said to have no influence on:

- the eating habits at home (60%);
- the householding (63%);
- the use of leisure (66%);
- the contacts with the parents' extended families (70%).

1e. *How the parents see the future*

One third of the parents (33%), especially the fathers, are convinced that, if faced with the same problem again in the future, they would be more strict and severe and that both parents together would take a more consistent attitude toward it. Sixteen percent say that they would intervene earlier (i.e., consulting a specialist), 13% would not change their attitude, 11% would take more time off for family life, 10% would consider special changes (e.g., not to take grandfather into the home, change from school), 10% do not know what to change, 7% would be less authoritarian or would try to have a closer contact with the patient.

Most parents feel insecure when thinking about the possibility that the eating problems would emerge again in the future. This shows a clear need for counseling. Faced with the idea that eventually there would never come a real solution or considerable improvement in the problems, the majority believes that this would induce no important change in the family, nor in the marital relationship. Only 13% of the mothers would become "sick" and for 6% of them the idea of a chronic eating disorder would be unbearable (a "catastrophe"). A surprising finding is that 80% of the parents are rather optimistic as to the future. They still believe a complete recovery is possible. For 13% only a partial recovery seems possible, and only 6% of the parents (always the mothers) are rather skeptical.

2. Questions about Child-Rearing Issues

2a. *In general*

Faced with the choice between three conceptions of parenting, for the majority of the fathers "child-rearing" means:

- first, to teach knowledge and life values;
- second, to feel intimately attached to the child;
- third, to be always ready to help the child, to take care of him/her and to sacrify oneself for the child.

For the mothers, however, this last meaning is the most important followed by the first and second. Fathers and mothers do largely agree about the "ideal" role of the parent. For them it means:

- first, considering the child as an equal person (it is giving and receiving of help, love and affection);
- second, being a clear model to the child;
- third, letting the child become oneself by giving him/her the freedom to experience and explore.

2b. *The given education*

- *Characteristics.* It is striking how much parents consider they have been too indulgent toward their children, the fathers being more demanding than the mothers. Most of the parents admit that the fathers are regularly absent from home (as a consequence of professional occupation?). The majority also agrees that the fathers do not have sufficient contact with their children. In general, the parents claim that there is practically no interference by others (grandparents, neighbors) in the regular family life.
- *The responsibility for the child-rearing.* Here, the parents differ from each other in their answers. The fathers say that the mothers have more responsibility while the mothers say they both have. Only in 50% of the families do both parents agree on this point. In none of the families was the responsibility taken by the father alone. Contrasting with these findings, are the answers to the question of who is making the most important decisions about the children. In the majority of families, both parents make them together. In one third it is up to the mother to decide on her own.
- *Contact with the children.* Before the eating problems emerged, it was the mother — without any exception — who had the most contact with the children. Thereafter, this situation did not change in 73% of the families. In 13% of the families the father became more closely involved with the children, while in 13% there was little or no contact left. In the great majority of families, the anorexic or bulimic daughter as well as the other children are most attached to the mother alone.
- *Agreement between both parents.* Most parents (50%) say that they did always agree about the handling of the children, before as well as after the eating problems emerged. About 35% of the parents say they usually agreed, and only 8% almost never agreed. Concerning possible differences in parenting, two thirds of the fathers assert there are almost no differences. One third of the fathers mention as differences the attitude toward the other children, the amount of presence at home, and their own (received) education. Two thirds of the mothers notice as differences that the fathers show less comprehension, are more authoritarian and more performance-oriented, and that they are usually too much involved in their job.

2c. *The received education*

  ●*Characteristics.* An important finding is that the fathers as well as the mothers evaluated their own education as too demanding. The parents of the fathers as well as of the mothers were not absent from home and yet they had insufficient contact with them.

  ●*Difference between received and given education.* The majority of the parents (70%) assert that their own (received) education is clearly different from the education they give their children. These differences are said to be relatively detached from the different time-context (only 10% of the parents ascribe the differences to the changing time-context). For only 10% of the parents there is no difference. They give their children almost the same type of education they received from their parents. Finally, about 10% cannot form any idea about this issue. For the parents who do really report a difference, 52% attribute this difference to the degree of strictness in child-rearing; they were raised more strictly than their own childen. Some parents (14%) think that the amount of prosperity makes the biggest difference. The children now are more spoiled, they have more goods and freedom, and work less. Among the other differences reported, the parents themselves were more often sent to a boarding-school, had less voice and were more tied to home. These results are true for both the fathers' and the mothers' received education.

3. Questions About the Marital Relationship

3a. Marital satisfaction

The majority of the parents (83%) perceive their marital relationship as satisfactory. But for half of them (and especially for the mothers) this changed with the onset of the anorexia or bulimia problem of their daughter. They became more nervous, depressive and irritable. Similarly, most couples (83%) report no specific problems with their partner. The couples who do mention conflicts (16%) ascribe these to drinking problems, clashing characters, illnesses or the presence of a grandparent at home.

3b. Psychological well-being of the parents

As far as the fathers are concerned, 40% of them experienced (after marriage) stress symptoms, especially from work. Twenty percent had a depression and another 20% had anxiety disorders. Only three fathers are said to have had a health problem before marriage. As for the mothers, 20% reported a period of marked slimming before marriage. After marriage, half of the mothers (53%) demonstrated a depression and 27% symptoms of stress. Serious psychological or psychiatric problems were reported in 40% of the first-degree relatives of the fathers and in 30% of the mothers' relatives. Most parents still have a lot of contact with their own parents, and more with the parents of the mothers than with the fathers'.

Table 1. EMBU (average scores)

	Father Figure			Mother Figure		
	Rejec-tion	Emotional warmth	Over-protection	Rejec-tion	Emotional warmth	Over-protection
Fathers*	34.5	51.3	35.0	36.4	53.8	38.7
Mothers*	37.0	48.0	40.5	38.0	49.6	42.3
Patients*	36.6	47.0	33.1	39.5	53.1	38.6
Controls**	34.4	49.8	32.1	35.2	52.2	35.3

*Own research sample (N = 15)
**Normative data from 277 non-patient normals (Arrindell et al., 1983 c; see also Perris et al., 1985)

Results of the Questionnaires

EMBU

As already mentioned, this questionnaire was filled out in each case by both parents as well as the patient. This gives us the opportunity to see how the parents experienced their own education and how the patient perceives the way in which she was raised by her parents (see Table 1).

As Arrindell et al. (1983c) noted for their sample, our results only partially support the cultural stereotype that mothers compared with fathers are experienced as less rejecting, more affectionate and more overprotective.

For *rejection,* we can say that, in general, the results of the mothers and the patients are close to each other, whereas those of the fathers resemble more the normative data of the (nonpatient) control sample. Both mothers and patients experienced more rejection especially from their mothers.

Regarding *emotional warmth,* all subjects as well as controls perceived mother as more affectionate than father. This difference in the experience of emotional warmth is the greatest for our hospitalized patients.

For *overprotection,* our sample shows higher scores than did the control group. The mother is experienced by all our subjects (but particularly by the mothers) as more overprotective than the father. Here again, we see that the patients notice the greatest distinction between both parents.

PBI

Our own Dutch version of the Parental Bond Instrument was filled out by both the patients and their parents, and compared with normative data from an Australian population (see Table 2).

Comparing the results of the fathers, the mothers and the patients with each other and with the normative data, we can highlight the following findings:

- with regard to the *maternal* dimension, the patients experienced the most care and the mothers the least, while the fathers' results are in

Table 2. PBI (average scores)

	Fathers*	Mothers*	Patients*	Controls**
Maternal Care	25.9	21.7	28.1	27.0
Maternal Protection	16.7	17.4	12.6	13.5
Paternal Care -	23.5	21.0	21.7	24.0
Paternal Protection	13.2	15.9	11.2	12.5

*Own researchsample (N = 15)
**Normative data from non-clinical subjects (Parker, 1983, 1984)

between. Again the mothers experienced the most protection and the patients the least.

●with regard to the *paternal* dimensions, the fathers are the ones who experienced the most care from their fathers; the mothers' and daughters' results are almost similar. The fathers' perception of care resembles the normative data. Remarkably, again the mothers experienced the most protection from their fathers; the fathers' results for perceived protection are the closest to the normative data.

Parker (1984) notes that the scales of the PBI can be used together in order to compare four general styles of parenting: "neglectful parenting," "optimal parenting," "affectionate constraint" and "affectionless control." Quadrants may be created by intersecting the care and the protection scales at their means or medians.

Applied to our own results (see Figures 1 and 2), this demonstrates that the mothers experienced the most extreme "affectionless control:" the lowest care combined with the highest protection scores. The fathers perceived their mothers as overprotective but evaluate the attitude of their own fathers as rather "neutral" (moderate care and protection). The patients, on the contrary, experienced a rather "optimal" parenting style from their mothers and a more clearly "neglectful" parenting on the part of their fathers.

MMQ

The Maudsley Marital Questionnaire assesses marital, sexual and general life adjustment. The parents' results may be compared with data from distressed and nondistressed or "happily married" couples (Arrindell et al., 1983 a and b).

It is clear from our results (Table 3) that the parent couples describe themselves as more similar to normal couples than to distressed ones. Comparing the scores of the fathers and the mothers, it appears that the latter are more dissatisfied with their marriages (this applies to ratings of marital adjustment, sexual adjustment and general life). The mothers tend to score intermediately between happily and unhappily married wives.

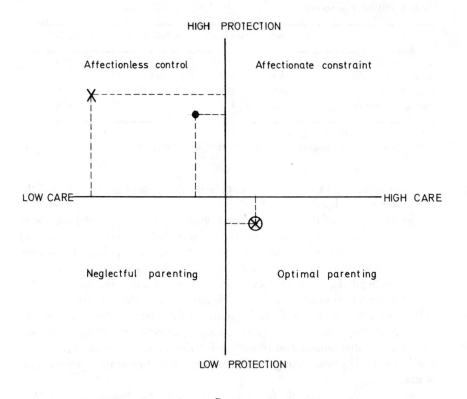

● Fathers, ✗ Mothers, ⊗ Daughters/Patients

Figure 1. Maternal dimensions

Table 3. MMQ (average scores)

	Husbands			Wives		
	Parent*	Normal**	Distressed***	Parent*	Normal**	Distressed***
Marital Adjustment	12.2	9.4	32.6	21.6	10.8	36.8
Sexual Adjustment	10.9	6.7	16.3	13.3	7.3	17.3
General Life	8.0	7.9	12.0	11.2	7.2	14.3

*Own research sample (N = 15)
**Non-distressed volunteers (N = 250) studied by Arrindell et al. (1983a)
***Distressed, unhappily married subjects (N = 100) studied by Arrindell et al. (1983a)

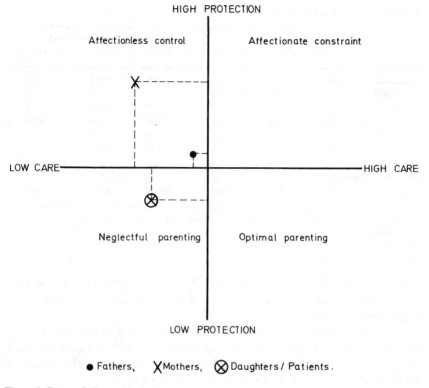

Figure 2. **Paternal dimensions**

SCL-90

The Symptom Checklist assesses the psychological well-being of the parents as individuals, compared with a normal Dutch population (Arrindell, 1986). A study of 432 men and 577 women yielded normative data for comparison with, respectively, the fathers and the mothers of our sample (Table 4). The Dutch version utilized a 7-point appreciation-classification, with the following classes: very high, high, more than average, average, less than average, low, and very low.

A total score (degree of psychoneuroticism) is an indication of the overall level of psychological as well as physical (dys)functioning over a recent time period. For both the fathers and the mothers, this score is high (Pc 80-95) in comparison with a normal population. The mean score of the mothers (164.9) is higher than that of the fathers (138.4).

Other high scores for both the fathers and the mothers are found on the depression scale (26.4 and 33) and the sleeping-problems scale (6.7 and 9.7). Again, the mothers scored higher than the fathers.

Table 4. SCL-90 (Dutch version)

	Fathers (N=15)			Mothers (N=15)		
	Mean	(SD)	Appreciation*	Mean	(SD)	Appreciation*
Anxiety	16.0	(6.0)	> average	18.6	(6.9)	high
Agoraphobia	8.4	(2.3)	> average	10.1	(4.7)	high
Depression	26.4	(9.2)	high	33.0	(8.7)	high
Somatization	18.2	(5.2)	> average	22.6	(8.6)	high
Insufficiency[a]	16.9	(5.4)	high	16.3	(4.9)	> average
Distrust[b]	26.6	(7.1)	> average	33.0	(9.1)	high
Hostility	7.5	(2.7)	> average	8.6	(2.4)	> average
Sleeping problems	6.7	(4.0)	high	9.7	(3.0)	high
Total[c]	138.4	(35.3)	high	164.9	(35.5)	high

*Comparison with normative data from a general population (Arrindell, 1986)
[a]Insufficiency in thinking and acting
[b]Distrust and interpersonal sensitivity
[c]Psychoneuroticism scale

On the following scales, the mothers show a high score and the fathers a greater than average score: anxiety, agoraphobia, somatization, distrust and interpersonal sensitivity.

On the remaining scales, the mothers do not present a higher score than the fathers (in comparison with the "normal" controls): on "insufficiency in thinking and acting" the fathers are scoring higher, and on "hostility" they obtain the same appreciation as the mothers (more than average).

In summary, these results show that the parents in our sample deviate clearly from the general population: they report more complaints and symptoms and, hence, may be considered as dysfunctioning neuroticly on a more than average level.

Case Vignettes

In the previous sections parents and patients are discussed as a group whose characteristics are expressed in terms of "average" results. In order to illustrate more vividly the aforementioned data from our study and to emphasize the heterogeneity of the families we are working with, we will describe the individual findings for three cases.

Family A

Father is a 52-years-old bus driver, a quiet background-figure within his family. Mother, also 52 years old, works at home and is very preoccupied with the patient (a 17-year-old student) but also with the other children (a 24-year-old married daughter and her 20-year-old sister). When meeting this family we had the following impression: both parents act in an overprotecting way toward their children and the mother especially is very controlling. The eating disorder symptomatology of the patient reflects, on the one hand, an adolescent crisis including problems with sexual identity, building up social contacts and leaving home. This separation individuation process, on the other hand, seems to be hampered by an over protecting parenting style.

Can we confirm these impressions on the basis of the results obtained by the investigation procedure? According to the standardized interview, both parents are still very involved with their family of origin. They both answer all questions in a very similar way. Their reaction to the eating problems was very empathic — they helped each other to cope with it. Concerning child-rearing issues, the parents say they always agree and share the responsibilities, though mother has a central position in this family.

Both parents characterize their child-rearing practice as too indulgent; they were also brought up like this. They experience their marital relationship as satisfying, without any special problems. This is also the case for their psychological well-being. Mother mentions she had a nervous breakdown after the birth of the patient, but it disappeared after a few weeks with medication.

On the EMBU, the patient notices a great difference between the parents, namely with respect to mother: more rejection and control but also more emotional warmth and overprotection. With regard to her own parents, mother did experience less rejection and more than average overprotection as well as emotional warmth. The father does not perceive any great difference between his father's and mother's attitude toward him. The PBI shows the same tendencies. On the MMQ, the parents confirm their answers in the interview: they are satisfied with their marriage. Finally, it is clear from the SCL-90 that both parents function psychologically quite well (only mother presents a high score on sleeping problems).

In summary, we seem to be faced here with an ordinary average family.

Family B

Father is a 39-year-old manager almost completely absorbed by a busy professional life. Mother is a 37-year-old teacher. There are two children: the patient (17 years old) and a younger brother (14 years). Again, the eating disorder appears to be linked with a problematic growing-up process. On the other hand, the symptomatology is connected with a family dysfunctioning: the over-involvement from father's family of origin does not allow enough psychological space and privacy for a harmonious family development.

During the first years of marriage, the parents lived in the same house with fathers' parents. Later on, they built a house just next door. As a little child, the patient was brought up by her grandparents because her parents both worked. A strong enmeshment of both families grew. The standardized interview revealed little agreement between both parents, especially on child-rearing issues and their marital relationship. Both parents reacted more empathically than confrontationally on the eating problems. Mother reports as the most important eliciting factor the conflicts she had with her husband about the interference of his mother in their family life. Father does not even mention this and he claims that concerning child-rearing issues there was never a disagreement between himself and his wife. But the latter says they often did disagree, because he seemed to be only interested in the daughter's achievement at school, while mother had to take most of the responsibilities and decisions.

About the characteristics of their education, father admits he was too indulgent but mother denies this. The greatest difference concerns the influence by others: father denies such an influence whereas mother complains of much interference from her mother-in-law.

Both parents perceive their marital relationship as satisfying but father notices that their sexual relationship changed since the anorexia: his wife enjoys sex less. She feels her husband is too often absent from home because of his job and his hobby, hunting.

Several years ago, father had a depression due (in his opinion) to overburdening in his job. But, according to his wife, his mother was the real cause of his problems: she did not allow him much independence — and she still cannot.

On the parenting questionnaires (EMBU, PBI) the patient notices a great difference: in contrast to her father, she perceives her mother as more affectionate and overprotecting. Concerning her family of origin, the mother did not experience such a great difference between the attitudes of her own parents, although compared with a normal sample she mentions more rejection and less emotional warmth. Father, on the contrary, perceived a greater difference between his parents, especially noting more protection from his mother.

Concerning the marital relationship (MMQ) father confirms what he mentioned in the interview (less satisfying sexual relationship) whereas mother now reports she is dissatisfied with her marriage and also with her life in general. Both parents admit personal problems on the SCL-90 with a high and very high total score for father and mother respectively.

In summary, this family resembles more the "classical" picture of the anorexia family: an absent father, an overinvolved mother, a dissatisfying marriage and an ill psychological health of the parents.

Family C

Father is a 54-year-old successful engineer who built up his own company while his 50-year-old wife was always living in his shadow. They have five children: three sons (29, 28 and 21 years old) who left home, the patient (18 years old) and her younger sister of 13 years. From the first contact on, the father appears as an authoritarian man whose reactions toward his children and especially his daughters are rather extreme: from a radical, sometimes hurting attitude, to an overinvolved approach. Mother is French-speaking and, after 30 years of marriage, she still does not speak Dutch and refuses to integrate in the Flemish community where she is living.

There are many problems in the marital relationship and father often considers the prospect of divorce. He demonstrates overt aggression toward his wife, whom he frequently humiliates in the presence of others. The children, especially the daughters, seem to stand between both parents. They were born against father's will. Nevertheless, he is very engaged with his daughters, probably because of guilt feelings. The patient's anorexia (with bulimia and vomiting) is only one of a series of behavioral problems. She was rather promiscuous in her sexual contacts, abused soft drugs and showed many problems at school. Her behavior reflects continuing conflicts regarding freedom and authority, limitations and autonomy. On the other hand, a lack of positive contact within a stable family milieu seems responsible for her chaotic lifestyle.

The standardized interview reveals that father — as only son — still has much contact with his parents (his father was his business-partner). Mother is the eldest of three daughters; her mother died two weeks before the patient's birth and recently her father moved to another country.

Both parents disagree on almost all issues, especially concerning their child-rearing practices and their marital relationship. Mother reacted with empathy in response to the eating problems of her daughter; father tried very hard to be confronting, but he was too much absorbed by his job to keep contact with the daily family life, and this gave him personal guilt feelings.

Father cannot agree with his wife's child-rearing ideas and with her lifestyle because, in his opinion, she is not able to handle problems at all. Mother says they are always blaming each other for what happened. Father admits he did not have enough contact with his children. He thinks he was too demanding while he himself received a too-indulgent education. Mother has much more contact with her sons than with her daughters. She thinks she was too indulgent because her own parents were too demanding.

Both parents give a competely different view of their marital relationship: he would never marry "this woman" again, whereas she would marry him again. He stresses they have a lot of marital problems while she denies them. Father believes that the birth of the youngest daughter induced an important change within the family, especially for the patient, because, from that moment on, mother neglected "his nice little girl."

In contrast with these findings during the interview, the patient herself does not mention (on the EMBU and PBI) any great difference between her father's and mother's attitude toward her. Maybe this response pattern is symptomatic for her position in the family: a buffer between her parents. Mother did not fill in the questionnaires because of language problems and father refused to complete the MMQ (though he had stressed the existence of a series of marital problems during the interview).

In summary, we are confronted here with a seriously distorted family, the basis for which is a fundamentally disturbed relationship between the parents. The childrens' healthiest reaction in such a milieu is to escape from it.

DISCUSSION

The limitations of this study, which had a predominantly exploratory purpose should be stressed. The small sample (together with the absence of a control group for the interview data) does not allow general conclusions. Therefore, this discussion should be viewed as a consideration about impressions and tendencies which may serve as guiding hypotheses for further research. One major conclusion, however, is quite obvious: there is a great diversity in the eating disorder families we encounter in our clinical work (cf. case vignettes). This has at least one important implication as to treatment, a thesis that is underscored repeatedly in the following discussion: not every family needs specific therapy, but many do need counseling, and all of them expect some guidance.

Parents Faced with an Eating Disorder

A considerable part of our standardized interview (see Appendix) was aimed at investigating the parents' reactions toward the eating disorder of their daughter.

First, most parents mention they felt the patient to be different from her siblings, even before the onset of the eating disorder. Were these patients really different as young children, i.e., psychologically more vulnerable, and did they thus elicit other attitudes from their parents (e.g., more protection and indulgence)? Or is this a typical kind of retrospective deformation of perception colored by the actual problematic situation? Have the symptoms been a special burden to the parents' educational abilities? Is their usual way to cope with developmental conflicts insufficient with regard to these "special" kids? Or do the parents perceive and treat them differently for personal reasons (individual or marital problems)? The issues that are discussed next may give some hints for answering these questions.

The parents see as eliciting factors of the eating problems:
- discontentment with weight and physical appearance (87%);
- problems at school or work (53%);
- changes due to puberty (47%).

This is somewhat surprising, because these are problems that almost all developing adolescents encounter once in a while. So the causes, as they are perceived by the parents, are not viewed in proportion to the consequences (serious eating disorder). The parents' interpretation or conceptualization of the eating problem is skewed in the same direction: both parents see the disorder, first, as an obsession or an addiction their daughter was not able to master and, second, as something she did to herself because she wanted to lose weight.

Now, it is striking to see how much *ambivalence* these parents show: on the one hand, they place all problems outside the nuclear family (at first sight it has nothing to do with intrafamilial relationships) and they do not even question their own interaction with the child as a possible etiological factor. On the other hand, there is the ever-returning guilt issue in counseling these parents ("What did we do wrong?"). Finally, the hypotheses they put forward are not very workable as to family interactions; they seem only to imply that the patient must be treated as an individual. The reactions of the parents to the eating problems have been more empathic than confronting: they did react, for instance, more with concern and worry than with authority or control. This appears to correspond to their general parenting style, as described in the following section.

In our study, apparently parents only admit their responsibility indirectly: most of them would act differently if they could do it over again; they would be more strict and consistent.

Concerning the impact of the eating disorder on the family life, the parents report a negative influence on the parent-child relationship, the interactions between the siblings and – as far as the mothers are concerned – also on the marital relationship. But they do not ask for direct help in order to restore these interactions; they seem to suppose that these disturbances will disappear once the eating disorder is cured. It is a typical way of linear causal thinking, since parents appear to minimize or overlook any influence of the family life on the eating disorder. This contains the danger that the patient becomes, directly or indirectly, a kind of scapegoat in the family. However, referring to what Selvini Palazzoli mentioned (see Chapter 11), "the child cannot be blamed, because she is sick." The parents indeed adopt an empathic attitude: they do not want to attack their daughter as a person but rather usually conceptualize the disorder as something she cannot help.

Here again, we can observe the ambivalence or double messages on the part of the parents especially concerning blame and guilt: "She disturbed our family life, but she cannot help it because of her illness. Why did we deserve this? What did we wrong?" This very unhealthy situation of confusing communications can become a vicious circle, resulting in a greater isolation of the patient and a growing helplessness in the parents. That is why, in counseling these parents, the whole *guilt-problem* must be unmasked as soon as possible. The parents have strong guilt feelings, sometimes highlighted by grandparents, friends or neighbors who declare that "such a thing" would never happen with their children.

We try to convince the parents that the real matter is not their feeling guilty but their taking on responsibilities. An efficient treatment in this case will be, first of all, a matter of co-responsibility between parents, patient and therapist (see part C in this book). Our interview data showed that parents not uncommonly avoid taking on their responsibilities: they delay getting (professional) help, they continue to blame each other, and so forth, in order to postpone a direct confrontation with their own helplessness.

Parental Rearing Behavior and Attitudes

The attitude toward the eating problems seems to reflect a general parenting style: more protective than confronting. Parents characterize their child-rearing practices as too indulgent and overprotective. This parenting style is clearly influenced by their own education (EMBU, PBI) which was too demanding (action-reaction). This phenomenon, probably not uncommon in many families, may reflect important *intergenerational issues*. Although the majority of the parents still live close to their own parents, we cannot conclude on the basis of our data that grandparents had a lot of direct influence, not only on the parents' own rearing practice but especially on their handling of the eating problem. The influence on parenting is an indirect one. The same may apply to separation-individuation issues. Unfortunately, we did not ask the parents how they experienced their own process of leaving home and becoming independent (in fact, do they really feel to be independent from their own parents?). This topic requires closer attention in future research.

Most parents say they usually agree upon child-rearing issues (cf. interview), while it is remarkable how the patients experienced clearly different attitude's from father and mother (cf. EMBU and PBI). Apparently, the so-called basic agreement between the parents was not experienced as such by their daughter.

Another striking observation is the *central position of the mothers* within the family, while the fathers are regularly absent from the family-life (usually because of their job). The latter have insufficient contact with the children, who are most attached to their mother. The fathers generally attribute most of the responsibility for the child-rearing to their wives, whereas the mothers claim it is a joint responsibility. In one third of the families the mothers make the most important decisions about the children on their own, without any help from their husbands.

Parents as Individuals and as Partners

Concerning the marital relationship and the psychological well-being of the parents, it is obvious that they try to present themselves better — socially desirable response pattern — in the interview than they do in the questionnaires. In the latter, both parents (but especially the mothers) reveal more dissatisfaction (MMQ) and more psychoneurotic complaints (SCL-90) than do normal controls. It is remarkable that the mothers report having experienced themselves the most unfavorable parenting atmosphere in their family of origin, and now, having their own nuclear family, they complain of individual as well as marital problems! This might be a consequence of the central position the mothers occupy in their family: alone, they could hardly bear the burden of major responsibilities, but they had chosen to do it without support from their husbands. On the other hand, it is also possible that the overinvolvement in the mother-role enabled them to partially escape from their own individual and/or marital problems. The fathers on their part could have reinforced this situation, since it allowed them to avoid direct interpersonal issues.

Perhaps, these two interpretations are interwoven into a never-ending vicious circle, which is known in the literature – be it in an overgeneralized stereotyped picture – as the strong, "pathological" relationship between the anorexic daughter and her mother, with the father being the absent outsider in this triangle. But again, this description is more a matter of interpretation than observation. As the case vignettes clearly illustrate, our impressions do not imply that parents of anorexics or bulimics always need marital therapy. What this study intends to emphasize is that all too often clinicians tend to assume a stereotyped attitude toward parents of eating disorder patients: either they are considered as antitherapeutic figures which must be excluded from the treatment process, or they are "disturbed" and need special therapy. Instead, we believe parents must be, first and foremost, approached in their *parental role* which has led them to ask for help in coping with their child's problem.

REFERENCES*

Anderson, C.W. (1981), Parent-child relationships: A context for reciprocal developmental influence. *The Counseling Psychologist,* 9(4):35-44.

Arrindell, W.A., Boelens, W. & Lambert, H. (1983a), On the psychometric properties of the Maudsley Marital Questionnaire (MMQ): Evaluation of self ratings in distressed and "normal" volunteer couples based on the Dutch version. *Personality and Individual Differences,* 4:293-306.

Arrindell, W.A., Emmelkamp, P.M.G. & Bast, S. (1983b), The Maudsley Marital Questionnaire (MMQ): A further step toward its validation. *Personality and Individual Differences,* 4:457-464.

Arrindell, W.A., Emmelkamp, P.M.G., Brilman, E. & Monsma, A. (1983c), Psychometric evaluation of an inventory for assessment of parental rearing practices. A Dutch form of the EMBU. *Acta Psychiatrica Scandinavica* 67:163-177.

Arrindell, W.A. & van den Ende, J. (1984), Replicability and invariance of dimensions of parental rearing behaviour: Further Dutch experiences with the EMBU. *Personality and Individual Differences,* 5:671-682.

Arrindell, W.A. & Ettema, J.H.M. (1986), *SCL-90: Handleiding bij een Multi-Dimensionele Psychopathologie-Indicator.* Swets & Zeitlinger, Lisse.

Belsky, J. & Vondra J. (1985), Characteristics, consequences and determinants of parenting. In: L.L'Abate (Ed.), *The Handbook of Family Psychology and Therapy.* Homewood (Ill.), Dorsey Press, pp. 523-556.

Bowlby, J. (1977), The making and breaking of affectional bonds. I. Aetiology and psychopathology in the light of attachment theory. *British Journal of Psychiatry,* 130:201-210.

Crowe, M.J. (1978), Conjoint marital therapy: A controlled study. *Psychological Medicine,* 8:623-636.

---

* This list contains only secondary literature, whereas the other references are mentioned in the final section of this book: "Bibliography on Family Aspects of Eating Disorders."

Derogatis, L.R. (1977), *SCL-90: Administration, Scoring and Procedures Manual (revised version)*. Baltimore: Johns Hopkins University School of Medicine, Clinical Psychometrics Research Unit.

Maccoby, E.E. & Martin, J.A. (1983), Socialization in the context of the family: Parent-child interaction. In: Mussen, P.H. (Ed.), *Handbook of Child Psychology. Vol. IV.* New York: John Wiley.

Parker, G. (1983), *Parental Overprotection. A Risk Factor in Psychosocial Development.* New York: Grune & Stratton.

Parker, G. (1984), The measurement of pathogenic parental style and its relevance to psychiatric disorder. *Social Psychiatry,* 19:75-81.

Parker, G., Tupling, H. & Brown, L.B. (1979), A parental bonding instrument. *British Journal of Medical Psychology,* 52:1-10.

Perris, C., Jacobsson, L., Lindstrom, H., von Knorring, L. & Perris, H. (1980), Development of a new inventory for assessing memories of parental rearing behavior. *Acta Psychiatrica Scandinavica,* 61:265-274.

Vandereycken, W. & Meermann, R. (1984), *Anorexia Nervosa. A Clinician's Guide to Treatment.* Berlin/New York: Walter de Gruyter.

APPENDIX

Parenting and Eating Disorders — Standardized Interview

Name: Educational level:
Age: Age at marriage:
Occupation: Years of marriage:
Date: Children (age):

Family of origin

- Residence with regard to own parents:
(1) living together, (2) in direct neighborhood, (3) nearby (same city), (4) at distance, (5) at great distance (more than 50 kms).

- Number of children in the family of origin (place of subject in birth order):

A. Questions about the eating disorder

1. Did your daughter had a special position, compared with the other children? And if yes, why?
2. When did you notice for the first time that she had eating problems?
3. Did you have special problems with the other children? If so, what kind of problems?
4. Whose initiative was it to consult a physician or another health care professional?
5. What kind of treatment did you consider as necessary?
6. How did you react to the eating/weight problem?
7. How did your partner react?
8. What attitude (and in which degree) did you/your partner assume? (1 = little or none; 2 = moderate; 3 = much) (a) patience, (b) support, (c) comprehension, (d) rage, (e) concern and worry, (f) authority (power, force), (g) helplessness, (h) pain and sorrow, (i) personal guilt-feelings, (j) threat with separation, (k) distrust and control.
9. What kind of influence (change) was caused by the eating disorder upon:
   (a) the interaction between you (and/or your spouse) and your children
   (b) the interaction between the children
   (c) the interaction between you and your spouse
   (d) the contact with your own (extended) family
   (e) the householding (shopping, cleaning...)
   (f) the use of leisure (friends, family visits, parties)
   (g) the eating habits at home

10. What are, in your opinion, the most important factors that caused the eating problems?
    (a) problems at school or work
    (b) conflicts between you and your spouse (marital problems)
    (c) conflicts between you (and/or your spouse) and your daughter
    (d) conflicts with siblings
    (e) puberty and associated physical changes
    (f) problems with a boy-friend
    (g) a discontentment about body weight and physical appearance
    (h) a medical reason (illness, operation)
    (i) another factor
11. To what extent do the following explanations of anorexia and bulimia apply to your daughter? (1 = not at all; 2 = maybe, to some extent; 3 = definitely)
    (a) Anorexia or bulimia is a physical illness, one is not responsible for.
    (b) It is purely psychological and a consequence of negative experiences in childhood.
    (c) It refers to a "lack of character" or a personality weakness.
    (d) It is something she has only herself to blame since she wanted to lose weight.
    (e) It is an obsession or an addiction, she is not able to control.
    (f) It is only a matter of fashion, following the culture of slenderness.
    (g) It means not being able to accept a feminine body shape.
    (h) It is a fear of adulthood, of growing up and taking responsibility.
    (i) It is a reaction upon tensions and problems within the family.
    (j) It is an expression of sexual problems (like fear for a sexual relationship).
    (k) It is a way of getting attention and care from others.
12. If you had the opportunity to do it all over again, would you act differently?
13. How can you as a parent help parenting that the eating disorder reoccurs in the future?
14. What could happen to your family or your marital relationship if no real solution or considerable improvement is to be expected?
15. Do you believe that a complete "recovery" is possible and why (not)?

B. Questions about child-rearing issues
1. What does child-rearing mean to you (in order of importance):
    (a) to teach knowledge and values of life
    (b) to be always ready to help the child, to take care of him/her
    (c) to feel intimately attached to the child
2. What is an "ideal" education in your opinion (following order of importance)?

(a)   letting the child become oneself by giving him/her enough freedom to learn and experience

(b)   giving a clear model to the child

(c)   considering the child as an equal person; it is giving and receiving help, love and affection

3.   To what extent do the following characteristics apply to the education you (and your partner) gave to the children? (1 = not at all; 2 = a little; 3 = moderately; 4 = much; 5 = completely)

(a)   regular absence of the parent(s)

(b)   insufficient contact with the children

(c)   being too indulgent

(d)   being too demanding

(e)   influence from others (family, neighbors, grandparents)

4.   Who takes the responsibility for rearing the children?

5.   Who is making the most important decisions about the education of the children?

6.   Who has the most contact with the children (before and after the eating problems emerged)?

7.   To whom is the patient the most attached? And the other children?

8.   Did you agree with your partner about child-rearing issues before and after the eating problems emerged?

9.   On what issues do you mostly agree/differ?

10.   Which of the following features apply to your own childhood (the education you got from your parents) and to what extent (see question B3)?

11.   Does the way you bring up your children differ from the rearing practice of your own parents? What are the differences/similarities?

C. Questions about the marital relationship

1.   Do you experience your marital relationship as satisfying? Did this change since the eating disorder of your daughter?

2.   Are there specific problems between you and your partner?

3.   Did you go through an episode of (before marriage and after marriage):

(a)   obesity

(b)   marked slimming

(c)   loss of appetite or disorders of digestion

(d)   alcohol or drug abuse

(e)   depression, nervous breakdown

(f)   fears, phobias, obsessions

(g)   confusion, being out of reality

(h)   symptoms of stress

4.   Did you notice specific problems in your family of origin?

5. Do you have contact with your own parents and your parents- in-law?
    (1 = none; 2 = little; 3 = moderate; 4 = enough; 5 = much; 6 =
    too much). Did this change due to the eating disorder of your child?

Chapter 8

The Perception of Interpersonal Relationships in Families of Anorexia Nervosa Patients Compared with Normals

M. Elisabeth Houben, Roland Pierloot and Walter Vandereycken*

A review of the extensive literature about anorexia nervosa shows the importance attached to family functioning as a "pathogenic" factor (see Chapter 2). It is widely believed that the basis of anorexia nervosa is a conflict between the girl and her family. In particular, the mother-daughter relationship is stated as being very important in the etiology. This relationship is often described as a peculiarly close one, the mother being very dominant, overprotective and not allowing her daughter freedom to develop. The father, on the other hand, is said to be weak, absent and living in the background of his family. In short, the family of the anorexic girl is usually conceived as one where the patient cannot cope with problems of adolescence: the family inhibits development of autonomy, personal growth, identity and sexual maturation.

In the light of these considerations a program was set up to investigate those characteristics of intrafamilial relationships, that reflect the presence or absence of a basic attitude that allows each family member to be oneself. Hence, our attention is focused on *subjective aspects of the relationships* within a family as the individuals perceive it.

Rogers (1966) described some aspects of the therapist's attitude and stated that they are necessary and sufficient conditions for personality change. These basic attitudes are considered to be not only an agent of therapeutic change, but also to be present in every constructive interpersonal relationship (e.g., marital or parent-child relationship). They are considered basic conditions that provide the individual the opportunity of personal growth and autonomy. We intended to investigate to what extent those relationship variables — as defined

* We wish to thank Prof. Dr. G. Lietaer (Department of Clinical Psychology, University of Leuven) for his valuable help.

Table 1. Composition of the groups.

	Anorexics	Normals
DAUGHTERS		
Daughters only	20	---
Together with parent(s)	23	18
MOTHERS		
Participation	22	18
No participation	1	---
FATHERS		
Participation	18	18
No participation	5	---

Table 2. General characteristics of the groups.

	Anorexics (N=43)	Normals (N=18)
AGE (years)		
Daughter	19.6 + 3.3	19.5 + 2.8
Mother	48.0 + 7.6	48.1 + 4.5
Father	50.3 + 8.6	50.3 + 4.6
SOCIAL CLASS* (%)		
Higher	41.9	22.2
Middle	34.9	33.3
Lower	23.2	33.3
Unknown	-	11.2
DAUGHTER'S EDUCATION (%)		
Higher	25.6	72.2
Secondary	72.1	27.8
Primary	2.3	-

*The social class was defined by father's social status according to the classification system of Nuttin (1956), which is based on the occupational level.

by client-centered therapy—are present or absent within the relationships between anorexic girls and their parents, as compared with normal girls.

SUBJECTS

The experimental group consisted of 43 female patients hospitalized at the University Psychiatric Center St. Jozef in Kortenberg, Belgium. All patients met the diagnostic criteria for anorexia nervosa according to Feighner et al. (1972). In a preliminary phase of the project, only the daughters were investigated (20 cases) whereas later on we also included the parents. In 6 cases only one parent could be contacted: the other parent was either deceased or refused to cooperate (see Table 1).

The control group consisted of 18 "normal" girls (mostly college students) and their parents who volunteered for participation in the study. The following selection criteria were used: (1) the girl and her parents must be functioning normally socially, i.e., studying or working regularly; (2) neither the parents nor any of their children have undergone psychiatric treatment; (3) the girl involved in the investigation has not been ill nor has she lost weight during the last year. Compared with the experimental group, there is one basic difference: the relationship between the girl and her parents has not been interrupted by hospitalization. With regard to the selection of the control group, the factors of age, social status and educational level have been matched, as much as possible, to the anorexia nervosa group (see Table 2).

METHOD

Client-centered therapists developed instruments that provide measures about constructive interpersonal basic attitude variables. We presented one of them to our subjects, namely a form of Barrett-Lennard's (1962) "Relationship Inventory" (RI), in a Dutch version revised by Lietaer (1974). On the basis of factor analysis it distinguishes five subscales or relationship-variables: *empathy* (E) is the extent to which one person recognizes the immediate awareness of the other and understands his or her emotions and feelings; *transparency* (T) means the degree to which one is willing to be known as a person by another, according to the other's desire for this; *directivity* (D) refers to an authoritarian attitude toward the other and involves such aspects as overprotection and intrusion; *positive regard* (P) concerns the feelings of respect, sympathy, liking and appreciation; negative feelings include e.g., impatience and lack of trust; *unconditionality* (U) means a constancy of regard felt by one person for another. Each subscale consists of 10 items. The subjects can indicate on a 6-point scale how appropriate each statement is as a description of their relationships. The total scores for each variable may thus vary from 10 to 60.

There are two forms of the Relationship Inventory: (1) the *Perception-form* or the way one perceives that the other is feeling or behaving toward oneself (P-form), and (2) the *Self-form*, or the way one feels toward the other (S-form).

Concerning the quality of the relationship between mothers, fathers and their daughters, measures were gathered about the five mentioned variables in both forms of the RI and from the viewpoints of each of the three family members:

   • Daughter: P-form = mother toward me, father toward me;

     S-form = as I feel toward mother/father;

● Mother: P-form = daughter toward me, husband toward me;
  S-form = as I feel toward daughter/husband;
● Father: P-form = daughter toward me, wife toward me;
  S-form = as I feel toward daughter/wife.

It is important to note that all the subjects involved in the study were asked to describe the quality of their "actual usual" relationships, i.e., their relationships as experienced during the last year. It was conceived that in the case of families with an "ill" child the perception of earlier relationships would be contaminated by the psychological and interpersonal difficulties they were now involved in. We wanted to avoid the possibility that they would idealize the interpersonal relationships before the period of "illness" of the girl.

Regarding the statistical analysis of the data, we carried out two-tailed Mann-Whitney U-tests (determined by computing the z-value when $N > 25$), two-tailed Willcoxon matched-pairs signed-ranks tests (determined by computing the z-value when $N > 25$) and Spearman rank-correlation coefficients (one-tailed significance; determined by computing the t-value when $N > 30$).

HYPOTHESES

Considering the previously mentioned clinical descriptions of the anorexic family, we first expected that results on the RI within the anorexic group would differ from the normal control group. Furthermore, the relationship of the anorexic girl and her mother is said to be a very close and intimate one. We thus expected that, compared with normal families, the anorexic girls would describe a higher degree of empathy and transparency in their own attitudes (S-form of RI) toward their mother, and perceive to a higher degree both of these characteristics in their mother's attitude (P-form of RI).

The anorexic's mother is often described as excessively controlling of her child's life. Therefore we presumed that the others' descriptions of their own attitudes (S-form of RI) toward their anorexic daughter would be more loaded on the directivity variable than within the control group.

Since fathers are described as interacting with their families in an unemotional way and as being aloof, we expected that, compared with normal controls, fathers of anorexics would obtain a lower score on the transparency variable when describing their own attitude toward their family members (S-form of RI) and will be perceived as such by both their daughter and wife (P-form of RI).

Finally, it would be interesting to verify not only if each of the interpersonal relationships indeed shows differences between both groups as just stated, but also if they are felt as being differentiated from each other. For example, does the daughter have different feelings toward her mother, compared with those toward her father? It concerns the *differentiation felt in the relationships*. A first but more general question has therefore to be answered: do the members of the family triad have a tendency to describe in common certain features of the relationship among the family members? If so, this similarity in descriptions may reflect either a basic attitude in their emotional (close) relationships, or a kind of rigidity in their response patterns (e.g., due to the procedure of being confronted with the rather numerous repetitive items of the RI). Further, we would like to address the following questions: do anorexic girls perceive their mother's relationship with them as different from their fathers? If so, is this differentiation felt in their relationships more or less pronounced than the differentiation felt by normal girls? In other words: does a member of the anorexic family (e.g., the daughter) perceive the relationships with the other family members (e.g., mother and father) as significantly more different from each other, than do of normal controls who might show a similar differentiation but to a lesser degree.

RESULTS

Before describing our results, we would like to note that a statistical comparison showed that the mean scores obtained on the RI by the normal control youngsters correspond almost completely with the normative data obtained in a student population (Lietaer, 1974). This makes our control girls a quite representative group.

In addition, the subjects show a marked similarity in their descriptions of certain common features in their relations with other family members. Two thirds of the correlation coefficients between the scores concerning the relations with both other family members are significant (see Tables 3 to 8). This tendency is found as much in the experimental as it is in the control group. Notwithstanding this tendency of similarity in the descriptions, several significant differences are found between the descriptions of both family relationships. It may suggest that they are all the more relevant.

Finally, a few more words about the statistical procedure concerning the aspect of felt difference (which we call "differentiation") between the relationships: in order to know if family members of one group are showing more differentiation than the other group, the differences (d) between those scores obtained by one person for each group (e.g., differences in the anorexic's perception of empathy from mother and from father) and then compared, using the Mann-Whitney U-test, with the other group (e.g., with the differences in the normal girl's perception of empathy from mother and from father).

Perceived Relationships

The daughter's perception of her parents' relationships with her (Table 3).
It is apparent that, as far as the father's relationship is concerned, no differences are found between anorexics and normal girls. We may observe a slight

Table 3. Daughter's perception of both parents' relationship with her

(A) Variable (P-form)	FATHER Anorexics (N=38)	Normals (N=18)	p*	MOTHER Anorexics (N=42)	Normals (N=18)	p*
E	38.4 + 13.4	35.9 + 11.4	NS	43.3 + 11.3	38.1 + 9.1	.05
T	40.4 + 10.4	39.9 + 8.05	NS	43.3 + 10.3	42.4 + 7.1	NS
D	38.1 + 8.9	34.1 + 7.6	NS	37.4 + 8.7	37.2 + 6.5	NS
P	48.2 + 10.4	49.2 + 7.1	NS	50.7 + 7.5	48.8 + 6.9	NS
U	39.6 + 9.2	39.7 + 9.5	NS	39.9 + 9.1	37.5 + 6.9	NS

(B)	CORRELATION** between perceived relations		(C) DIFFERENTIATION* between perceived relations (d)
E	.01	NS	NS
T	.01	.05	NS
D	.01	.05	NS
P	.01	NS	NS
U	.01	NS	.05

*Mann-Whitney U-test (two-tailed)
**Spearman Rank Correlation Coefficient (one-tailed)
 E=Empathy, T=Transparency, D=Directivity, P=Positive regard, U=Unconditionality

tendency to experience fathers as showing more directivity in the group of anorexics (Mann-Whitney U-test significant at .10 level). Mothers, on the other hand, are experienced as more empathetic and understanding by the anorexics than by the normal group. No further differences are found between these groups. The results suggest a closer and more open attitude in terms of a desire to share experiences in the case of anorexics' mothers, as perceived by their daughters. In short, the anorexic and normal daughters' experiences of their parents' relationships with them are much alike (Table 3A). Anorexic girls show a tendency to give similar descriptions of their fathers' and mothers' relationships with them on all relationship variables (correlation coefficients: Table 3B). Such a pronounced similarity in response pattern was not found in the experimental group. As compared with the anorexics, the normal girls show a bit more pronounced differentiation in the way they perceive both parents (Table 3C). They feel a significant difference between their parents' attitudes toward them with respect to the variable "unconditionality" (they experience, to a greater extent than anorexics, more unconditionality from their father than from their mother).

*The mother's perception of the relationship of her daughter
and her husband with her (Table 4).*

There is high agreement between the anorexic and normal group regarding the mothers' perceptions of their daughters' relationships with them. But, compared with normals, mothers of anorexics perceive their husband as being significantly less transparent (Table 4A). Regarding a possibly similar tendency in the descriptions of both relationships, mothers of anorexic girls apparently do not show a similar basic attitude of rigidity in the perception of their daughter's

Table 4. Mother's perception of daughter's and husband's relationship with her.

(A) Variable (P-form)	DAUGHTER Anorexics (N=18)	Normals (N=18)	p*	HUSBAND Anorexics (N=16)	Normals (N=18)	p*
E	38.4 + 13.1	40.8 + 7.9	NS	43.4 + 8.5	45.5 + 7.5	NS
T	40.1 + 9.7	41.7 + 8.7	NS	37.6 + 9.6	45.7 + 7.9	.05
D	34.4 + 8.5	33.6 + 5.9	NS	37.6 + 7.2	35.8 + 5.3	NS
P	46.4 + 12.3	48.3 + 8.7	NS	46.4 + 9.0	50.9 + 9.2	NS
U	38.9 + 10.8	38.9 + 6.7	NS	40.7 + 9.9	40.4 + 7.4	NS

(B)	CORRELATION** between perceived relations		(C)	DIFFERENTIATION* between perceived relations (d)
E	NS	.05		NS
T	NS	.05		NS
D	.05	NS		NS
P	NS	.01		NS
U	.01	.01		NS

*Mann-Whitney U-test (two-tailed)
**Spearman Rank Correlation Coefficient (one-tailed)
 E=Empathy, T=Transparency, D=Directivity, P=Positive regard, U=Unconditionality

and husband's relationship with them (Table 4B). We found rather a fluctuating pattern: at one point there would be a common basic attitude in the experience, and at another point there would be a different one. Mothers of normal girls, however, generally describe more similarity in their feelings about the attitudes of their daughters and husbands. Notwithstanding this difference, one cannot say that the differentiated feelings the anorexics' mothers show are significantly different from the control mothers (Table 4C).

Table 5. Father's perception of daughter's and wife's relationship with him.

(A) Variable (P-form)	DAUGHTER Anorexics (N=15)	Normals (N=18)	p*	WIFE Anorexics (N=12)	Normals (N=18)	p*
E	37.3 + 6.5	38.6 + 6.8	NS	39.9 + 4.4	46.6 + 5.7	.002
T	39.1 + 8.7	38.3 + 6.5	NS	43.7 + 8.0	46.4 + 6.5	NS
D	37.1 + 7.6	31.6 + 6.2	.05	39.0 + 4.7	37.6 + 7.2	NS
P	46.1 + 9.9	47.6 + 8.0	NS	47.5 + 8.1	51.3 + 8.0	NS
U	39.3 + 7.2	36.9 + 5.3	NS	37.0 + 5.6	41.8 + 7.9	NS

(B)	CORRELATION** between perceived relations		(C)	DIFFERENTIATION* between perceived relations (d)
E	NS	.05		NS
T	NS	.05		NS
D	.01	.01		NS
P	.05	.01		NS
U	.01	NS		.02

*Mann-Whitney U-test (two-tailed)
**Spearman Rank Correlation Coefficient (one-tailed)
 E=Empathy, T=Transparency, D=Directivity, P=Positive regard, U=Unconditionality

Table 6. Daughter's own attitude towards her father and mother.

(A) Variable (S-form)	FATHER Anorexics (N=39)	Normals (N=18)	p*	MOTHER Anorexics (N=42)	Normals (N=18)	p*
E	40.1 ± 8.1	38.4 ± 6.4	NS	43.0 ± 6.8	40.3 ± 6.1	NS
T	39.3 ± 11.8	39.0 ± 7.6	NS	43.7 ± 10.0	42.0 ± 8.3	NS
D	32.3 ± 9.3	29.5 ± 4.2	NS	33.7 ± 9.0	32.9 ± 5.3	NS
P	49.1 ± 9.6	48.4 ± 8.0	NS	50.6 ± 7.9	47.9 ± 5.9	NS
U	40.8 ± 10.0	40.1 ± 7.1	NS	40.9 ± 9.9	37.1 ± 7.0	NS

(B)	CORRELATION** between perceived relations		(C)	DIFFERENTIATION* between perceived relations (d)
E	.01	.01		NS
T	.01	.01		NS
D	.01	NS		NS
P	.01	NS		NS
U	.01	.05		NS

*Mann-Whitney U-test (two-tailed)
**Spearman Rank Correlation Coefficient (one-tailed)
E=Empathy, T=Transparency, D=Directivity, P=Positive regard, U=Unconditionality

The father's perception of the relationship of his daughter and his wife with him (Table 5).

Fathers of anorexics (Table 5A) feel a more directive, authoritarian or intrusive attitude within their daughter's relations with them, compared with the normal groups from which they do not differ on the other dimensions. When looking at their wife's relationship to them, anorexics' fathers perceive their spouse as significantly less empathic than within the normal group. No differences were found on the other dimensions. They show nearly as many significant correlation coefficients between the perceived dimensions in both relationships do as fathers of normal girls (Table 5B). We note here a significance in the differentiation between the relationships that we did not observe in the group of mothers. There is a clear trend within the father of the normal control group to experience "unconditionality" from their wives rather than from their daughters (Table 5C).

Own Attitudes

The daughter's attitude toward her parents (Table 6).

The anorexic daughters show no differences on any of the five dimensions of their own relationships toward their parents when compared with normal girls (Table 6A). As in the P-form of the RI, here too the anorexic girls show a significant correlation, on all dimensions, between their own relationships with their parents, whereas this tendency of similarity fluctuates is more within the normal group (Table 6B). Regarding the differentiation, no significant differences concerning this aspect of the experienced attitudes are observed between both groups (Table 6C).

Table 7. Mother's own attitudes towards her daughter and husband.

(A) Variable (S-form)	DAUGHTER			HUSBAND		
	Anorexics (N=22)	Normals (N=18)	p*	Anorexics (N=20)	Normals (N=18)	p*
E	45.4 ± 9.7	44.6 ± 6.4	NS	42.7 ± 9.0	44.6 ± 6.0	NS
T	42.6 ± 9.3	43.6 ± 6.9	NS	40.5 ± 9.0	43.2 ± 8.9	NS
D	40.7 ± 8.7	36.3 ± 5.4	.05	37.7 ± 9.9	34.9 ± 5.6	NS
P	50.1 ± 6.3	52.0 ± 5.5	NS	47.3 ± 8.0	52.7 ± 7.6	NS
U	43.0 ± 11.6	40.1 ± 8.9	NS	37.9 ± 9.9	40.8 ± 8.4	NS

(B)	CORRELATION** between perceived relations		(C) DIFFERENTIATION* between perceived relations (d)
E	.01	.05	NS
T	NS	.01	NS
D	.05	.05	NS
P	.05	.05	NS
U	.01	.01	NS

*Mann-Whitney U-test (two-tailed)
**Spearman Rank Correlation Coefficient (one-tailed)
 E=Empathy, T=Transparency, D=Directivity, P=Positive regard, U=Unconditionality

The mother's attitude toward her daughter and her husband (Table 7).

The mothers' attitudes toward their daughters are quite similar in both groups. The one noteworthy difference is that mothers of anorexics describe themselves as more "directive" in the relationship with their daughters. The attitude toward their husband does not differ between the anorexic and the normal control group (Table 7A). We may mention a slight tendency in anorexics' mothers to show less "positive" feelings toward their husband than mothers in the control group (Mann-Whitney U-test significant at .10 level). The mothers of both the anorexic and normal groups show a highly similar tendency in the description of their attitudes toward both husband and daughter (Table 7B).

Table 8. Father's own attitudes towards his daughter and wife

(A) Variable (S-form)	DAUGHTER			WIFE		
	Anorexics (N=18)	Normals (N=18)	p*	Anorexics (N=15)	Normals (N=18)	p*
E	42.7 ± 5.3	42.9 ± 5.1	NS	43.5 ± 6.2	45.1 ± 6.2	NS
T	43.6 ± 6.9	40.9 ± 7.1	NS	42.2 ± 9.5	45.9 ± 8.0	NS
D	38.7 ± 5.3	36.7 ± 8.5	NS	39.1 ± 5.4	36.1 ± 7.4	NS
P	49.4 ± 7.3	49.9 ± 5.6	NS	47.5 ± 8.7	52.6 ± 6.3	.05
U	44.4 ± 9.1	42.7 ± 6.1	NS	44.7 ± 7.2	45.2 ± 6.9	NS

(B)	CORRELATION** between perceived relations		(C) DIFFERENTIATION* between perceived relations (d)
E	NS	NS	NS
T	.01	.01	.05
D	NS	.01	NS
P	.05	NS	.05
U	.05	NS	NS

*Mann-Whitney U-test two-tailed)
**Spearman Rank Correlation Coefficient (one-tailed)
 E=Empathy, T=Transparency, D=Directivity, P=Positive regard, U=Unconditionality

The felt differentiation between their feelings toward their husband and daughter does not show any difference at all between the two groups (Table 7C).

The father's attitude toward his daughter and his wife (Table 8).

Fathers in the anorexic group do not differ from the normal group with regard to their attitude toward their daughter. An equivalent observation is obvious concerning the marital relationship, except for the same variable as mentioned in the case of their wife's attitude toward them, namely "positive regard," which is lower in the anorexic group than in the normal controls (Table 8A). In both groups, fathers show a significant correlation, on several dimensions, between their attitudes toward their wives and daughters (Table 8B). Concerning the differentiation, fathers in the normal group do acknowledge rather different feelings toward their daughter as compared with their attitudes toward their wife: in contrast to the anorexic group, they show more "transparency" and "positive regard" toward their partner than toward their daughter. At the same time it means that fathers of anorexics do not show as much differentiation in feelings (Table 8C).

DISCUSSION

When both groups of findings are reviewed together, we see first each family member's perceptions of how the others feel or behave toward her/him (P-form of RI) and, second, the perception of his/her own attitude when relating with both of the other persons (S-form of RI). The results appear to support a few of our hypotheses, but give little evidence for the other ones.

Maybe the most striking conclusion of our investigation is that relationship variables that are experienced by anorexic family members as compared with those of normal families show far more similarity than expected. When between-group comparisons are made with regard to the emotional qualities as measured by the five variables, the anorexic girls and their parents relate to each other in a way which is more in line with normal families than was hypothetically expected (only 6 out of the 60 Mann-Whitney U-test values are significant).

A more detailed analysis of the significant differences between RI results supports the clinical observations that the *relationship between the anorexic girl and her mother* is indeed a very close one. As expected, anorexic girls view their mothers as more understanding of their (the daughter's) emotions and feelings, or as more able to discriminate and sense what is going on within them, than in the normal girls' experience. But, they do not perceive their mothers as more willing to be known by them (the daughters) than do normal girls. Inspecting the mother's description of her own attitude toward her daughter, we see that she does not describe herself as more understanding than do mothers of the normal control group. We found, however, a more pronounced directive atti-

tude toward their daughters. Even if we hypothesize that the mothers of anorexia nervosa patients relate in a more authoritarian or directive way as a reaction to their daughter's pathology, it still remains noteworthy that anorexic girls,
in comparison with normals, do not perceive more directivity in the attitude of
their mothers who, on the contrary, describes herself as responding so. Maybe
because of the crisis period she is in, the anorexic girl experiences her mother
as concerned instead of authoritarian or intrusive.

The results concerning the *father-figure* are quite interesting. The anorexic
girls perceive him in a way similar to the way normal girls do. But they describe
him as showing not as much "empathy" and "transparency" or openness in his
attitudes as they experience from their mother, while normal girls do not show
this difference (AN: Willcoxon test is significant at .01 level for empathy and .05
for transparency). Compared with the normal group, the anorexic's mother perceives her husband as being not so transparent or open toward her, and he perceives her as not so empathically understanding toward him.

All these results seem to suggest that fathers of anorexic girls relate to others
with a lack of emotions, or at least without showing it. This may be the reason
their wives complain of a lack of openness. It seems to support clinical descriptions of the anorexics' fathers as rather "cool" persons: they do not show their
affection to others, or they have difficulties in expressing their feelings. This may
explain why they view their daughter as being directive and intrusive: her rather
normal demands to him might be felt as too emotional and therefore too intrusive.

Another rather unexpected observation is the *similar tendency* in the *anorexics' descriptions of the parental-relationship dimensions* (anorexic girls are the
only subgroup where all the correlation coefficients are significant). As stated
before, this could reflect a rigidity in their response pattern or a common basic
attitude in their emotional relationships. However, that much similarity was not
found in the other family members (except for normal mothers), nor within the
group of normal girls. It may imply that the anorexic daughters, because they
are hospitalized and thus separated from their parents, are giving answers more
in line with a common basic attitude toward their parents than normal girls do.
Or, it might indeed reflect an existing rigidity in their overall feelings within their
parental relationships. From an individual intrapsychic and psychodynamic
point of view it could suggest that they do not show a differentiation in their
feelings to the same extent as normal girls do and thus as normally would be expected. It does not imply, however, that the anorexic daughter does not feel any
differentiation at all in her relationships with her parents. As a group they show
more transparency toward mother than toward father and they experience their
mother as more empathically understanding and open toward them in comparison with their father.

Comparing the *differentiation* in relationship variables between both groups,
a striking and unexpected result concerns the *marital relationships of anorexics'*

parents. In the control group, fathers show significantly more transparency and positive feelings of sympathy and appreciation toward their wives than toward their daughters, and they perceive more unconditionality in their wives' relations to them than in their daughter. These kinds of differentiation are significantly more pronounced in fathers of the normal group than in anorexics' families where such a differentiation is far less obvious. This may be seen as a lack of intrafamilial boundaries. In other words, it may reflect an emotional "enmeshment" which, according to Minuchin et al. (1978), is a typical characteristic of the psychosomatic family structure especially observed in anorexia nervosa patients (see Chapter 2).

A final remark concerns the question of comparability of our study. Therefore, we note some of its restrictions. We studied only the family triad: father-mother-daughter. This does not mean that the influence of other family members (e.g., grandparents, siblings) would not be important. We had to restrict ourselves to this classic triad because of methodological reasons: in view of (1) the instrument we used, and (2) the comparability of the groups studied. With regard to the latter factor, the composition of the families was too variable to include, for instance, other siblings. Moreover, the problem of group matching (for example as to age) would be practically impossible to resolve unless there is a very large sample selected. The other restriction concerns the instrument we used. Barrett-Lennard's (1962) "Relationship Inventory" (RI) is well-known in psychotherapy process research. Originally designed for measuring personal dimensions of therapist response in individual psychotherapy, this questionnaire has undergone several revisions and has also been adapted for a variety of relationships, e.g., family interactions and friendship relations (Barrett-Lennard, 1978; Lietaer, 1974). It is, however, best kown as one of the major instruments used in assessing the patient's perception of the therapeutic relationship (Gurman, 1977). Therefore, through the use of RI our study can in part be considered as an assessment of the family relationships as experienced by the family members themselves, i.e., the *subjective insiders' perception of family interaction.* Moreover, the instrument we used (RI) focuses on those experiential dimensions of intrafamilial relationships which are supposed to be of special importance for the development of autonomy and self-esteem in adolescents.

Another important restriction of this study could be that the subjects, when asked to fill in a questionnaire (such as the RI), give a socially desirable picture of themselves and their relationships, whereas their actual behavior might be quite different. This stresses the importance of carrying out family research from various viewpoints (see Chapter 5), i.e., including the insiders' perception (the subjective way family members feel and think about their family) as well as an outsiders' observation (the "objective" assessment of family functioning).

We deliberately avoided the question of causality, because there is no substantial research evidence in support of any particular theory regarding family issues in the pathogenesis of anorexia nervosa (see Chapter 3). Anorexia nervosa is a multidetermined syndrome and as such only a multidimensional approach, both in research and treatment, seems appropriate. The intention of our study has been to elucidate just one aspect of the interactional dimension of the disorder.

REFERENCES

Barrett-Lennard, G.T. (1962), Dimensions of therapist response as causal factor in therapeutic change. *Psychological Monographs, 76* (whole no. 43).

Barrett-Lennard, G.T. (1978), The Relationship Inventory: Later developments and adaptations. *JSAS Catalog of Selected Documents in Psychology,* 8.

Feighner, J.P., Robins, E., Guze, S.B., Woodruff, W.A., Winokur, G. & Munoz, R. (1972), Diagnostic criteria for use in psychiatric research. *Archives of General Psychiatry,* 26:57-63.

Gurman, A.S. (1977), The patient's perception of the therapeutic relationship. In: Gurman, A.S. & Razin, A.M. (Eds.), *Effective Psychotherapy.* New York, Oxford: Pergamon Press, pp. 503-543.

Lietaer, G. (1974), Nederlandstalige versie van Barrett-Lennard's Relationship Inventory: Een faktoranalytische benadering van de student-ouder-relatie (Dutch version of Barrett-Lennard's Relationship Inventory: A factor analytic approach of the student-parent relation). *Nederlands Tijdschrift voor Psychologie,* 29:191-212.

Nuttin, J. (1956), De verstandelijke begaafdheid van de jeugd in de verschillende sociale klassen en woonplaatsen (The intelligence of youngsters in different social classes and geographic areas). *Mededelingen van de Koninklijke Vlaamse Academie voor Wetenschappen, Letteren en Schone Kunsten van Belgie* (Klasse der Letteren), 7:25-27.

Rogers, C.R. (1966), Client-centered therapy. In: Arieti, S. (Ed.), *American Handbook of Psychiatry, Volume III.* New York: Basic Books, pp. 183-200.

Chapter 9

The Influence of a Family-Oriented Inpatient Treatment on Individual and Familial Factors in Eating Disorders: An Outcome Study

Johan Vanderlinden and Walter Vandereycken

INTRODUCTION

It is quite astonishing, in view of the ever increasing popularity of family therapeutic approaches in eating disorders, that research on the effectiveness of family therapy in anorexia nervosa or bulimia is almost completely lacking. Nowadays family therapy in eating disorders is recommended by a growing number of clinicians. Some even claim that it must be considered as the treatment of choice for young anorexics living at home (Garfinkel & Garner, 1982; Vandereycken & Meermann, 1984).

Apart from the famous study by Minuchin and co-workers (1978), who reported more than 80% of successful outcome results, we have not been able to find other published investigations. Although we do not want to minimize the importance of Minuchin's study, some critical remarks must be mentioned: their sample consisted of fairly young anorexics (average age of 14 years) with a short duration of illness (average of 6 months), living at home in intact families who were willing to come to therapy. None of these characteristics apply to the clinical population we are faced with.

Research on the effectiveness of family therapy is spare. One possible explanation for this phenomenon is the exceptional dedication and commitment needed from all team members to constantly motivate the families to collaborate in the research procedure. Moreover, research on family functioning is difficult when practical and reliable investigation instruments are still lacking.

The purpose of our study was to assess family functioning in eating disorder patients at the beginning of inpatient treatment, after six months and after one year. Besides the assessment of the family functioning, we were also interested in the evolution and changes in individual symptomatic and psychosocial adjustment of the eating disorder patient. Finally, though we hoped to find some guidelines for the choice of treatment type (e.g., family therapy or not), the present investigation was not aimed at measuring differential effects of family therapy. Such a goal would require a totally different and more complex research design (see Szmukler, 1983).

RESEARCH PROCEDURE

Our investigation consists of a prospective study of 24 families with an eating disorder patient who was hospitalized in our special treatment unit (see Vandereycken, 1985). Data were gathered at admission, after six months and after one year. The patient and her family were invited each time to engage in a clinical interview and to fill in some self-report questionnaires.

Twenty-four families consented to our study: 15 families with a restricting anorexic, 4 families with a bulimic anorexic, 2 families with a normal-weight bulimic and 3 families with an atypical eating disorder patient. Because we were interested in the functioning of patients within their family of origin, married patients were excluded from the study. The age of our patients averaged 19 years with a mean duration of illness of 22 months. In addition to the eating disorder symptoms, many patients (42%) showed overt psychopathological characteristics such as obsessive-compulsive behavior, impulse-control disorders, and borderline personality. All patients were treated before, most commonly having received individual outpatient therapy (67%), whereas 21% had received family therapy. All patients were admitted in our specialized inpatient treatment program (see Vandereycken, 1985), which can be defined as a multidimensional, pragmatic and eclectic approach integrating interactional (structural, strategic) and behavioral elements (including group- and family-oriented therapeutic strategies). The average duration of hospitalization of our sample was about 18 weeks.

The patients were asked to fill in the *Eating Disorder Inventory* or EDI (Garner et al., 1983) which assesses typical behavioral and attitudinal dimensions of anorexia nervosa and bulimia. For each patient the therapist judged the severity of symptoms and psychosocial dysfunctioning by means of the *Eating Disorder Evaluation Scale* or EDES (Vandereycken, 1987) which yields a global clinical score: the lower the score, the more serious the disorder (> 80 normal range, 65-80 partially dysfunctioning, 50-65 moderately disturbed, 35-50 seriously disturbed, < 35 extremely disturbed). Finally, our investigation focused on the triadic relationship between father, mother and identified patient. Each of them had to complete the *Leuven Family Questionnaire* (Kog et al., 1985) measuring conflict, cohesion and disorganization within the family.

Table 1. General psychosocial functioning (N = 24)

	At admission	After six months	After one year
Weight (% of ideal weight)	76	91	92
Regular menses (%)	0	4	30
Eating behavior (%)			
– food faddishness	100	37	48
– vomiting	21	8	17
– bulimia	17	12	17
– purging	33	0	4
Mean global clinical score *	34	49	56
Satisfying sexual contacts (%)	4	22	39
Being engaged (%)	4	17	33
Living together with parents (%)	92	83	62
Satisfying contact with peers (%)	17	49	74
Follow-up judgement (%)			
– recovered	–	0	13
– much improved	–	62	48
– slightly improved	–	30	35
– unchanged	–	8	4
– worsened	–	0	0

*Eating Disorder Evaluation Scale (see Table 2)

We've made several subgroup comparisons based on clinical features (restricting anorexics, bulimic anorexics, normal-weight bulimics and atypical eating disorder patients), duration of illness (less or more than 2 years), age (less or more than 18 years), and application of separate family therapy sessions during inpatient treatment (yes or no).

With regard to the perception of family interactions we compared the results of our sample with the average scores of a group of 220 normal families.

RESULTS

Several family members did not complete the self-report questionnaires after six months or one year. This "dropping-out" (missing data) has been taken into account in the statistical analysis of our findings (means, standard deviations and t-tests). For practical reasons, we limit ourselves to the description of those findings that have practical implications for the clinician, and those that focus on the perception of family functioning.

General Functioning

Table 1 summarizes the results of the clinical data. An interesting finding is the almost similar evolution, after one year, of the variables of menstruation, sexual contact and being engaged. Likewise we see that about 30% of our patients are launching, or changing their residences away from their family of origin. Hence, we suppose that return of menstruation is not only caused by

Table 2. Eating Disorder Evaluation Scale* in three subgroups (average score).

	Restricting Anorexics (N=15)	Bulimic Anorexics (N=4)	Atypical Eating disorder (N=3)
At admission	37.5 + 7.2	25.0 + 5.3	28.7 + 9.0
After six months	56.5 + 7.3	47.5 + 9.7	45.3 + 20.1
After one year	66.5 + 11.4	51.5 + 21.4	54.0 + 22.5

*
A global clinical judgement of both symptomatic and psychosocial functioning. The lower the score the more severe the dysfunctioning : > 80 normal range, 65-80 partially dysfunctioning, 50-65 moderately disturbed, 35-50 seriously disturbed, < 35 extremely disturbed (Vandereycken, 1986).

weight restoration and concomitant normalization of certain hormones patterns, but that all the aforementioned psychosocial variables are influencing each other mutually.

The follow-up results of the eating behavior show an obvious decrease of the symptoms after six months, but after one year we notice a rise for all eating behaviors. Bulimia seems to be a particularly therapy-resistant behavior and represents a serious challenge to our actual treatment potential when generalization to the outside world is targeted. On the other hand, it is our experience that some restricting anorexia nervosa patients may evolve toward bulimic patterns after treatment. The general psychological condition, a judgment based on an interview with the patient, seems to improve remarkably, as reflected by the global clinical score (EDES). About two thirds of all patients (61%) can be considered as "recovered" or at least "much improved" after one year. Recovered (13%) means that the patient is doing well not only symptomatically, but also with regard to intimate relationships, work or study, and that she has obtained a stable autonomy regarding her family. Forty-eight percent have made a strong improvement after one year, but some problems still necessitate psychotherapeutic guidance (once or twice a month). None of our patients worsened during out treatment.

When analyzing the global clinical scores of the symptomatic subgroups — the normal-weight bulimic patients are omitted, because of their small number — (see Table 2), several significant differences emerge (t-tests have only been carried out in the restricting anorexics because of the small number of patients in the other subgroups).

The restricting anorexic patients have the highest (= most normal) clinical score at admission and also after one year (a significant improvement: $p = .000$). The atypical eating disorder patients and the bulimic anorexics present a significantly longer duration of illness (respectively, 3.7 and 2.9 years), when compared with the restricting anorexics (1.7 years), and a lower (= more severe) clinical score at admission and after one year.

Table 3. Eating Disorder Inventory (average scores)*

Subscales	At admission	After six months	After one year	t-test[b] p
Drive for thinness	10.1 + 6.7	5.5 + 6.9	3.2 + 5.8	***
Bulimia	2.1 + 4.0	1.4 + 2.4	0.9 + 2.4	NS
Body dissatisfaction	9.7 + 7.8	5.6 + 7.1	4.2 + 6.3	***
Ineffectiveness	10.3 + 7.0	5.8 + 5.0	5.7 + 7.0	**
Perfectionism	0.2 + 3.9	4.8 + 3.6	4.5 + 3.1	NS
Interpersonal distrust	8.0 + 5.4	4.5 + 5.8	3.0 + 4.2	***
Interoceptive awareness	8.9 + 7.9	5.6 + 7.7	3.1 + 5.6	***
Maturity fears	6.7 + 5.5	3.2 + 3.8	2.7 + 4.6	**

[a]Only 16 patients completed the questionnaire at the three moments of assessment.
[b]* = p <.05, ** = p <.01, *** = p <.001, NS = non significant.

In summary, we can conclude that, generally speaking, our multidimensional family-oriented inpatient treatment results in a considerable improvement, both with regard to general psychosocial and symptomatic variables, in two thirds of our patients after one year. Prognosis seems to be worse in patients with a longer duration of illness and a more severe symptomatology (bulimia, vomiting, laxative abuse).

Behavioral and Attitudinal Characteristics

Table 3 summarizes the results on the *Eating Disorder Inventory* (EDI). Sixteen patients completed this self-report questionnaire at the three assessment points (at admission, after six months of after one year).

Our patients judge themselves as improving significantly on 6 of 8 variables of the EDI: they evolve toward the normal range after six months and even more obviously after one year. When analyzing the results reported by the several subgroups, we found that the longer the duration of illness and/or the more complex or severe the eating disorder (bulimia, vomiting, abuse of laxatives), the more the patients appear to deny or to minimize problems, especially during follow-up.

Perception of Family Relations

When overviewing the mean scores on the *Leuven Family Questionnaire* of *all family members* (parents and patient taken together), the following results are the most striking (see Figure 1). Families with an eating disorder patient situated in the launching phase (the average age of our patients is about 19 years) experience more conflict, more cohesion and more disorganization (at admission) when compared with normal families. After six months (i.e., shortly after inpatient treatment, since the mean length of hospitalization is about 4 months)

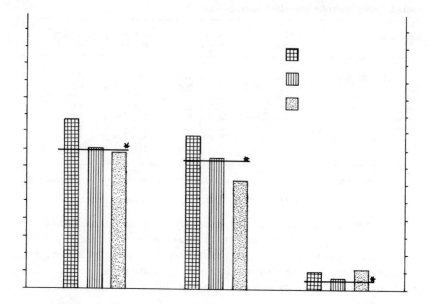

Figure 1. The Leuven Family Questionnaire: results of father, mother, and daughter together.

all families evolve on all subscales toward the scores of normal families: they experience almost as much conflict and cohesion and only a bit more disorganization. After one year the scores on conflict remain almost the same, but cohesion is further decreasing, while disorganization is increasing.

The evolution on the variables "cohesion" and "disorganization" can be interpreted as an exaggerated reaction of the family members. Indeed, we often remark that the discharge from the hospital and the returning home of the daughter provokes a period of crisis within the family system. We believe that this crisis is a necessary process of growth the family has to endure on their way toward a new equilibrium. The evolution on the variable "conflict" gives further evidence for the fact that family functioning improves regardless of the increased tension, because they can better handle conflicts after one year.

The results of the *separate family members* (see Table 4) show that father, mother and patient are perceiving their family life very differently, not only at admission but also after six months and one year follow-up. At admission the patient experiences the highest conflict and the lowest cohesion, but both variables change significantly after one year, moving more toward the scores of normal families. Another interesting finding in the eating disorder families (with adolescents in the launching phase) are the high scores on cohesion of both parents at admission. After one year both father and mother experience significantly lower cohesion in the family. Cohesion is indeed the only variable which significantly decreases after one year for all family members. The fathers experience the lowest conflict at admission, when compared with the scores of their wife and daughter. But they are still perceiving more conflict compared with normal families. Disorganization tends to increase in the perception of the patients and to decrease in the perception of the fathers, but the differences are not significant.

The *scores of the four clinical subgroups* can be summarized as follows: the families with a restricting anorexia nervosa patient differ at admission only on one variable from the scores of normal families: they experience even higher cohesion! They probably tend to give an idealistic and socially desirable view of their family and deny or minimize the presence of conflicts. On the other hand, we see that the restricting anorexics evolve the most toward the normal scores, a finding that corresponds with the best global clinical score for this group after one year. The atypical patients differ the most from the normal group on the variables conflict and disorganization, not only at admission but even after one year.

Finally, we were wondering whether the *addition of separate family therapy* sessions to our inpatient treatment program did have an influence on the outcome. Therefore, we made a comparison between those families who attended separate family therapy sessions during inpatient treatment (16 families) and those who did not (8 families). An interesting and important finding is that both groups differed already on several characteristics at admission: the patients of the family therapy group had a longer duration of illness with a different treatment history (more individual therapy, less family therapy) and a more disturbed general clinical score. Hence the family therapy group seems to present a more severe pathology. This makes comparisons as to the differential effect of family therapy very difficult, since the choice for adding family therapy to the standard treatment program was not made at random. The follow-up results on the global clinical score do not show significant differences between the two groups, but rather only some tendencies. The family therapy group appears to improve faster on interaction variables (engagement, positive interaction with other family members and peers, satisfying sex) but not on symptom variables. After one year, however, the no-family-therapy group evolves more clearly toward normality, while the family therapy group is improving rather slowly.

The scores of the patients on the *Leuven Family Questionnaire* elicit some interesting tendencies although the differences are not significant (see Table 5). The follow-up results of the family therapy group after six months asks for special attention. The patients of this group then report more conflict, less cohesion and more disorganization than at admission, while the no-family-therapy group experiences less conflict and less disorganization after six months. This is, in our opinion, an interesting finding because an important treatment goal of the separate family therapy sessions was to provoke a crisis within the family system in order to break through rigid interaction patterns. The provocation of this crisis did probably increase the patient's experience of conflict

Table 4. Leuven Family Questionnaire (mean scores of separated family members)

	Patients (N=15)			Fathers (N=13)			Mothers (N=17)		
	Conflict (94)*	Cohesion (80)	Disorgan. (55)	Conflict (84)	Cohesion (90)	Disorgan. (50)	Conflict (85)	Cohesion (92)	Disorg. (49)
Admission	109.4	85.7	55.0	90.3	97.4	53.9	95.9	96.5	52.4
6 months	107.0	75.8	61.9	85.0	90.8	50.4	89.5	89.5	55.0
1 year	96.1	77.2	59.7	79.2	85.9	49.7	84.1	83.6	53.5
t-test (p)	<.05	<.01	NS	NS	<.01	NS	<.05	<.001	NS

*The numbers between brackets refer to the average score in normal families (see Kog et al., 1985).

Table 5. Evolution of the patients (with or without family therapy) on the Leuven Family Questionnaire

	With Family Therapy[b]			Without Family Therapy[c]		
	Admission	Six Months	One Year	Admission	Six Months	One Year
Conflict (94.5)[a]	101.0	103.9	97.7	115.6	98.4	96.7
Cohesion (80.4)	89.0	78.6	80.1	83.3	80.6	76.8
Disorganization (55.2)	51.8	61.2	58.8	56.8	55.4	64.0

[a] The numbers between brackets refer to the average score in normal controls (see Kog et al., 1985).

[b] N=17

[c] N=17

and disorganization and decrease the presence of cohesion after six months. After one year all variables evolve toward the scores of normal families – perhaps toward a new equilibrium? Surprisingly enough these changes are only reported by the patients and not by the parents.

One last interesting finding is that the number of rehospitalizations after one year is much lower in the group with separate family therapy sessions (12.5% versus 25% in the no-family-therapy group) although the former group appeared to have a more complex pathology before treatment.

DISCUSSION

This investigation consisted of a prospective study of 24 families with an eating disorder patient who was hospitalized in our special treatment unit. The purpose of this study was to assess the evolution of family functioning as well as individual symptomatic and psychosocial adjustment of the eating disorder patient before and after treatment, and at follow-up (up to one year after admission).

The results of the *clinical assessment* show that, generally speaking, our multidimensional family-oriented inpatient treatment induced a considerable improvement, both with regard to general psychosocial and symptomatic variables, in 61% of our patients after one year (13% were judged as "recovered"). It is interesting to note that this group was already functioning quite well after six months (62.5% were judged at that time as being clearly improved but none were considered recovered). This finding gives evidence that short-term follow-up results probably have prognostic value. We further found the evolution after treatment to be worse in patients with a longer duration of illness and a more severe symptomatology (bulimia, vomiting, purging).

A detailed analysis of the results reveals high differences among the clinical subgroups not only on the clinical evaluation but also on the self-report questionnaires. This finding stresses the importance and absolute need for a differentiated diagnosis in the early assessment of the eating disorder against the background of the family system.

Bulimia seems to be a very therapy-resistant behavior at least in our sample and with our treatment program. Almost all bulimic patients can stop bingeing and vomiting quite soon during inpatient treatment but many flee back into their disturbed eating pattern as soon as they are confronted with the outside world. Hence, partial hospitalization (day treatment), where the bulimic patient is daily confronted with the outside world, might be the treatment of choice in severe cases where outpatient therapy alone has failed.

We further postulate that different psychological conditions mutually influence the presence or absence of menstruation: namely, leaving the family of origin, becoming engaged, experiencing satisfying interactions and sexual relationship, and so forth.

The results of the *Eating Disorder Inventory* (Garner et al., 1983) show that our patients evolve significantly toward the normal scores after treatment. However, data gathered by self-report questionnaires may be colored by important denial mechanisms or the tendency to give socially desirable answers (Vandereycken & Vanderlinden, 1983). Indeed, we established that several patients gave a more positive image of their condition on the questionnaires than during interview for clinical assessment. The longer the duration of illness and/or the more complex and severe the eating disorder, the more the patients tend to deny or minimize the presence of eating problems, in particular at follow-up, when information is gathered by self-report questionnaires.

When summarizing the results of the *Leuven Family Questionnaire* (Kog et al., 1985) we see that families with a restricting anorexia nervosa patient, although they tend to deny very strongly the presence of conflicts at admission, evolve the most toward the scores of the normal families. This finding corresponds with the best global clinical score for this group after one year. The atypical eating disorder patients differ the most from normal controls. We are wondering whether a combination of high scores on conflict and disorganization and low scores on cohesion, as in these atypical cases even after one year, have to be considered as an indication or contraindication for family therapy?

Although we need clearer indication and contraindication criteria for family therapy with severe eating disorder patients, the addition of separate family therapy sessions during inpatient treatment seems to accelerate, at least over the short-term, improvement of the interactions inside and outside the family (becoming engaged, having sexual contact, etc.). It appears, however, not to enhance the general treatment effect on the typical eating problems, although patients who also received family therapy, showed fewer relapses after discharge. Our research design, however, does not allow conclusions about the specific value of family therapy within the treatment package, since there was not a random allocation of family therapy. Anyway, this investigation demonstrates the complex interplay between individual and familial factors, which necessitates a multifaceted assessment and, accordingly, a multimodal treatment approach.

REFERENCES

Garfinkel, P.E. & Garner, D.M. (1982), *Anorexia Nervosa. A Multidimensional Perspective.* New York: Brunner/Mazel.

Garner, D.M., Olmsted, M.P. & Polivy, J. (1983), Development and validation of a multidimensional eating disorder inventory for anorexia nervosa and bulimia. *International Journal of Eating Disorders,* 2 (2):15-33.

Kog, E., Vertommen, H. & De Groote, T. (1985), Family interaction research in anorexia nervosa: The use and misuse of a self-report questionnaire. *International Journal of Family Psychiatry,* 6:227-243.

Minuchin, S., Rosman, B. & Baker, L. (1978), *Psychosomatic Families. Anorexia Nervosa in Context.* Cambridge (Mass.): Harvard University Press.

Szmukler, G. (1983), A study of family therapy in anorexia nervosa: some methodological issues. In: Darby, P.L., Garfinkel, P.E., Garner, D.M. & Coscina, D.V. (Eds), *Anorexia Nervosa: Recent Developments in Research.* New York: Alan Liss, pp. 417-425.

Vandereycken, W. (1985), Inpatient treatment of anorexia nervosa: Some research-guided changes. *Journal of Psychiatric Research,* 19:413-422.

Vandereycken, W. (1987), The management of patients with anorexia nervosa and bulimia — Basic principles and general guidelines. In: Beumont, P.J.V., Burrows, G.D. & Casper, R. (Eds.), *Handbook of Eating Disorders. Part 1: Anorexia and Bulimia Nervosa.* Amsterdam: Elsevier-North Holland Biomedical Press, pp. 235-253.

Vandereycken, W. & Meermann, R. (1984), *Anorexia Nervosa. A Clinician's Guide to Treatment.* Berlin-New York: Walter de Gruyter.

Vandereycken, W. & Vanderlinden, J. (1983), Denial of illness and the use of self-reporting measures in anorexia nervosa patients. *International Journal of Eating Disorders,* 2(4):101-107.

Chapter 10

Eating Disorders in Married Patients: A Comparison With Unmarried Anorexics And An Exploration Of The Marital Relationship

Stephan Van den Broucke and Walter Vandereycken*

INTRODUCTION

The widespread assumption that eating disorders, especially anorexia nervosa and bulimia, typically occur during teenage years has diverted the attention from exploring the specific characteristics of these disorders in adult patients (Vandereycken, 1988). As pointed out by Garfinkel and Garner (1982), the average age at onset of anorexia nervosa seems to be gradually increasing, approximating the boundary between adolescence and early adulthood. Consequently, the number of patients who develop anorexia nervosa at or after the time of their marriage is growing considerably. Research concerning married anorexics, as reported in the literature, is mostly restricted to descriptive case studies or to clinical impressions regarding their backgrounds, treatment and often unfavorable prognosis (see Chapter 17). Moreover, in spite of the noted interference of anorexia nervosa with the patient's sexual and relational life, very little is known about the interaction between eating disorders and marital relations.

Dally (1984) has conducted an exploratory survey of the backgrounds and personalities of married anorexics and their husbands. His findings suggest that the "anorexia tardive" (developed during the engagement period, after marriage or after childbirth) represents a maladaptive solution to a growing marital conflict between, in general, a dependent and insecure wife and an im-

* The authors wish to thank Martine Van Regenmortel and Prof. Dr. Paulette Van Oost (University of Gent) for their cooperation in the research project.

mature husband. This is in line with Lafeber's (1981) and Palmer's (1980) earlier conclusions regarding the repercussions of recovery from anorexia nervosa
through psychotherapy on the relationship between the patient and her marital
or sexual partner. Dally's study, however, appears to be based on rather general
clinical impressions and data from medical records.

In spite of the growing number of older patients, the literature on anorexia
nervosa in married patients remains very scarce and a systematic comparison
with representative groups of unmarried anorexics is still lacking. In this chapter, such a comparison of demographic and clinical features in married and
single patients is presented. Moreover, no systematic investigation has been
done, as far as we know, of the interaction between eating disorders and marital relations, in contrast to the elaborate research on the connection between
other psychopathological syndromes and patients' marriages (e.g., phobias;
Vandereycken, 1983). For this reason, we also carried out an explorative pilot
study, which should guide more extended future research by generating specific
hypotheses.

METHOD

Comparative Study

To obtain as large a subject sample as possible, a consecutive series of 200
female patients, who met the diagnostic criteria for anorexia nervosa as proposed by Feighner et al. (1972) and who were treated as inpatients at the Anorexia Nervosa Unit of the University Psychiatric Center St. Jozef in Kortenberg,
Belgium was involved in this study. In line with the more current DSM-III criteria for the diagnosis of anorexia nervosa, Feighner's age limit criterion of 25
years was not applied. Of the total group of 200 subjects, 34 were married. In
order to make the married and unmarried patient groups more comparable with
respect to age, all subjects under 18 years (i.e., the minimum age observed in
the married group) were excluded from the unmarried sample, leaving a total
of 102 unmarried patients. Twenty-three (or 22.5%) of the single and 6 (or
17.6%) of the married patients evidenced bulimic episodes.

Data of both the married and the single patient groups concerning the course,
symptoms and outcome of the illness, as well as demographic data, were
gathered in a similar, standardized manner. Comparisons between the two
groups were made using t-tests for the continuous variables (with separate or
pooled variance estimates according to the variance equality as indicated by an
F-test) and chi-square-tests for the noncontinuous variables.

Explorative Study

Ten couples, the female partners of which were diagnosed as suffering from
anorexia nervosa, bulimia or atypical eating disorder acccording to the DSM-

III criteria, were involved in this part of the study. Nine of the couples were married, the mean duration of their marriages amounting to 11 years. The tenth couple was engaged, living together for one year and planning marriage. Ages ranged from 22 to 50 for the women (mean age 30.7) and from 25 to 62 for the men (mean age 34.8). The number of children varied between 0 (in 3 cases) and 8 (in 1 case). Five of the patients were anorexic, three were bulimic and two were classified as atypical. The mean duration of the illness was 6 years, with a minimum of 4 months and a maximum of 17 years.

Each couple was subjected to a *standardized interview* (see Appendix) which lasted approximately two hours and focused on the following issues: eating or weight problems experienced by the husband, partner choice and onset of the relation, course of the eating disorder, the partner's reaction, the couple's attributions of the problem, their way of coping with the disorder and their way of dealing with disagreements in general.

Measures of the quality of the relationships between the spouses were gathered by a form of Barrett-Lennard's (1962, 1978) *Relationship Inventory,* in a Dutch adaptation by Lietaer (1974). Two forms of the Relationship Inventory were used, each one consisting of 50 self-report items: (1) the Perception-form or the way one perceives the other is feeling or behaving toward oneself (P-form), and (2) the Self-form, or the way one feels toward the other (S-form). On the basis of a factor analysis, five subscales may be distinguished: empathy (E) is the extent to which one person recognizes the immediate awareness of the other and understands his or her emotions and feelings; transparency (T) means the willingness to be known as a person by the other; directivity (D) refers to an authoritarian attitude toward the other and involves such aspects as overprotection and intrusion; positive regard (P) concerns the feelings of respect, liking and appreciation as opposed to negative feelings include such as impatience and lack of trust; unconditionality (U) means a constancy of regard felt by one person for another. Each subscale consists of 10 items. The subjects can indicate on a 6-point scale how appropriate each statement is as a description of their relationships. The total scores for each variable may thus vary from 10 to 60. The five variables were measured in the P-form and S-form from the viewpoints of patient and spouse.

Finally, the couples' interactional structures as well as those of their families of origin were measured by means of a Dutch version of the *Herbst Questionnaire,* which consists of 56 items concerning different activities, decision-making instances, and tensions occuring within the relation (Herbst, 1952). For each partner an index of tension is obtained which refers to the percentage of disagreement each observe within their own marital relations and, looking back at their family of origin, between their parents. The questionnaire allows one to identify three basic interaction types: an autonomous pattern (one person both makes the decisions and carries out the activities on his own); an autocratic pattern (one person makes the decisions regardless of who is carrying out the activities); a syncretic pattern (there is a cooperation between the partners regarding decisions and activities).

RESULTS

Comparative Study

The characteristics of anorexia nervosa in married patients show a close resemblance to those observed in single patients, yet a number of differences should be noted (see Table 1).

On the average, the married patients of our sample were significantly older than the unmarried ones at the onset of the illness as well as at their assessment (admission in the hospital). Whereas neither their presenting weight nor the loss from their premorbid weight differed significantly from that of the unmarried patients, a greater loss from their ideal weight (as a function of age and length) was presented. Also, a longer duration of the illness was observed in the married sample. Conversely, no significant differences were found between the two groups regarding the age of menarche, duration of amenorrhea, symptom pattern and treatment history.

Married and single anorexia nervosa patients differed significantly with respect to professional occupation and educational level. As compared with the single patients, a greater percentage of married subjects were working on a regular basis, and had received professional (as opposed to a high school level) education. Like the unmarried ones, the married anorexia nervosa patients predominantly belonged to the middle class.

Due to the large number of drop-outs in the follow-up part of our study (a research problem we discussed elsewhere: Vandereycken & Pierloot, 1983) our findings regarding the long-term outcome of these patients can only be stated tentatively. At follow-up averaging four years after admission, it appears that on most variables measured (including weight fluctuations, preoccupation with weight, menstruation and psychosocial adaptation) married and unmarried patients presented a similar picture. However, the continuation of dieting behavior following treatment occurred significantly more often among the married patients, and their overall outcome was rated as considerably (yet not significantly) less favorable.

Whereas in the previous analysis a difference in presenting age between the married and the single patients may have contaminated the results (although the minimum age of the patients in the two groups had been leveled), the specificity of the married-patient group has unexpectedly been confirmed by the results of a cluster analysis performed on the data of the original sample of 200 patients. This analysis (with a fixed maximum of three clusters) yielded clusters of 127, 43 and 30 patients, respectively. For each clinical and demographic vari-

Table 1. Comparison between married and unmarried anorexia nervosa patients.

	Married (N=34)	Unmarried (N=102)	P
Age (years)	26.7 ± 5.3	22.3 ± 3.8	.001
Age at onset (years)	21.1 ± 6.0	18.3 ± 3.0	.05
Duration of illness (years)	5.8 ± 4.5	4.0 ± 3.3	.05
Age at menarche (years)	13.6 ± 2.1	13.5 ± 1.6	NS
Duration of amenorrhea (years)	2.8 ± 3.1	3.3 ± 2.8	NS
Weight (kg)	36.9 ± 5.0	38.9 ± 5.9	NS
Actual weight loss (kg)	15.6 ± 5.5	15.4 ± 7.3	NS
Loss from ideal weight (%)	34.3 ± 8.7	30.1 ± 9.9	.05
Previous treatment (%)			NS
general hospital	63.6	43.6	
psychiatric hospital	18.2	25.7	
outpatient	6.1	10.9	
none	12.1	19.8	
Symptoms (%)			NS
vomiting	21.2	16.0	
bingeing	18.2	23.0	
constipation	6.1	3.0	
laxative or diuretic abuse	36.4	28.8	
hyperactivity	9.1	7.0	
none of the above	9.1	23.0	
Educational level (%)			.05
lower education	9.1	1.2	
high education	9.1	31.4	
professional education	48.5	29.4	
university-college	33.3	37.3	
Professional occupation (%)			.01
attending school	3.0	37.3	
unemployed	12.1	8.8	
regular job	51.5	34.3	
unable to work	12.1	8.8	
no occupation	21.2	10.8	
Social class* (%)			NS
lower	40.6	27.0	
middle	50.0	48.0	
upper	9.4	25.0	

*According to father's occupation.

able it was then verified if the clusters differed significantly from each other. The variables for which significant differences between the clusters were found are presented in Table 2.

The main differences between the clusters concern the presenting age, duration of the illness, problem seriousness, symptoms, personality type and professional occupation (which is probably connected with the age difference). The majority of the subjects are found in the first cluster, and correspond with the "typical" adolescent anorexia nervosa patient. The other two clusters contain relatively older and chronic patients. The main difference between the latter two clusters, then, concerns the marital status of the subjects: approximately

Table 2. Major differences among three clusters of anorexia nervosa patients.

	cluster 1 (N=127)	cluster 2 (N=43)	cluster 3 (N=30)	P 1/2	1/3	2/3
Presenting age (years)	19.3	23.1	25.4	*	*	–
Age at onset (years)	17.0	18.1	19.6	–	*	–
Duration of illness (yrs)	2.4	5.0	5.8	*	*	–
Duration of amenorrhea (yrs)	2.0	3.1	4.2	–	*	–
Weight loss (kg)	15.6	12.3	16.7	*	–	*
Loss from ideal weight (%)	30.7	25.6	35.3	*	–	*
Symptoms (%)				*	–	–
vomiting	6.4	38.1	20.7			
bulimia	18.4	21.4	17.2			
constipation	7.2	0.0	6.9			
hyperactivity	12.8	2.4	17.2			
laxative abuse	21.6	23.8	27.6			
Personality (%)				*	*	*
undifferentiated	36.0	14.6	0.0			
schizoid/introvert	30.4	24.4	14.3			
passive dependent	11.2	7.3	17.9			
hysterical/hystrionic	20.8	41.5	32.1			
obsessional	1.6	7.3	35.7			
antisocial	0.0	4.9	0.0			
Marital status (%)				–	*	*
unmarried	96.0	90.5	23.3			
married	4.0	9.5	76.7			
Professional occupation				*	*	–
attending school	64.3	28.6	10.0			
unemployed	7.9	0.0	13.3			
regular work	23.0	21.4	53.3			
unable to work	0.8	21.4	10.0			
none of the above	3.4	28.6	13.3			

–=not significant ; *=P <0.05.
Significance was determined with ANOVA (Tuckey procedure) for the continuous
variables and with chi-square tests for the percentual distribution of subjects in each cluster for the categorical variables.

90% of the patients in the second cluster are single, whereas more than 75% of
the ones in the third cluster are married. Furthermore, the patients in the
"married" cluster suffered a greater weight loss and predominantly manifested
a different type of personality as compared with the "unmarried" ones. So, the
results of this cluster analysis suggests that, *in addition to* the age difference the
marital relationship influences the onset and/or the course of the eating disorder.

Explorative Study

The information resulting from the standardized interviews can be summarized as follows. With regard to the husbands' problem history, it appeared
that none of the male partners had ever experienced eating or weight problems.
One husband had suffered from a depression prior to entering his present relationship. Two husbands reported marital problems in their parents' relation-

Table 3. The patient's and husband's conceptualization of the eating disorder.

The eating disorder may be viewed as	Patients	Husbands
A physical illness for which the patient cannot be responsible :	2.6	2.1
A form of obsession or addiction :	3.2	3.4
A sequela of early childhood experiences :	3.6	3.2
A reaction to marital problems :	2.6	2.1
A means to receive more attention :	2.1	2.5

*During the interview, each subject had to estimate on a 5-point scale the degree of applicability of each conceptualization (0= most unlikely, 5= most likely).

ship. None of them had known about the existence of eating disorders before their marriage.

As to the reasons for being attracted to their partner, the men stressed the importance of physical attractiveness, friendliness, sociability, femininity and the partner's need for support. The women, on their side, reported gentleness, friendliness and good physical appearance as determining their choice of partner. None of the subjects in our sample had had much sexual or relational experience before entering their marriage relationship. Four of the couples claimed to have experienced no problems upon starting their relationship; in three cases the female partner had known feelings of being "too fat" and one patient reported inferiority feelings during the engagement period. In two cases the contacts between the patient and her parents were referred to as problematic.

On the average, the men did not notice their wives' eating problems until three years after their marriage. In six cases the patients had not openly admitted their eating habits. Professional help was sought on the initiative of the husband and/or parents, but never by the patients themselves.

Partners sometimes differed with regard to their explicit conceptualization of the eating disorder (see Table 3). In general, both spouses were more inclined to view the disorder as something separate from the relationship than as having a special function within the marriage. Except for one of them, all the husbands claimed to believe that a complete recovery from the eating disorder was possible.

More eliciting factors were mentioned by the male partners than by the female patients. Among them, dissatisfaction with physical appearance or weight (mentioned by five men and five women) and conflicts between the patient and her parents (mentioned by four of the men and two of the women)

Table 4. The husband's reaction to the eating problem*

Type of reaction	According to husband	According to patient
Worry	4.4	4.6
Patience	4.3	4.6
Sadness	4.1	4.1
Support	4.0	4.4
Understanding	4.0	4.0
Control or distrust	1.8	2.3

*During the interview, both husband and wife had to judge the degree of the
way the husband reacted to the eating problem (0= absent, 5= extreme).

were the most common ones. Two patients referred to marital conflicts as eliciting anorexia nervosa, as opposed to none of the husbands.

The disorder was reported to have influenced the quality of the relation (in nine cases), the conversation between the partners (in eight and nine cases according to the men and women, respectively), sexual life (nine cases), childrearing (six cases), family contacts (seven and eight cases according to men and women, respectively), leisure activities (six and eight cases), household activities (four and three cases) and family eating habits (two cases). The husbands' reaction to the eating problems as inferred from ratings by both spouses on a 5-point scale, was mostly judged in a similar way by the husband and the patients except for control and distrust (see Table 4), which was generally overrated by the patients.

The satisfaction of the patients and their partners with their present relationship can be compared using their scores on the Barrett-Lennard Relationship Inventory (see Table 5).

Patients and spouses alike perceived their relationship as favorable. The self- and the partner-ratings of patients and spouses on the five relationship scales show a similar pattern, with positive regard receiving the highest scores, and directivity and unconditionality the lowest. A comparison of the global relationship satisfaction rates (as measured by the sum of the P, E and T scores) indicates that the patients perceived their partners' relational attitude as more favorable than the partners themselves (147.5 vs 138.3). The opposite is seen for the patients' relational qualities, which were rated lower by the husbands than by the patients themselves (127.4 vs 140.9).

The predominant interaction type as well as the respective tension indexes for each couple and their families of origin, as inferred from the Herbst Questionnaire, are presented in Table 6.

Table 5. Mean scores of patients and spouses on the Barrett-Lennard Relationship Inventory.

	Self-rating		Partner-rating	
	Men	Women	Men	Women
Empathy (E)	43.8	42.0	39.7	47.8
Transparance (T)	43.4	45.8	40.0	47.8
Directivity (D)	38.3	34.0	36.9	35.4
Positive regard (P)	51.0	52.4	47.7	53.3
Unconditionality (U)	40.6	40.6	35.8	39.4
Global satisfaction (P.E.T.)	138.3	140.9	127.4	147.4

Table 6. Tension index and interaction type of the marriage and of the family of origin, as inferred from the Herbst Questionnaire.

Case number	1	2	3	4	5	6	7	8	9	10
MARITAL RELATIONSHIP										
interaction type										
husband	S	S	S	S	S	S	A(W)	A(W)	A(W)	-
wife	S	S	A(H)	S	S	S	-	S	S	-
tension index										
husband	5.9	6.3	16.7	60.6	36.4	0	47.1	66.0	59.6	-
wife	11.8	14.6	45.2	18.2	35.5	43.4	-	40.0	25.0	-
FAMILY OF ORIGIN										
interaction type										
husband	S	D(M)	A(M)	S	A(M)	S	A	A	A(M)	-
wife	S	A	A(M)	A	S	S	-	A(M)	S	A(M)
tension index										
husband	6.7	2.4	17.7	35.3	0	0	33.3	46.0	19.1	-
wife	14.7	0	22.0	41.9	5.0	23.2	-	42.0	0	18.8

S= syncratic structure ; D= autocratic structure ; A= autonomous structure ; M= mother ;
W= wife ; H= husband

In the majority of the couples, both spouses described their relationship as a syncratic structure whereas an autocratic structure did not occur. In three couples, however, the husband and wife presented a different view of the relationship. Tension indexes varied considerably between and within couples, but were often high for at least one of the partners. As to the families in which the subjects had been raised, an autonomous structure prevailed in both the patients' and their husbands' families, followed by the syncretic interaction type. Only one subject had been raised in a family characterized by an autocratic structure. The tension indexes for the families of origin showed a considerable variability, but they were generally lower than those observed in the couples' relationship. There was only a minor resemblance between the interaction structure in one's family of origin and in one's own marriage.

DISCUSSION

The *clinical* correspondence between the anorexia nervosa syndrome as observed in married and in unmarried (mostly adolescent) subjects has been described earlier (Dally, 1984), but has not yet been determined systematically. In the current study, a statistical comparison of married and single anorexia nervosa patients of a comparable age confirms that both groups are indeed strikingly similar with respect to most clinical variables. The widespread assumption of a greater seriousness of the disorder among married subjects is only partly corroborated: we only noticed a more pronounced loss from the ideal weight and a longer duration of the illness in our married sample. The fact that the married patients evidenced a significantly greater loss from their ideal weight, yet not from their premorbid weight, seems to indicate that married patients, as compared with unmarried ones, are more likely to be underweight prior to the onset of the disorder. This observation stresses the importance of considering the loss from ideal weight rather than from premorbid weight as an index of the problem seriousness, as has been suggested before (Vandereycken & Meermann, 1984). The greater seriousness and longer duration of the disorder may then result in a less favorable prognosis for married patients, as is suggested by the greater frequency of continued dieting behavior and by the worse overall outcome judgments at long-term follow-up. However, one must be careful when interpreting these outcome findings on account of the large number of missing data which thwarted the follow-up part of our study. In spite of the alleged gravity of the problem in married patients, more time has been spent before assessment took place, as can be inferred from the greater difference between age at onset and presenting age. Again, this may add to the unfavorable prognosis.

As to *demographic* aspects, the main distinction between married and single anorexia nervosa patients concerns their educational and professional background. Yet, this distinction may at least partly be explained by the highly significant difference in presenting age, which, notwithstanding the fact that the minimum age of the two groups was leveled for the purpose of this study, remains the most prevailing distinguishing characteristic. Indeed, this age difference probably reflects the fact that in most populations, married subjects, on the average, are likely to be older than single ones. A more important finding with respect to our research question, however, is the fact that for the married subjects the onset of the disorder is situated at an older age, i.e., their early twenties on the average. Despite the tendency of married patients to be underweight already before the actual onset of the disorder, as was pointed out above, the comparatively late age at onset suggests that the relationship with the marital partner may have influenced the development of the problem, and contradicts the theory that anorexia nervosa in married life is merely a continuation of an eating disorder which began in adolescence.

The distinctiveness of anorexia nervosa in married subjects, which became apparent from this comparative study, invited us to further investigate *the role of marital interaction* in the development and/or maintenance of eating disorders in married patients. An initial exploration into this matter, by way of interviewing eating disorder patients and their partners and applying two inventories assessing aspects of their marital interaction, yields a number of interesting observations.

First, the eating disorder is generally developed after the start of the relationship, although either partner may have experienced other problems before. Again, this supports the view that anorexia nervosa or bulimia in married patients is not simply a relapse into a previously existing eating problem.

Second, on a conscious level marital conflicts seem relatively unimportant as eliciting factors of the eating disorder. Dissatisfaction with one's own physical appearance is most often seen as a trigger for the problem. Interestingly, physical attractiveness is mentioned as one of the important factors determining the partner choice in both patients and husbands.

Third, the marital relationship is mostly described as satisfactory and cooperative (syncretic and nondirective), which may seem at odds with the drastic impediment of the couple's interaction and of the family life due to the wife's illness. However, much credit for this accord is awarded to the husband, whose relational qualities are praised (as opposed to those of the patient) and whose reaction to his wife's problem is generally characterized as worried yet very supporting. Evidently, husband and wife reinforce each other's role as protective caretaker and dependent patient, respectively. A strong mutual interdependency, similar to the one often observed in the patients' original families (see Chapter 3), is thus maintained.

Further, it should be considered that the items of the Herbst Questionnaire, on which the interaction style is assessed, focus on the activities and decisions of the partners rather than on the meaningful communication between them. Also, in the majority of the couples at least one partner senses a considerable degree of tension. It is possible, then, that the couple's interaction is cooperative on a very superficial level only, whereas more intimate communication between the spouses is strictly avoided. A similar inability to communicate about intimate matters has also been described in the relationship between anorexia nervosa patients and their families (see Chapter 3).

The intention of this exploratory study regarding the marital interaction of eating disorder patients was to generate hypotheses for future research rather than to investigate well-defined theories. To serve this purpose, the use of qualitative (as opposed to quantitative) procedures yielding information about very diverse aspects of the interaction was justified. From our survey, it appears that the interaction between the eating disorder patient and her marital partner merits further attention. More specifically, the superficial nature of the communication between the spouses and the interdependent interaction pattern seem worthy of a further examination. Future research, then, should apply the application of more elaborate and quantifiable methods to investigate the connection between marital interaction and the occurrence (development, maintenance) of eating disorders in married subjects.

REFERENCES

Barrett-Lennard, G.T. (1962), Dimensions of therapist response as causal factor in therapeutic change. *Psychological Monographs,* 76 (nr. 43).

Barrett-Lennard, G.T. (1978), The Relationship Inventory: Later developments and adaptations. *JSAS Catalog of Selected Documents in Psychology,* 8.

Dally, P. (1984), Anorexia tardive-Late onset anorexia nervosa. *Journal of Psychosomatic Research,* 28:423-428.

Feighner, J.P., Robins, E., Guze, S.B., Woodruff, R.A., Winokur, G. & Munoz, R. (1972), Diagnostic criteria for use in psychiatric research. *Archives of General Psychiatry,* 26:57-93.

Garfinkel, P. & Garner, D. (1982), *Anorexia Nervosa. A Multidimensional Perspective.* New York: Brunner/Mazel.

Herbst, P. (1982), The measurement of family relationships. *Human Relations,* 1:3-35.

Lafeber, C. (1981), Wisselwerking tussen herstel van anorexia nervosa en de partnerrelatie (Interaction between recovery from anorexia nervosa and marital relationship). *Tijdschrift voor Psychiatrie,* 23(supplement): 97-103.

Lietaer, G. (1974), Nederlandstalige revisie van Barrett-Lennard's Relationship Inventory: een factoranalytische benadering van de student-ouderrelatie (Dutch revision of the Barrett-Lennard Relationship Inventory: A factor analytical approach of the student-parent relationship). *Nederlands Tijdschrift voor de Psychologie,* 29:191-212.

Palmer, R. (1980), *Anorexia Nervosa. A Guide for Sufferers and their Families.* London: Penguin Books.

Vandereycken, W. (1983), Agoraphobia and marital relationship: Theory, treatment and research. *Clinical Psychology Review,* 3:317-338.

Vandereycken, W. (1988), Anorexia nervosa in adults. In: B.J. Blinder et al. (Ed.), *The Eating Disorders.* New York: PMA Publications.

Vandereycken, W. & Meermann, R. (1984), *Anorexia Nervosa. A Clinician's Guide to Treatment.* New York: Walter de Gruyter.

Vandereycken, W. & Pierloot, R. (1983), Long-term outcome research in anorexia nervosa. The problem of patient selection and follow-up duration. *International Journal of Eating Disorders,* 2(4):237-242.

APPENDIX: Anorexia/Bulimia Nervosa and Marital Relation – Standardized Interview

Identification Data

- Name:
- Age:
- Education:
- Profession:
- Age of cohabitation:
- Age of marriage:
- Age of first AN/bulimia symptoms:
- Number and age of children:

Questions With Reference to the Spouse

1. Did the spouse ever experience one of the following symptoms *prior* to the marriage? And *after* the marriage?
    (a) obesity (> 20% overweight), (b)severe weight loss, (c) loss of appetite, (d) digestive problems, (e) alcohol or drug abuse, (f) depression, (g) neurotic symptoms, (h) psychotic symptoms, (i) psychosomatic problems.
2. Was the spouse familiar with the syndrome of anorexia nervosa *before* the marriage?
    (a) never heard about it, (b) heard or read about it, (c) learned about it through the spouse's condition, (d) learned about it through another patient.
3. Were there ever any serious problems in the spouse's family? If so, which ones?

Questions Regarding the Partner Choice and Onset of the Relationship

4. At what age did each partner start dating members of the opposite sex?
5. Did they have a relationship prior to the present one?
    (a) platonic love, (b) loose relationship without sexual contact, (c) loose relationship with petting, (d) loose relationship with intercourse, (e) steady relationship without sexual contact, (f) steady relationship with petting, (g) steady relationship with intercourse, (h) none of the above.
6. If the answer was "yes" on item e, f or g of the previous question:
    (a) was the previous partner younger/same age/older? (b) was the previous partner experienced/unexperienced? (c) did he/she or the previous partner breakup the relationship? (d) what was the reaction of the parents to the previous relationship and its breakup?

7. Who took the initiative for the following steps in the present relationship? (a) for the first contact, (b) for the engagement, (c) for sexual approach, (d) for sexual intercourse, (e) for marrige.
8. What in particular attracted the partners to each other?
9. Was there any evidence of eating/weight problems on the part of the patient at the start of the relationship?
10. What was the parents' attitude toward the relationship?

Questions Regarding the Present Status of the Marital Relationship

11. How do the partners evaluate the time they spend together as a couple?
12. What topics do the partners agree about most?
13. What topics do the partners disagree about most?
14. Do the partners tell each other what they like or dislike?
15. Do they consider their partner as attractive? In what sense (physical or other)?
16. Do they consider themselves as attractive for their partner? In what sense?
17. Were there ever extramarital sexual contacts?
18. What are the main qualities of a good spouse? (a) in general, (b) socially, (c) sexually.

Questions Regarding the Impact of the AN/Bulimia on the Relationship

19. When did the partners become aware of the eating or weight problem?
20. Did the patient try to hide the eating habits or symptoms?
21. When was the term anorexia nervosa or bulimia first used in order to describe the problem or as a diagnosis?
22. When, why and on whose initiative was professional help called in?
23. Which form of treatment was considered appropriate at the moment of the first consultant?
24. How did the spouse *overtly* react to the eating/weight problem?
25. How did the spouse *emotionally* react to the eating/weight problem? Rate: 1 = not at all; 2 = not very; 3 = fairly; 4 = very; 5 = extremely). (a) patient, (b) supportive, (c) understanding, (d) worried, (e) helpless, (f) sad, (g) guilty, (h) authoritative, (i) angry, (j) distrusting/controlling, (k) threatening with divorce.
26. In what respect did the eating disorder influence the interaction between the partners (e.g., communication, disclosure of feelings, mutual trust)?
27. In what respect did the eating disorder influence the physical and sexual interaction between the partners?
28. In what respect did the eating disorder influence the relationship with the children (if any) and/or the wish for children?

29. In what respect did the eating disorder influence the relationship with the extended family?
30. In what respect did the eating disorder influence the arrangement of household tasks?
31. In what respect did the eating disorder influence the spending of free time?
32. In what respect did the eating disorder influence the eating habits at home?
33. In what respect did the eating disorder influence the quality of the marital relationship?

Questions Regarding the Conceptualization of the Disorder

34. Which factors are considered to have elicited the eating disorder? (List one or more of the following).
(a) problems at school/work, (b) moving, (c) conflict between parents, (d) conflict between patient and parents, (e) conflict with brother/sister, (f) first sexual contact, (g) engagement, (h) cohabitation/marriage, (i) pregnancy/miscarriage/giving birth, (j) marital conflicts, (k) education of children, (l) dissatisfaction with appearance, (m) medical reason, (n) other (list).
35. What is the conceptualization of the eating disorder?
(Rate: 1 = not true at all; 2 = probably not true; 3 = perhaps; 4 = probably true; 5 = definitely true).
(a) the eating disorder is a physical disease for which one is not responsible, (b) the eating disorder is of psychological nature and is rooted in experiences of early childhood, (c) the eating disorder represents a lack of willpower, (d) the eating disorder is something the patient has done to him/herself by trying to lose weight, (e) the eating disorder is a form of obsession or addiction, (f) the eating disorder represents an inability to accept the female body, (h) the eating disorder represents a fear of the responsibilities of adulthood, (i) the eating disorder is a reaction to marital distress, (j) the eating disorder is a way to avoid sexual intercourse, (k) the eating disorder is a way to gain attention, (l) other (list).
36. In which way would the partners react differently if they had the change to do everything over again?
37. In which way would they want their spouses to react differently if they had the chance to do everything over again?
38. How do they think the *spouse* can help to solve the problems and to avoid relapses in the future?
39. What will happen to the marriage and family if there would be no real improvement of the eating disorder?
40. Do they believe that a complete recovery from the eating disorder is possible?

Chapter 11

Overview of the Family Therapy Literature*

Johan Vanderlinden and Walter Vandereycken

PATHWAYS TO A FAMILY-ORIENTED TREATMENT

There are few disorders that have, like anorexia nervosa, stimulated so many researchers and therapists to engage in a trial-and-error search for new and promising therapeutic approaches. Before 1970, these therapeutic attempts were mostly individual-oriented: anorexia nervosa was considered as an intrapersonal matter, a paradigm of psychosomatic disease (Kaufman & Heiman, 1964). The family, especially the parents, had to be separated from the patient (*parentectomy*) because of an implicit belief that faulty parenting could cause or at least aggravate this otherwise therapy-resistant disorder. The historical roots of this point of view go back to Gull and Lasègue in the 19th century.

For Gull (1874) the role of the parents was quite clear: "The patients should be fed at regular intervals and surrounded by persons who would have moral control over them, relatives and friends being generally the worst attendants." But it was Lasègue (1873) who depicted so accurately how "the dispositions of those surrounding her (the patient) undergo modification as the disease becomes prolonged." He recognized very soon a typical pattern in the family of anorexics: "The family has but two methods at its service which it always exhausts — entreaties and menaces — and which both serve as a touchstone. The delicacies of the table are multiplied in the hope of stimulating the appetite; but the more the solicitude increases, the more the appetite diminishes. The patient disdainfully tastes the new viands, and after having shown her willingness, holds herself absolved from any obligation to do more. She is besought, as a favour,

---

* Parts of this chapter have been published in an article by Walter Vandereycken: "The constructive family approach to eating disorders" (*International Journal of Eating Disorders*, 1987, 6:455-467).

and as a sovereign proof of affection, to consent to add even an additional mouthful to what she has taken; but this excess of insistence begets an excess of resistance.... The anorexia gradually becomes the sole object of preoccupation and conversation. The patient thus gets surrounded by a kind of atmosphere, from which there is no escape during the entire day." Lasègue soon realized the pathological interplay between patient and family, ending up in the situation "that the disease becomes developed and condensed so much the more as the circle within which revolve the ideas and sentiments of the patient becomes more narrowed." For Lasègue, and especially Charcot, hospitalization was the best therapeutic means to escape from this vicious circle. Hence, from the early medical history, parentectomy became a generally accepted guideline in the treatment of anorexia nervosa, thus reinforcing a long tradition of individual-oriented therapies, from which other family members were completely excluded as if they could only exert anti-therapeutic influences.

By the early 1950s, child psychoanalysts in Europe and the United States began to recognize the role of parental psychopathology in the development of childhood disorders. "They saw that despite the successful analysis of underlying conflicts, the patient's progress was severely limited if the family environment was unchanged" (Benson & Futterman, 1985, p. 156). Some psychoanalysts started experimenting with direct *parental involvement in the treatment*. Like Benedetti (1956a + b) in the case of anorexic children, Melitta Sperling (1950, 1978) began to include mothers in the treatment of adolescent anorexics. Depending upon the degree and nature of the pathology in the daughter and/or the mother, she either did a full psychoanalysis with the mother or just engaged in occasional contact with her. In the same period, Berlin and co-workers (1952) published a lengthy case report on "adolescent alternatives of anorexia and obesity." These authors in their introduction expressed the hope that they "may contribute in some way to a further understanding of the intrafamilial nature of conflicts which may be expressed in the symptoms of a child" (p. 387). Surveying the available literature on anorexia nervosa and obesity, the authors were struck that the family milieu and the character of the parents, as reported, looked very much alike. These clinicians, then, engaged in a collaborative psychotherapy with the hospitalized anorexic, her mother and her father, each one being seen individually in treatment by three different therapists (who had the same supervisor). "This is one of the few reports in the literature that describes the simultaneous treatment of three principal family members and the only account in the literature, to our knowledge, that describes this type of process with an anorexia nervosa patient" (Benson & Futterman, 1985, p. 156). Berlin and co-workers honestly described their problems with this treatment format but did not seem to realize that it was the individual-oriented intrapsychic approach which prevented them from recognizing important interactional dynamics within this family. Strikingly enough, they concluded their vivid case description as follows: "We believe an approach which looks upon the illness as *a family problem* to be of value, especially since anorexia nervosa has classically been proved to be extremely difficult to treat" (Berlin et al., 1951, p. 418, italics added).

The authors cannot be blamed for not having engaged in family therapy since it did not really exist at that time. What they did, however, was then extraordinarily new and hazardous. It was, at the same time, a symptom of an emerging new paradigm, since in the early 1950s an important confluence of forces led toward the "birth" of the family therapy movement (Kaslow, 1982). But we had still to wait another two decades before family therapists began treating anorexic patients. In the meantime, the old idea of parentectomy kept on prevailing in the therapeutic climate although several clinicians more often including the parents in the treatment process. A team, for example, at the Children's Hospital Medical Center in Boston with a large experience in treating anorexics (Blitzer et al., 1961; Blackwell & Rollins, 1968; Rollins & Blackwell, 1968) utilized different therapists for parents (separate or joint interview) and for the anorexic child. Later on, in the 1970s, influenced by the family therapy movement and Minuchin's ideas, these clinicians incorporated family treatment into their multimodal approach (Piazza et al., 1980; Rollins & Piazza, 1981).

Although only a small number of therapists reported successful treatment outcome with these patients, it did not lead to questioning the common individual-oriented therapeutic approach. It only induced a strong conviction that anorexia nervosa was a highly treatment-resistant condition. But as Seltzer (1984) remarks: "The treatment resistant character of anorexia nervosa may not be a property of the condition itself; instead, it may be contingent on the various methods employed in treating it" (p. 196). The widespread pessimistic view, nevertheless, provoked some researchers and therapists to explore new pathways in their search for refreshing and inspiring ideas about the etiology and treatment of the anorexic condition. In the meantime, the individual approach had fallen somewhat into disfavor due to several changes in the psychiatric field (Vandereycken & Meermann, 1984a): hospitalization was sharply criticized by antipsychiatrists while systems theories replaced linear models of causation. Hence, child psychiatry turned away from parent-blaming and enthusiastically joined the family therapy movement.

The year 1970 may be viewed as the start of a new era in the treatment history of anorexia nervosa. A talented American clinician, Salvador Minuchin (1970), reported for the first time on the application of structural family therapy in anorexia nervosa under the title: "The use of an ecological framework in the treatment of a child." At about the same time, but on the other side of the Atlantic, the Italian child psychiatrist Mara Selvini Palazzoli (1974) was considering a radical change in her conceptualization of anorexia nervosa: from an intrapsychic to a transpersonal approach to self-starvation. Surprisingly enough, these two clinicians independently from each other developed approaches with many similarities: their respective theoretical conceptualizations of the disorder were remarkably congruent (Lagos, 1981). Their common idea is that anorexia nervosa is not an individual mental illness, but reflects a dysfunctioning of the family system for which it, at the same time, fulfills a homeostatic, stabilizing role.

Minuchin (1970), therefore, stated that according to a systems theory approach the therapist must focus on the family system, i.e., on the characteristic ways of relating to each other, rather than on the individual child. He redefined the crazy symptom of food refusal as an interpersonal problem. Selvini Palazzoli (1974) developed distinctively a similar approach. In her view, anorexia nervosa must be considered as the only possible adaptation by a given subject to a given type of family functioning. Adopting the cybernetic view that a family is a self-regulating system based on certain rules, the therapist must do his utmost to unearth the secret rules (often unconscious and unverbalized) by which the family perpetuates its own dysfunctioning. The publication of these new ideas soon provoked a considerable shift in the theoretical and therapeutic approach to anorexia nervosa patients.

Around these two leaders, two popular schools of family therapy were formed: the structural family approach of the Philadelphia school (Minuchin) and the cybernetic systems model of the Milan school (Selvini Palazzoli). They would dominate the literature on family therapy in anorexia nervosa during the 70s. The ideas developed by Minuchin and co-workers (1978) in particular enjoyed a great popularity, especially in the United States (see e.g., Fishman & Rosman, 1986). Both their theoretical family models and their treatment strategies (in particular the famous "lunch sessions") were welcomed as great innovations. But ten years later, this enthusiasm is still in high contrast with an almost complete absence of methodologically proper research on Minuchin's and Selvini's approach (see also Pinsov, 1981). The defense of the family models as well as the claims regarding treatment efficacy seem still to be largely based on semireligious beliefs instead of on solid research data (Kog & Vandereycken, 1985).

Around 1980, a new movement in family therapy emerged – "the second generation" – integrating concepts and elements from different models (behavioral, structural, strategic, systemic and even psychodynamic). Many clinicians and therapists are now making a plea for a multifaceted – usually eclectic but flexible – family-oriented approach to the treatment of anorexia nervosa (see Vandereycken & Meermann, 1984a). The decade of the 80s will be known for the suddenly growing popular and scientific interest in eating disorders. A decade that started with the official recognition of a "new" syndrome: bulimia (also referred to as bulimia nervosa, bulimarexia, binge eating etc.). Albeit that their existence is not so new (see Casper, 1983), bulimic disorders seem to be emerging in epidemic proportions among young women, especially in the United States. This phenomenon is reflected by the enormous proliferation of scientific literature on the subject. But again, as in the case of anorexia nervosa before, practically all the reports concern the bulimia patient as an individual.

Aside from a few case studies, no systematic family approach has been described with the exception of the work by Schwartz and co-workers (1985) who strongly advocated that bulimia treatment must also focus on the family context. We conclude this short historical excursion by stressing the striking parallelism in the growth of the family therapy movement on the one hand, and the increasing interest in (together with the rising incidence of) eating disorders. Whether there is a connection between these phenomena remains a matter of speculation (see Vandereycken & Meermann, 1984b).

FAMILY THERAPY AND ANOREXIA NERVOSA

Until the 1980s family therapists appeared to be divided into three major groups: (1) *insight-oriented* therapists (such as Boszormenyi-Nagy, Framo and Stierlin) whose goals are to lead the family to an understanding of its problems (hence their connection with the psychoanalytic tradition), and enhance communication of thought and affect; (2) *structural* therapists (Minuchin and the Philadelphia school) who seek to change dysfunctional transactional patterns within the family system using active and straightforward directives around the symptom (i.e., action instead of insight); (3) *strategic* therapists (a rather heterogenous group including Haley, Madanes and Selvini Palazzoli) who are also symptom-oriented but situated within a circular systemic conceptualization according to which it is necessary to uncover the hidden "family game" and attempt to stop the maladaptive cycle by using indirect, seemingly illogical and paradoxical interventions. Since the first group has not made a specific contribution to the treatment of eating disorders (except for Stierlin), we will confine ourselves to an extensive discussion of the contributions from the second and third groups of practitioners who belong to the "first generation" of family therapists. Finally, we will describe the more recent work (from 1980 on) of the "second generation" family therapists, whom one may also call the integrationists or eclecticists.

Minuchin and the Structural Approach

Structural family therapy has become very popular in the treatment of anorexia nervosa, especially after the publication of the book *Psychosomatic Families — Anorexia Nervosa in Context* (Minuchin et al., 1978). Before going into detail concerning the specific therapeutic strategies used by Salvador Minuchin and co-workers, we will first summarize the most important theoretical concepts which apply to families with an anorexia nervosa patient (see also Chapter 2). Based on clinical observations and interactional investigations, Minuchin developed his well-known structural model of psychosomatic families, identifying five predominant characteristics of interactions encountered in families with an anorexic member: enmeshment, overprotectiveness, rigidity, lack of conflict resolution, and involvement of the symptomatic child in the unresolved marital and family conflicts (Liebman et al., 1983).

Enmeshment refers to an extreme form of proximity and intensity in family interactions leading to poorly differentiated subsystem boundaries. *Overprotectiveness* is a relationship in which highly intensive interactions predominate. In anorexic families a feedback system exists in which the patient is often as highly protective toward her parents as they are toward him or her (Liebman et al., 1983). *Rigid* families are heavily committed to maintaining the status quo. When events require change (for example, when a child reaches adolescence), family members insist on retaining accustomed methods of interaction while denying any need for change within the family. Hence, conflicts between family members are often denied or avoided. Normally, such *lack of conflict resolution* within a rigid, overprotecting family system where boundaries are poor due to intensive but enmeshed transactional patterns would lead to an explosive situation if there was no kind of "lightning-rod" within these families. This fifth factor, *involvement of the symptomatic child* in parental (marital) conflicts, forced Minuchin to move from a linear to a systems explanation for the etiology and maintenance of anorexic symptoms: "Parents unable to deal with each other directly unite in protective concern for their sick child, avoiding conflict by protective detouring. Or a marital conflict is transformed into a parental conflict over the patient and her management.... The effectiveness of the symptom bearer in regulating the internal stability of the family reinforces both the continuation of the symptom and the peculiar aspects of the family organization in which it emerged" (Minuchin et al., 1978, p. 32).

Applying this model to anorexia nervosa patients, the structural family therapist starts from the principle that an elimination of the anorexic symptoms is a first and necessary, but insufficient step which must be followed by a basic restructuring of the family system. Usually, structural family therapists are quite active in this process and prefer straightforward directives and interventions to accomplish their goals.

General Principles and Guidelines

Minuchin and his (former) co-workers developed a structural family systems approach to the treatment of anorexics at the Philadelphia Child Guidance Clinic and the Children's Hospital of Philadelphia. Working mainly with children and young adolescents, this child psychiatric-pediatric team prefers an outpatient setting whenever possible. Once the diagnosis of anorexia nervosa is confirmed, the family and the patient have to be prepared for psychotherapeutic intervention. This is done by both the pediatrician and child psychiatrist working in a mutually supportive collaborative fashion. The results of the initial evaluation will determine the need for *inpatient versus outpatient therapy*. Indications for short-term pediatric or psychiatric hospitalization are (Liebman et al., 1983):

- the need to rule out an organic etiology for the weight loss,
- correction of severe metabolic-physiological complications of the disorder,
- the presence of suicidal or (non organic) severe psychotic symptoms in the patient,
- situations in which prior or current outpatient psychotherapy has been ineffective,
- those patients who have repeatedly gained weight in the hospital only to relapse after discharge.

The percentage of patients referred to the Philadelphia group who need hospitalization, has gradually diminished from 57% (Minuchin et al., 1978) to less than 25% (Hodas et al., 1982), and is currently averaging 10-15% (Liebman et al., 1983). This trend may reflect a change in the patient population they are seeing (e.g., earlier referrals, younger or more "benign" cases) as well as a change in the attitude of the treatment team based on growing clinical experience.

The inpatient program is congruent with a family-oriented systems approach to therapy. The general goals of the short-term (3-4 weeks) psychiatric or pediatric hospitalization are to interrupt dysfunctional (but resistant) family coalitions and alliances, and to neutralize the problem of food refusal or threatening weight loss. Further treatment is aimed at stimulating the disengagement process by decreasing symptom severity and at increasing the patient's and parents' sense of competence and effectiveness by the acquisition of new problem-solving skills. Basically, the same strategies are used in both inpatient and outpatient treatment. Hospitalization, however, includes the risk of reinforcing the patient's role as symptom-bearer for the family and, therefore, parents are strongly stimulated to participate in the development and implementation of the treatment plan (Liebman et al., 1983).

In order to initiate weight gain, a behavior therapy program is used in combination with family lunch sessions. As a direct means to decrease the target symptoms of anorexia, an *operant reinforcement paradigm* is used (outpatient example: see Liebman et al., 1983; inpatient example: see Hodas et al., 1982). Usually, the therapist will gradually shift the focus from the individual symptom to the family functioning by assigning anorexia-related but interaction-oriented tasks which establish generational boundaries and clarify differentiation of the roles of the family members. This shift from eating to interpersonal issues is particularly emphasized in the *family lunch session*. This is a rather dramatic meeting in which the patient, the other family members and the therapist(s) eat together (Rosman et al., 1975). If the anorexic eats uneventfully, the therapist will reframe the symptoms as a problem of growing up, communication or other interpersonal issues. If the patient refuses to eat, the parents are given the responsibility of getting their child to eat and they are told to continue working together until the patient cooperates. Occasionally, this can mean that a parent physically forces food into a resistant patient's mouth (Collins et al., 1983). If the parents, however, fail in their attempts to get the patient to eat, the therapist underlines their failure as strongly as possible and points out how the patient has "won" again. The parents are told, then, that they will continue to fail unless they work more effectively together (Hodas et al., 1982). So, in fact, each possible outcome of these lunch sessions can be made useful as a catalyzer within the family-oriented treatment approach.

The lunch sessions may:
- accelerate the process of weight gain;
- enable the patient to eat with her parents without the development of a power struggle; this provides an entirely new experience for the family with respect to eating;
- induce a crisis within the family by bringing the parents to the point of admitting failure or impotence and thus to the point of accepting therapeutic interventions;
- redefine the presenting symptom by dismantling the family's myth that they are fine except for the presence of their "medically sick" child; this formulation is transformed into a recognition of the intrafamilial conflicts and thus decreases the patient's centrality and the manipulative power of the anorexic symptoms;
- provide exceptional opportunities for the therapist to observe family members' transactions around eating and to make on-the-spot interventions to change the patterning of the transaction.

The use of lunch sessions was very popular among structural family therapists and its creation of high drama in the family was often seen as a condition sine qua non for change. Minuchin himself (1984) does not currently stress the need for these lunch sessions, although they remain an interesting diagnostic and therapeutic tool. Miller (1984) even states that Minuchin no longer employs them, finding that he can achieve the same results through less dramatic means (see also Chapter 12 on outpatient treatment).

Once the treatment program starts, the child psychiatrist/family therapist assumes primary responsibility; the family therapy starts while the pediatrician is functioning as consultant. The general goals of the treatment are (Liebman et al., 1983):
- to eliminate the symptom of food refusal and weight loss on which the family concentrates as a way of avoiding or detouring intrafamilial (marital) conflicts;
- to elucidate the dysfunctional patterns in the family that reinforce and maintain the patients' symptoms;
- to change the structure and functioning of the family system in order to prevent relapses or the appearance of a new symptom or a new symptom-bearer.

Once the treatment starts, the family therapist becomes an active intruder, changing the family field by his very presence (Hoffman, 1981). Based on the structural model of normal functioning, the family therapist snaps the family organization and hierarchy and tries, first of all, to create a stable coalition between both parents to take charge over the process of eating, which is defined as an interpersonal task (see also Compernolle, 1982). The patient has to gain a certain amount of weight every week (= responsibility of the patient), and if this does not happen, planned consequences have to be executed (= responsibility of the parents).

During the first weeks of the treatment program, many anorexic patients will test their parents by not reaching the weight goal. The therapist, then, must support the parents to follow and execute the arrangements as they had previously agreed upon. Once the weight starts to progress, the therapist concentrates on trying *to influence the different subsystems of the family and change the family structure.* For this purpose, he starts by accepting and respecting family hierarchies and values, supporting family subsystems and confirming individual members in their self-esteem. He assumes the leadership of the system by presenting himself as an expert, establishing rules of the system, controlling the flow of transactions, organizing and balancing family dyads, supporting or stressing family members and, in general, exploring family members' distorted views of reality and offering them alternatives which promise hope (Minuchin et al., 1978). The therapist joins the family and tries to gain the family's acceptance of his leadership.

The structural family approach to the treatment of anorexia focuses on:
- undermining the family reality or belief system about the anorexic behavior;
- challenging those family patterns (enmeshment, overprotectiveness, etc.) that inhibit the individual growth of family members (especially the anorexic child);
- supporting family members as they struggle with the uncertainties of change;
- giving tasks or directives, modeling and encouraging family members in an effort to establish new, more satisfying patterns of relationship.

Specific Therapeutic Interventions

Beside the aforementioned strategies of operant reinforcement and lunch sessions, many other techniques (also used for other types of problems) are recommended by structural therapists. The challenge to the family members' *experience of reality* is the first step in the process of change (Minuchin et al., 1978). The anorexic family's framing of reality is very often a strong belief that their daughter is sick and suffers from a strange, incurable illness. An often-employed reframing of this reality by structural family therapists is redefining the eating or weight problem as a fight for control between parents and child. The anorexic behavior is then relabeled as a voluntary act and, hence, placed within the triadic-relationship among parents and child (examples: Minuchin, 1984, p. 107; Minuchin & Fishman, 1981, p. 138).

When *challenging enmeshment,* Minuchin et al. (1978, p. 98) point out three different operations: supporting the individual's life space, strengthening subsystem boundaries and supporting the hierarchical organization of the family system. These operations are aimed to promote autonomy and individuation of the different family members. Challenging enmeshment means, for example:

- blocking mind-reading acts, every family member has to speak for himself or herself (in the first person) and cannot answer for another;
- reinforcing competent acts, especially of the anorexic patient;
- seeing the different subsystems (parents as well as children) separately;
- modeling respect for generational boundaries by not allowing a child to intrude in discussions between the parents.

Many of these operations do *challenge overprotectiveness as well.* In addition, it is important that the therapist supports coping behavior of the anorexic child (example: Minuchin, 1984, p. 99). *Conflict-avoiding transactions* are very often deeply embedded in the anorexic system. Most of these families present themselves as "ideal," without any significant problem except for their daughter's anorexia. Interventions are needed that create boundaries and help the disagreeing family members to discuss and resolve their conflicts. The therapist acts as a "gatekeeper," preventing intrusion and escape, and maintaining the dialogue longer. It is not uncommon for the child to be involved in parental conflicts — and, therefore, for family therapy to end marital therapy for the spouses. Challenging conflict avoidance means also stimulating the development of conflict resolution (negotiation) between the parents and the anorexic child in areas outside the issue of eating (examples: Minuchin et al., 1978, p. 320; Minuchin, 1984, p. 103). Minuchin (1984, p. 99) states: "In my work with anorectics, I have observed that a capacity for direct challenge in an area not related to food is a pre-requisite for improvement." Once family members engage in negotiating about conflicts, the therapist tries to encourage explicit conflict in areas of normal autonomy. Since "cure and growth" are the most important goals in the treatment of anorexics, Minuchin encourages the *process of individuation* and independence of the anorexic patient. It is interesting to remark here that Minuchin, in his reinterpretation of the Menotti family in his book *Family Kaleidoscope* (1984, p. 101) — a case report originally published in "Psychosomatic Families" (1978) — stresses more the importance of this "growth" process toward a higher degree of autonomy, and he seems to give more attention to typical individual-related issues such as the anorexic's strong negative self-perceptions and feelings of ineffectiveness.

To challenge *the rigid transaction patterns* in the anorexic family system the therapist has to force up intensity and drama by frequent repetition of his messages (see, e.g., Minuchin & Fishman, 1981, p. 122), increasing the duration of conflictful encounters between family members and creating no-exit boundaries. The structural family therapist often tries to provoke an enactment of the family conflicts within the therapeutic room (see, for example, the lunch sessions) and repeatedly creates a dramatic atmosphere.

Challenging the structures that keep the child involved as a *conflict-detouring* pathway is perhaps the hardest of the therapeutic strategies to discuss in the abstract, requiring, as it does, an ability "to run with the hares and to hunt with the hound" (Minuchin et al., 1978, p. 106). Sometimes the family therapist can block directly the intrusive maneuvers of parents and child, and other times he can enter into a coalition with (more than) one family member to imbalance the prevailing family structure. Often the therapist must block the conversation in order to prevent the patient from being triangulated between the parents and to shift focus of dialogue away from her (example: Minuchin et al., 1978, p. 258).

Though what has been said up to now about challenging these structural patterns of enmeshment, overprotectiveness, conflict avoidance, and rigidity may look quite simple and logical, it demands a high affective involvement and a lot of creative skills on the part of the therapist. Although the therapeutic process and strategy looks very simple and logical, the practice of structural family therapy is much more difficult. Moreover, family therapists must remain flexible and adapt their approach to the *developmental needs* of the symptomatic child and the family life cycle. The parental authority needs to be rational in the sense that it should be flexible and in harmony with the child's level of development (Compernolle, 1982). For preadolescents, the primary goal of therapy is increasing parental effectiveness (control) and strengthening the parental coalition especially around executive functions. When working with this age group, therapists use family sessions initially, shifting to parent-only sessions in the later phases, while the preadolescent patients are not seen individually.

When working with adolescents, the focus is on increasing their independence and, at the same time, decreasing parental control and overprotectiveness. Here, separate sessions with the different subsystems (individual, siblings, couple) are more common. Parents and children are, therefore, stimulated to discuss more typically adolescent conflicts associated with this developmental period. Frequently, parents and the adolescent patient are seen separately: the first to discuss marital issues, the latter to discuss age-appropriate issues. Only a small minority of the anorexia nervosa patients described by Minuchin and co-workers were between the age of 17 and 21. In older adolescents and young adults, the structural family therapist works only in the beginning with family therapy sessions, switching more quickly to separate individual sessions in order to promote self-differentiation and autonomy. The launching of the young adult into an independent life becomes the most important goal.

Some Adherents of the Structural Approach

We will just mention briefly those clinicians who preferred the structural family model in their work with anorexic patients, insofar as they published their research and theories. There are, of course, the people who had been trained by or worked with Minuchin and his team at the Philadelphia Child Guidance Clinic and the Children's Hospital of Philadelphia. In many of Minuchin's publications between 1975 and 1983 the same names appear (in varying order, see list of references): Ronald Liebman, Lester Baker, Bernice L. Rosman. Other co-workers were Lee Combrinck-Graham (1974), Leroy Milman and Thomas Todd (see Minuchin et al., 1973, 1975). Braulio Montalvo is acknowledged in the early reports (e.g., Liebman et al., 1973a + b) for his assistance in the analysis of the family lunch sessions.

Barcai (1971) was one of the first clinicians who was not directly affiliated with the Philadelphia group who endorsed Minuchin's ideas in a leading journal (*American Journal of Psychiatry*). But, at the same time, he warned against the existence of possibly negative effects of crisis-induced family therapy: "1. The family may be unable to sustain anxiety induced by the crisis approach and might thus choose to discontinue therapy. 2. An inadvertent, dangerous, and alarming reaction might occur in other family members as a result of confrontation and release of affects that have been put up for a long time" (p. 283). As an example of this second situation, Barcai mentioned the case report by Minuchin (1970) where, following the intervention in a family of a male anorexic, the father made a suicide gesture.

Minuchin's approach to anorexia nervosa seemed to be officially recognized in the field of family therapy by Aponte and Hoffman's (1973) well-known article in *Family Process*. It was a lengthy commentary on a videotape of an initial interview by Minuchin with a family of an anorexic girl. In fact, videotapes of this kind (e.g., Minuchin, 1982) became available for professional training and were shown all over the world (we would like to add here that in our opinion Minuchin exploited his success commercially to such an extent that he finally was more "on tour" than in a therapist's chair).

After Minuchin left Philadelphia, Liebman became the leading figure who continued to work according to the same principles but more within a collaborative child psychiatric-pediatric team approach (Collins et al., 1983; Hodas et al., 1982; Liebman et al., 1983; Sargent et al., 1985). Fishman (1979) too, became a prominent figure: he co-authored, with Minuchin, the book on *Family Therapy Techniques* (Minuchin & Fishman, 1981) and he attempted to apply the structural family model onto adult anorexics (see also Keeney & Ross, 1985, pp. 177-204). Other examples of the application of the structural family approach to the treatment of anorexia nervosa are reported by Compernolle (1981, 1982), Conrad (1977), Hendrickx (1981a), Hubschmid (1979), Lagos (1981), Miller (1984), and by Moore and Coulman (1981).

Conclusion

The structural approach relies upon a theoretical model of normal family structure and starts from a comparison between this normative model and the observed structure in the anorexic family. The latter is typified by the following structural characteristics: enmeshment, overprotection, conflict-avoidance, rigidity, and involvement of the child in parental conflict. When challenging these dysfunctional interactions, Minuchin acts as a strong, emotionally involved director of the family drama, focusing especially on the triadic relationship between the parents and the anorexic child (Keeney & Ross, 1985). This triadic structure is used as an entrance to the family system. The final goal is dismantling and changing this family structure in order to promote "cure and growth."

Structural family therapy as the main approach appears to be very useful in fairly young anorexics with intact families, on the conditions that the parents are relatively healthy emotionally, that the eating disorder has not lasting for too long a time, and that the index patient is not entangled in a chronically disturbed family pattern (Vandereycken & Meermann, 1984a). Although the results of this approach do look quite impressive, the outcome research (Minuchin et al., 1978) was too weak to allow overenthusiastic conclusions (see Chapter 3). In fact, team members of the Philadelphia group themselves state that they have found treatment to be more difficult and complicated:

- in patients having symptoms of eating disorder for more than one year prior to referral;
- for patients with prior significant delays or problems in psychosocial development;
- in families where the parents are separated or divorced, or where one parent is deceased;
- in families in which one or both parents display severe psychopathology (Liebman et al., 1983).

When we consider the patients and families we are treating in our center, they mostly correspond with the above conditions. It is our experience that restructuring interactions within these families does seldom suffice on its own in order to promote profound change on the long-term, not just with regard to the family functioning in general, but especially concerning the patient's physical and psychological well-being as an autonomous individual. Reaching this goal usually requires an intensive, multidimensional approach of which family therapy may be one of the major ingredients.

Selvini Palazzoli and the Systemic Model

The contributions of Maria Selvini Palazzoli and her co-workers Luigi Boscolo, Gianfranco Cecchin and Giuliana Prata at the Milan Family Center (Centro per lo Studio della Famiglia di Milano) received widespread interest and growing popularity in the field of family therapy (Campbell & Draver, 1985). The Milan approach is probably the one closest to orthodox systems theory, but viewed from a more pragmatic perspective they belong to the group of strategic therapists. Though the influence of the Milanese school on the family therapeutic approach to anorexia nervosa has not been as great as Minuchin's, its impact is considerable and unmistakable.

Selvini Palazzoli first began to work with anorexics from an individual-oriented psychoanalytic and existential-phenomenologic viewpoint. Disillusioned by her poor treatment results and impressed by the systems theory literature, she switched to a family approach (Selvini, 1974) which was mainly inspired by cybernetics and communication theory (Haley, Watzlawick, Jackson, Beavin and Bateson).

Two influential works highlight the basic ideas of the Milan approach: *Self-Starvation* (1974) which deals with Selvini's evolution from the intrapsychic to the transpersonal approach to anorexia nervosa, and *Paradox and Counter-paradox* (1978), which describes a new model for the therapy of families with schizophrenic transactions.

General Principles and Guidelines

Selvini developed and delineated a systemic view of anorexia nervosa, in which the symptom-bearer or index patient serves a homeostatic, stabilizing role in the family. We will summarize the fundamental characteristics of this model (see also Chapter 2). Like Minuchin's notion of "enmeshment," Selvini (1974, p. 242) noted that "the collective sense of the family is so pronounced that the individual is pushed into the background. There is a tendency to stick together like a brood of ducklings." She observed that in these families *self-sacrifice* is regarded as the most important of personal qualities, so much so that any form of personal interest has to be excluded.

Using Jay Haley's model about the pragmatic axioms of human communication, Selvini et al. (1976) further identified the following interactional characteristics within anorexic families:

- every member commonly rejects or disqualifies messages sent by others;
- all family members, and especially the parents, are reluctant to assume personal leadership overtly (i.e., proscription of individuality);
- although secret coalitions are very common, open alliances between two members against a third are forbidden;
- no one family member is really prepared to assume personal responsibility for error or insult; the anorexic symptom is accepted because the patient cannot help it ("she is ill").

Selvini (1974) further adds that "behind the facade of respectability and marital unit, the parents generally conceal a deep disillusionment with each other that they are quite unable to acknowledge, let alone resolve" (p. 213). The couple displays a "symmetry through sacrifical escalation" that urged them to join in secret alliances and to focus especially on the patient, who is secretly encouraged to side with the more persecuted of her two parents.

In summary, Selvini noted that anorexic families are characterized by a high degree of marital dysfunction, problems of leadership, a rejection of communicated messages, poor conflict resolution, covert alliances or "denied coalitions" between family members, blame shifting and extreme rigidity. Though she focused her attention on intrafamilial communication processes while Minuchin studied family structures, both views led to theoretical conclusions and concepts that have many similarities (Lagos, 1981; Miller, 1984). It is a pity that they did not use the same language, which makes communication between different family theorists and therapists at times very difficult and confusing.

Although Selvini and co-workers offer the reader a lot of information about the formal characteristics and process of their family therapy sessions (Selvini, 1974; Selvini et al., 1978, 1980a + b) they do not discuss indication criteria for eventually inpatient treatment* nor do they describe what kind of anorexic patients and families they have treated (duration of illness, previous treatment, age, intact families, etc.). Moreover, well-outlined follow-up data are completely absent.

Family therapy is carried out on an *outpatient* basis by a group of four therapists (two women and two men). The active pair meets with the family and the other pair observes through a one-way mirror (more recently, only one therapist conducts the interview, with one to three colleagues behind the screen). During the first meeting the family members are informed that the sessions will be videotaped and that the therapists work in a team together with colleagues observing the family from behind the one-way mirror. The family is also told that, in the course of the treatment, they will receive a number of directives, and that the overall success of the therapy depends on their implementation. The therapeutic observers intervene only "when things go terribly wrong:" they will then knock on the door, call the active therapist outside the room, and suggest a different strategy. All decisions about the assignment of tasks or the prescription of rituals are made by the team as a whole. Strategic decisions can be prepared before or during the sessions. In the latter case, the therapeutic team interrupts the sessions and goes into conference. The intervention or recommendation of the team can be a ritual, a task or a prescription. It will be given at the end of the session and must be shared by all family members. It can be in written form, in which case each member is given or sent a copy.

The family is invariably seen as a whole, but may from time to time be split up into different groups in order to stabilize, for example, intergenerational boundaries. The treatment should be completed in no more than twenty sessions within a certain time limit. There is also a tendency to fix a long interval

---

* Selvini (1974, p. 717) advises, for the sake of the patient's psychological health, against hospitalization if there is any alternative. She admits, however, that she has no personal experience with inpatient treatment and that her opinion may be influenced by the situation in Italy where "the hospital atmosphere is, with few exceptions, not conducive to psychotherapeutic treatment."

(monthly or longer) between the sessions, especially after the therapists feel they have made a good contact with the family. Ever since they have used longer intervals between the sessions, they have found that concrete instruction may have a much greater effect (Selvini et al., 1980b). Each family has its own time span for processing a complex set of information and, the more richly joined or enmeshed the system, the longer the time it will take for this process (Hoffman, 1981). The systemic approach seems to be, at the same time, a brief therapy considering the number of sessions, and a long treatment considering the length of time needed for change and family reorganization.

Specific Therapeutic Interventions

The Milan approach to anorexia nervosa differs in many aspects from the structural family therapy. Unlike Minuchin's approach, eliminating the symptom of food refusal and weight loss no longer has priority. Instead, the first step is detecting a hypothesis that will explain the symptom within the family system. *Hypothesizing* for the systemic family therapist refers "to the formulation of an hypothesis based upon the information he possesses regarding the family he is interviewing. The hypothesis establishes a starting point for his investigation as well as his verification of the validity of this hypothesis based upon specific methods and skills. If the hypothesis is proven false, the therapist must form a second hypothesis based upon the information gathered during the testing of the first" (Selvini et al., 1980, p. 4). This hypothesis must be systemic, including all components of the family, and must furnish a supposition concerning the total functioning of the family. So, the hypothesis underlines the function of the anorexic behavior for all family members. To gather all the information necessary to form a hypothesis that fits family systems, Selvini et al. (1980) advocate the use of *circularity* and *circular questioning*.

Circularity means "the capacity of the therapist to conduct his investigation on the basis of feedback from the family in response to the information he solicits about relationships and, therefore, about difference and change" (p. 8). Circular questioning, on the other hand, assumes that every member of the family is invited to tell the therapist how he or she sees the relationship between the two other members of the family. Through this type of questioning the family therapist breaks one of the secret rules of anorexic families.

The authors describe several interview techniques for soliciting information to form a systemic hypothesis. The therapist gathers information:

- in terms of specific interactive behavior in specific circumstances and not in terms of feelings or interpretations (*example:* "What does your mother do when your sister refuses to eat? How does your father react to what your mother does?");
- in terms of differences in behavior and not in terms of predicates supposedly intrinsic to the person (*example,* concerning the so-called

meddlesomeness of grandparents: "Who intervenes the most, your grandfather or your grandmother?");
- in terms of ranking or classification by various members of the family of a specific behavior or a specific interaction (*example:* "Who can cheer your mother up the most when she's sad—your grandmother, father, brother or you? Make a scale");
- in terms of (behavior indicative of) change in the relationship before and after a precise event, i.e., diachronic investigation (*example:* the therapist can ask if the patient started to eat less before or after a specific life event in the family);
- in terms of differences with respect to hypothetical circumstances (*example:* the therapist may ask "How both parents would go along when the children would leave the house and start to live on their own").

From the first session all these methods are used for the investigation of the symptom: "Rather than become enmeshed in the tedious listing of symptomatic behavior, the therapist conducts the investigation of *how* each member of the family reacts to the symptom" (Selvini et al., 1980, p. 10).

The goal of these circular techniques is to gather information about the sequential organization of the problem, other relevant behaviors and the actual family coalitions. But the Milan team also tries to make an analysis of the patterns of relationship within the referring contexts, and of past and future views of coalition patterns, particularly in association with the onset of the eating problem. As Keeney and Ross (1985, p. 206) point out: "The Milan approach is not primarily a symptom or problem-focused therapy, although it addresses these communications. Its emphasis is on the 'context of meaning' that phrases and organizes symptoms. The aim is to discover a pattern of contextual meaning for use in helping the troubled system reorganize itself."

Once such a systemic hypothesis is constructed, the next move is to encourage the family and the symptomatic member to continue with their problem behavior. Moreover, the symptomatic behavior is positively connotated and connected with the larger configuration of relationships surrounding the problem. *Positive connotation* (reframing, relabeling, restructuring) within the anorexic family means that all behaviors are considered as, for example, "expressions of love" or as "the result of the understandable desire to maintain the unity of the family exposed to so much strain and threat of dissolution." The therapist underscores that the entire group is engaged in a single pursuit, namely the preservation of the unity and stability of the family. He shows that the patient is so sensitive and generous that she cannot help sacrificing herself for her family, much as the others cannot help sacrificing themselves for the same ends.

The way is now open for the decisive therapeutic step: *the therapeutic paradox.* The symptom, defined as essential to family stability, is prescribed by the therapist, who advises the patient to continue limiting her food intake, at least for the time being. Simultaneously, the relatives are also instructed to persist in

their customary behavior patterns (Selvini, 1975, pp. 234-235). Positive connotation gives the symptom a positive function and puts all the members of the
family system, including the identified patients, on the same level. Within this
reframed context, the symptomatic behavior of all family members is prescribed. So, it is not just a matter of setting a paradoxical task, but to find interactional or transactional paradoxes involving all family members and thus linking the symptom to the rest of the system. All too often, the Milan approach is
erroneously viewed as simply paradoxical treatment, especially the use of ritualized prescriptions. Though rituals and paradoxes are major ingredients in the
approach (see Selvini et al., 1977, 1978), the crucial aspect is not the technique
but rather the systemic reconceptualization of the problem (for detailed discussion of the approach see: Campbell & Draper, 1985; Weeks & L'Abate, 1982).
Maybe the misunderstandings have been induced by the authors themselves,
especially Boscolo and Cecchin (1982), who appeared to pay special attention
to this part of the therapeutic work. Keeney and Ross (1985), however, remark
that this emphasis on "given prescriptions" has declined and that the Milan therapists moved to a seemingly simple kind of questioning, which, nevertheless, is
assumed to provide "invisible prescriptions" toward the family.

In fact, the Milan approach consists of other important aspects. A further
step in the therapeutic process can be described as a dialectical movement between the therapist's hypothesis and the reactions and responses of the family
members toward the questions and formulated hypotheses of the therapeutic
team. This process must be governed by *neutrality* on the part of the therapeutic team. It means that the family therapist tries to avoid alliances with any family
member (by having successive alliances with everyone and by neutralizing any
attempt toward coalition, seduction, or privileged relationships with him) and
that he abstains from moral judgments of any kind. The Milan group believes
"that the therapist can be effective only to the extent that he is able to obtain
and maintain a different level (*metalevel*) from that of the family" (Selvini et al.,
1980, p. 11).

Finally, there are some specific strategies aimed at altering the typical communication characteristics and transactional patterns that exist within the anorexic family system. In order to challenge the problem of *the rejection of messages,* the active therapeutic team can split into two parts: one therapist play the
"passive" part of the silent observer. When the family does not agree upon what
the "active" therapist says (rejecting his message), the "passive" observer can
overtly discuss with his partner in front of the family about what is going on
(metacommunication). Both therapists can agree then upon the family's view
by arguing that if every member of the family finds it so difficult to confirm what
the therapist says, there must be a good reason for it, and no attempt need be
made to change it. In more rigid and difficult cases showing a higly repetitive
pattern of rejecting messages, a similar preplanned splitting technique may be
useful: one therapist can attack a family member very sharply, while his co-ther-

apist openly disagrees and explicitly allies himself with the attacked member. The rejected therapist looks duly contrite and, by acknowledging his error, confirms his colleague's message.

To challenge the *problem of leadership* the therapist emphasizes to the family the natural right of each person to have desires of his own and to express them openly. He then asks each family member to state his or her likes and dislikes in the first person. One family member can assume the task of deserving the other family members and noting any failures to adhere to this rule.

When facing the *problem of coalitions* Selvini (1974) notes that the fathers in anorexic families are very often labeled as peripheric and unreliable. The mother tries to convince the therapist that father is totally incompetent as to family problems, a belief that is completely assented to by the husband. To challenge this problem of coalitions, it may be essential to draw father and daughter into a constructive alliance, be it only temporarily, and with great care that it is not destructive to the mother (example: see Selvini Palazzoli, 1974, p. 225). The final goal of this type of intervention is to disentangle the secret coalitions between one generation and the next, i.e., to open the generation gap, so that the daughter may at long last start having her own life.

Possitive connotation of the symptomatic behavior and the transactional patterns within the family system is a suitable technique with which to intervene into the problem of *blame shifting.* The therapeutic team, however, takes great care not to accuse anybody in whatever form or sense, and least of all the parents. Many anorexic patients are indeed experts in blaming their parents indirectly. The therapists try to short-circuit this behavior by positively connotating the parents' reaction, for example, as "self-sacrificing activities for the welfare of their daughter."

Some Adherents of the Systemic-Strategic Approach

The ideas and techniques emanating from Milan, first from the Center for the Study of the Family (with Selvini as leading figure) and later from the Center for Family Therapy (founded in 1983 by Boscolo and Cecchin) have inspired much enthusiasm and criticism on both sides of the Atlantic (see Campbell & Draper, 1985; Tomm, 1984). However, when we look at the publications from other therapists who apply the systemic-strategic model to the treatment of anorexia nervosa, the literature is scarce and mostly European. In the U.S., the Milan model appears to be erroneously identified with a specific type of ritualized paradoxical therapy and has been, as such, widely applied (see Weeks & L'Abate, 1982). The influence of the Milan group may be found in many family therapists of the "second generation" who integrated useful concepts and techniques within a more eclectic model. The few specific reports we found in the literature on the application of the Milan approach all came from Europe. Caillé and co-workers (1977) from Oslo described a Selvini-like systemic family therapy in a case of anorexia nervosa and they concluded that the systems theory approach provides neither explanations nor norms for the problematic situation: "After treatment is ended, the family will not have an intellectual explanation for how improvement occurred. In this way, the treatment process resembles the learning process of Zen-Budhism. The teacher challenges the student with unconventional answers to his questions until the student has no alternative but to discover his own truth" (p. 404). Pina Prata (1980) and Elkaim (1979), in a similar sense, describe systemic family therapy in anorexics. Buddeberg and Buddeberg (1979) stress a type of double-bind communication in anorexic families: the parents communicate to the patient that she must grow up but without leaving the family, whereas the patient seems to react that she will remain at home but that she will punish her parents for it. Anyway, these authors emphasize the paradoxical component together with the positive connotation as crucial elements in the treatment. Finally, Epple (1984) reports on the choice between Minuchin's and Selvini's approaches to anorexia nervosa. According to this author, the Milan method is to be preferred in families with great resistance to changes, in families with a predominantly irrelevant style of communication, and in families with an identified patient older than 18 years.

Conclusions

In 1974 Selvini emphasized that her data should be considered preliminary because of the smallness of her sample (p. 204) and that her conclusions are tentative "since only follow-ups can tell us, whether the improvements are either lasting, or, as we hope, stepping stones on the road to further progress" (p. 242). Now, more than ten years later, we are still waiting for well-outlined research and follow-up data demonstrating the effectiveness of the Milan approach to the treatment of anorexia nervosa. In the meantime the Milan Family Center published several reports with (unfortunately much of the same) absorbing, stimulating and fascinating casuistry.

Nevertheless we have learned a lot from their work, both for diagnostic purposes and therapeutic practice. Their unique interviewing procedure of the family, while collecting data to construct an hypothesis that underlines the function of the anorexic symptom within the family system, enlarged our diagnostic and assessment skills. Especially the formulation and presentation of a systemic hypothesis to the family, including an interactional but positive reframing of the problems, helped us to avoid the symmetrical fight with the family and to evade the high resistance for change, so common in these rigid family systems.

But the same point made regarding Minuchin's approach, is also applicable and appropriate to the systemic-strategic treatment model: in our experience, the more difficult (severe or chronic) cases of anorexia nervosa need more than just family therapy. Once again, we recommend a multifaceted approach, wherein family therapy — or better a family-oriented approach — is just one component of a total treatment program which also addresses the individual (psychological and biological) aspects of anorexia nervosa.

The "Second Generation" Search for Integration

By the late 1970s, a clear tendency toward developing an eclectic or integrated treatment approach to eating disorders began to stand out (Garfinkel & Garner, 1982). This current trend toward eclecticism and integration is recognizable, first, in the incorporation of family therapy within a multidimensional in- or outpatient treatment program, and, second, in the abandonment of orthodox adherence to one particular school of family therapy. Instead, more and more family therapists tend to combine concepts and strategies derived from different models (psychodynamic, behavioral, structural, strategic and systemic).

Integration and Eclecticism

In the German- and French-speaking parts of Europe, the development from individual to family therapy has been strongly influenced by and is still embedded to a great extent in the psychoanalytic tradition. A particular characteristic of this evolution, as reflected in the treatment of anorexia nervosa, is the tendency not to replace the individual psychotherapeutic approach by family therapy, but rather to combine or to integrate both. Though in 1976, a Germany medical journal for general practitioners summarized the treatment of anorexia nervosa in one telling headline: "rule out the parents" ("Magersucht-Therapie: Eltern ausschalten," *Praxis-Kurier,* May 26, 1976, p. 30), clinicians at the University Hospital of Heidelberg started to publish their experience with a "polypragmatic" approach to the treatment of inpatient anorexics including special sessions of what they called "family confrontation therapy" (Petzold, 1976; Petzold et al., 1976a + b; Petzold, 1979). These as well as other German publications in the 1970s (e.g., Buddeberg & Buddeberg, 1979; Overbeck, 1979; Sperling & Massing, 1972) clearly represent attempts to enlarge the scope on anorexia nervosa from an intrapsychic to an interpersonal view, thereby using a psychodynamic language for the translation of intrafamilial processes. Only recently, the same tendency is emerging in the French literature (e.g., Snakkers, 1984; Stelzer, 1984). In fact, the psychoanalytic therapist remains the same, but now the family is lying "on the couch" (Eiguer, 1983).

An important integrationist, who really succeeded in the development of a psychodynamic family model (a fruitful mixture of European traditionalism and American creativeness), is Helm Stierlin, head of what we may call the "Heidelberg school of psychosomatics" (Winawer, 1983; Wirsching & Stierlin, 1985; see also Chapter 2). Although Stierlin and co-workers seem to move progressively toward systemic thinking, basically they emphasize individual dynamics in dialogue with family dynamics. Another attempt at enlarging the scope on the part of family therapists is described by White (1983) who pays attention to cognitive aspects. He suggests a possible link between the anorexic symptoms and certain rigid but implicit family beliefs transmitted through the generations (transgenerational issues are discussed in Chapter 17). A more explicit cognitivistic approach is defended by Guidano and Liotti (1983). They focus on the patients' cognitive organization as shaped by their developmental history, especially in dyadic transaction with the parents. These authors, however, prefer an individual psychotherapy in order to challenge the maladaptive cognitive organization of anorexic patients. This brings us to the discussion of treatment preferences or, more specifically, the question of *compatibility of family therapy with individual therapy*. In fact, there seems not to exist a real incompatibility regardless the primary preference of the therapist: Bruch (1978), for example, included certain family tasks in her individual-oriented treatment, whereas Minuchin et al. (1978) consider the possibility of individual sessions depending on the developmental stage of the patient (see Lagos, 1981). Peake and Borduin (1977) express this need for flexibility as follows: "We would not like to treat an anorexic by having to choose only one theoretical approach. The classical analytic approach would neglect the family and the urgent need for symptom change; the behavioral approach can change the symptoms, but may leave unaltered the family dynamics and the explanation of the girl denying her femininity; and the family approach, alone...may fail to respond to urgent symptoms" (p. 55).

There's a strong tendency toward a multimodal eclectic approach that, to a varying degree and usually in a flexible way, combines individual and family therapy, often intertwining behavioral, psychodynamic, structural, strategic and other interventions (Batholomew, 1984; Dare, 1983; Hedblom et al., 1982; Koizumi & Luidens, 1984; Kwee & Duivenvoorden, 1985; Mirkin, 1983; Moultrup, 1981; Piazza et al., 1980; Schneider, 1981; Todd, 1985). Treatment is then aimed at different levels of functioning (Dym, 1985), but such a multidimensional approach requires an integrative way of thinking on the part of the therapist or the therapeutic team. This is necessary in order to avoid the unproductive "supermarket" treatment in which an accidental accumulation of techniques is used as a machine-gun to ensure that some targets are hit. The *ecosystemic* treatment perspective, described by Stachowiak and Briggs (1984), is a valuable alternative and a fruitful frame of reference. It is a multiple-level treatment perspective founded on principles of human ecology and systems theory. Diagnosis and treatment are focused on the most inclusive system context relevant to the problem situation: "The unit of treatment is the person-environment context, taken as a whole. This context is in turn composed of a series of interlocking system levels. Physiological and intrapsychic processes interact with dyadic and family dynamics all within a network of social relationships, role responsibilities, and community-cultural influences. From this matrix of interaction, the therapist selects relevant elements from each system level to compose a system context suitable for intervention" (Stachowiak & Briggs, 1984, p. 7). The authors illustrate this approach with the case of an anorexia nervosa patient who was treated by combining different treatment forms (including family therapy) within a residential setting. Their working-method is probably exemplary for many treatment centers in the area of eating disorders (see e.g., Andersen, 1985; Crisp, 1980; Garfinkel & Garner, 1982; Vandereycken & Meermann, 1984a).

Finally, as in the case of psychotherapy, one can no longer speak about *the* family therapy since so many forms have been developed and many other will be "invented." Again as in the field of psychotherapies, the expanding movement of family therapies is characterized by a tension between orthodoxy and flexibility, theoretical purity and technical eclecticism. "In everyday practice, the schools of family therapy tend to become synthetic and integrative. Therapists from technique-oriented schools, that focus on small sequences of interaction (behaviorists and strategists), have began to adopt the organizing frameworks of schools with more comprehensive understanding of family dynamics (Bowenian and structural). At the same time, certain techniques that have proven their potency have been adopted by many of the schools of family therapy. Family therapists of all persuasions are now likely to clarify communications, direct enactments, and prescribe resistance, no matter what their approach" (Nichols, 1984, p. 509).

In the next part, we will give an overview of those strategies and interventions in family therapy with anorexia nervosa patients that are born out of this "second generation" of therapists and which, in our clinical experience, proved to be quite useful particularly for family therapy in cases of severe or chronic eating disorders.

Direct and Indirect Interventions

In their inspiring book *Behind the Family Mask* Andolfi and his colleagues (1983) at the Family Therapy Institute in Rome describe a creative and highly dramatic systemic approach to promote therapeutic change in rigid family systems. Andolfi's family therapeutic approach to anorexia nervosa demonstrates quite convincingly, in our opinion, how concepts and strategies from different models — namely the structural approach of Minuchin, the strategic and paradoxical interventions of Watzlawick and Haley, the systemic model of Selvini Palazzoli, and the experiential teachings of Whitaker — can be integrated in a creative and effective way. The innovative element in Andolfi's approach lies in the combination and alternation of direct and indirect interventions: active provocation and strategic denial.

At one moment the family therapist becomes the director of the family drama and tries to provoke, in a most direct way, a crisis within the family, using the identified patient as entrance into the anorexic family system. The first objective is to induce a therapeutic crisis, but "we must be certain we have the strength to provoke one and to do it in such a manner that the intensity of the crisis is directly in proportion to the degree of rigidity present in the family system" (Andolfi et al., 1983, p. 46). The therapists further hypothesize that their counterprovocative response might use the anorexic patient as the point of attack in the system: "If the family provokes the therapist and controls the therapeutic system through the identified patient, the therapist, too, must try to provoke the family and to control the therapeutic system using the same channel" (p. 51). Andolfi et al. (1983, pp. 62-63) describe the first family session with a married anorexic (Donatella), both her parents, her husband and one brother. Donatella enters the room, sustained by her mother and her brother. She says nothing and the therapist immediately seats her behind his back, excluding her totally from the circle he has created with the rest of the family. He does not pay attention to her "because she'll never give an adult response!" He then goes on stressing to the rest of the family that she is absorbing all attention "with this story of not eating...."

This *active provocative* style or direct confrontation is regularly alternated with another seemingly opposite approach, namely anticipating and neutralizing the possible relapse of the family. In this paradoxical technique of *strategic denial*, the therapist "allies himself with the homeostatic element in the system, unearthing and amplifying the bases for the impossibility of change" (p. 71). In the very first session already, the therapist can, for example, deny the need for therapy, especially in cases where the parents "have searched everywhere for the right 'magician' who would work wonders, but every attempt at therapy has been flatly refused" (Andolfi et al., 1983, p. 76). The same strategic denial can be used later on when the first signs of improvement are observed or reported by the family. The therapist again denies this improvement and may even define it as dangerous. Andolfi et al. (1983, pp. 79-82) illustrate this paradoxical strategy in the case of a 15-year-old girl with serious anorexia nervosa. In the preceding session the therapist had provoked the patient in her function as the link between her parents. The therapy sessions have brought about noticable improvement in the girl's symptomatology, as well as in the relations between the family members. The therapist now organizes a lunch session in order to deny the improvement. During this session the patient stresses she is going better, but for the therapist it sounds like a strange miracle. By refusing her proof of improvement, he stimulates the girl to defend her successes and causes the parents to take a position which, at the same time, brings their difficulties into the open. For this type of interventions to be successful an intense and positive relationship between the family and the therapist must exist. Now encouraging changes in the family members and then warning them about the same changes is like the movement of a pendulum: a process of alternating the times of participation, where the therapist enters the emotional space of the family (provocation), with periods of separation, when he leaves (denial). The ultimate goal is to permit the family to become more flexible in such a way that they can find their own capacity for growth and change.

Similar to Andolfi's alternation strategy is Peggy Papp's (1980, 1983) technique of the *Greek Chorus*, which, in our experience, is very useful in the treatment of rigid families with a high resistance and fear of change. It consists of the creation of a therapeutic triangle between the family, the active therapist(s) and a consultation group behind the one-way mirror. This consultation group acts as a *Greek Chorus,* providing a commentary on the interaction between the family and the therapist, and on the phenomenon of systemic change: how it will come about, what the consequences will be (for whom and in what way) and what the alternatives are. While the active therapist encourages the family toward change, the consultation group regularly sends a message in the family therapy room to warn the therapist and the family for the danger of systemic change. The difference with Andolfi's alternation between active provocation and strategic denial lies in the fact that the paradoxical attitude is carried out by a third group: the consultation group takes the position of the antagonist of change while the family therapist, who has a direct and personal relationship with the family, functions as the protagonist of change. The family is given two opposite messages at the same time, confronted with an inevitable dilemma: if they change, they prove the therapist right, if they remain the same, they prove the group right (this resembles Selvin's splitinig technique described above.)

Papp (1983, pp. 97-98) illustrates this technique with the example of a 23-year-old anorexic woman, who had begun dieting four years before. The consultation group is advising her not to change (i.e., leaving home) for her own sake, while the therapist emphasizes he cannot endorse that opinion, since it would imply that she should be unhappy and should not make her life any better. The patient immediately agrees with the therapist, who then thanks her for this support of his viewpoint! One must bear in mind, however, that these techniques are not tricks but well-planned interventions within a therapeutic framework that comprises many other essential components. Peggy Papp's (1983) lengthy case description of "the daughter who said no" is a telling illustration of such a flexible, multiform attempt to change an anorexic family system.

Hospitalization as Therapeutic Strategy

Though hospitalization must be a heathenish idea in the mind of a rigid systems theorist, the "second generation" family therapist is no longer led by the sacred laws of orthodoxy but rather by the pragmatics of clinical practice. It is a matter of both the unavoidability of hospitalization in critically emaciated anorexics and also the growing clinical experience and flexibility which have shown that admission in a residential setting is far from irreconcilable with a family-oriented treatment (see Chapter 13). Hospitalization of the anorexic patient may then have several goals (Sargent et al., 1985):

1. clarifying the patients' diagnosis or monitoring the physical condition;
2. treating acute physical complications brought on by the weight loss or malnutrition;
3. helping the parents to recognize the seriousness of the condition and to initiate weight gain in the patient;

4. responding to complicating psychiatric symptoms, such as psychosis or suicidal ideation or behavior;
5. creating a crisis in the treatment or raising its intensity when outpatient therapy is not progressing.

Recently, several authors have shown the possibilities of a family-oriented approach within a residential (psychiatric) setting specialized in the treatment of severe eating disorders (Andersen, 1985; Combrinck-Graham, 1985; Hunter, 1985; Koizumi & Luidens, 1984; Mirkin, 1983; Sargent et al., 1985; Seltzer, 1984; Stern et al., 1981; Swift, 1982; Todd, 1985; Vanderlinden & Vandereycken, 1984). Stern et al. (1981) were the first authors to strongly advocate a family-systems model of hospitalization for anorexia nervosa, wherein the individual focus of inpatient care and the systems focus of family therapy are integrated. Hospitalization no longer functions as a first step toward family therapy, but becomes the major therapeutic intervention of a family-oriented approach.

One of the basic principles in order to make the treatment as effective as possible, is to work with a small team that speaks a common therapeutic language and wherein the family therapist has a central and coordinating position (see Chapter 15). The hospitalization itself often provokes a crisis within the family system and can be used therefore as a powerful intervention to challenge coalition patterns and hidden conflicts in the family. However, one should be aware of the eventually negative effects and possible pitfalls of the hospital environment which can function as a sort of homeostatic regulator, providing safety and protection both for the identified patient and the family. It may only consolidate the family with a member suffering of anorexia nervosa, hence cristallizing the identified patient's illness and, conversely, the family's "wellness" (Combrinck-Graham, 1985). In view of the systems model, ideally all family members should be admitted in the hospital, as Seltzer describes (1984), but this still is a very exceptional procedure.

Stern et al. (1981) identify five stages in the treatment team's interaction with anorexic families during hospitalization, resembling the developmental stages Whitaker has described in family therapy: holding, battle for structure, battle for initiative, availability, and separation. The therapeutic team should offer a "holding environment" not only for the patient but for all family members, i.e., "a combination of protection, firm structure, reliability, support of initiative, and tolerance of regression" (Stern et al., 1981). Seltzer (1984) also distinguishes five stages in his family hospitalization program: the observation phase, the care phase, the loosening-up phase, the individuation or oppositional phase, and the symptom-free phase. What characterizes both approaches is that the therapeutic model stimulates both the identified patient and the other family members, who are passing along various identifiable phases, to evolve toward personal growth and individuation. Several aspects of a family-oriented inpatient treatment of eating disorders will be highlighted further on in this book (see especially Chapter 13, 15 and 18).

Conclusion

The "second generation" of family therapists working with anorexia nervosa and bulimia has just been born. They have at least partially dissociated themselves from an implicit obedience toward their masters in a search for their "own identity." They may still echo the ideas of their teachers but they do not stand anymore in their shade. More and more therapists are experimenting with pragmatic eclectic and flexible models wherein concepts and strategies emanated from different (family) therapeutic approaches are combined or integrated. They have further discovered the potential of hospitalization as an effective therapeutic intervention within the family system especially since present-day clinicians are, more than ever before, confronted with complex cases of eating disorders, with older and married patients whose life and that of their families has been distorted for many years by anorexia or bulimia.

No doubt, family therapy has build up a solid reputation; therapeutic work with the family nowadays is considered as an indispensable component of the multidimensionally oriented approach to eating disorders. Unfortunately, most therapists still lack the "scientist-practitioner" spirit, i.e., the fructifying fusion of the creativeness of the artist, the skilfulness of the clinician, and the self-criticism of the researcher.

FAMILY THERAPY AND BULIMIA

General Considerations

Up until recently only a few therapists reported upon their experience with a family therapeutic approach to bulimia (Bologna, 1983; Haley, 1984; Madanes, 1981; Moley, 1983; Root et al., 1986; Schwartz, 1982; Schwartz et al., 1985). How can we explain why the family of the bulimic patient had to queue up such a long time until they got a ticket to meet the family therapist? The most likely explanation is that only in the 1980s has this peculiar eating disorder caught the general attention of psychiatrists and psychologists. This neglect may be attributed partially to the attitude of the bulimics themselves, who tend to conceal their problematic behavior from the outside world. The absence of the consideration of the family context in the literature on bulimia may also be explained by the higher average age of most bulimics compared with anorexics, and that therefore many no longer live at home or are already married (Schwartz et al., 1985).

The rather recent — though burgeoning — interest in bulimia explains that although different conceptual models abound, we do not as yet have an adequate knowledge of the etiology, development and maintenance of the disorder. The various theories are mostly variations upon the conceptualizations of anorexia nervosa. First, there is the *sociocultural viewpoint* defended mainly by feminist theorists. Bulimia is then considered: "As a desperate attempt to control one's weight in a society where low weight is closely tied with personal worth; as an example of the extremes in which women are willing to resort in order to please men in male-dominated society; or a symptom of the contradictory pressures facing contemporary women to be competitive and 'nice' at the same time" (Schwartz et al., 1985, p. 281). Next, there are several models that view bulimia as an *individual* disorder (Wilson, 1985) that may be interpreted in many different ways: as a form of affective disorder, as a variant of addictive behavior, as a symptom of borderline personality disorder, as an anxiety-reducing mechanism resembling obsessive-compulsive behavior, as the result of dysfunctional cognitions, and so forth.

Finally, bulimia may be explained against the *family* background (Schwartz et al., 1985, p. 281):

- As an excuse for not performing well or for being irritable or moody in a family where any of these behaviors are not acceptable.
- As the "passive" rebellion of a person who cannot rebel more directly against overprotective, intrusive parents, in a family where eating has special significance.
- As a way to protect the patient's parents or marriage by providing a focus that distracts them from their conflicts or their depression; to provide an upper threshold for overt conflict (e.g., "Stop fighting, we are upsetting her").
- As an attempt to get nurturant attention or to demonstrate the severity of one's problems in a family that denies any problem and/or in which siblings are extremely competitive.
- As the response of a family that has become extremely isolated and interdependent, due to the mobility and competitiveness of American culture or due to being detached from its kin network.

It is quite clear that no single theory may get a grip on something as complex as bulimia and, like in anorexia nervosa, one can conclude that "a procrustean model of family functioning uniformly applicable to all cases is clearly not acceptable" (Rakoff, 1983, p. 37).

From a practical point of view, the *involvement of the family* (the spouse or significant others) in the treatment of bulimic patients may not only be quite useful but sometimes even inevitable. For instance, in the cases where the bulimia causes stress or anger in a family (Bologna, 1983): Should the patient be wholly responsible for the expense and other problems of her binges? What aspects of the binges should family members tolerate? Should they have to continue filling the cupboard and refrigerator after the bulimic binges? Should they require the patient to eat normal meals together with the rest of the family ? Should they prevent her from vomiting afterwards? "Probably the most important goal of adjunct family therapy with bulimics is to help the significant others in the bulimic's life to set limits on their own responsibility toward the bulimic's binges" (Bologna, 1983, p. 131).

When there exists a positive attitude of family members toward the bulimic patient, they can be used as co-therapists. Including, for example, the husband will increase the chances that therapeutic directives will be followed and that the symptoms will be truthfully reported (Haley, 1984).

Schwartz et al. (1985), on the other hand, remark that they have observed similar interaction patterns as described by Minuchin in anorexic families: enmeshment, overprotectiveness, rigidity, lack of conflict resolution and involvement of the patient in parental conflict (see Chapter 2). Schwartz and co-workers add three other characteristics for bulimic families: isolation, consciousness of appearance, and a special meaning attached to food and meaning. As structural family therapists, they consider the bulimic symptom as a maladaptive solution for a family whose structure hampers adjustment to changing developmental tasks. Treatment, then, is aimed at helping the whole family evolve to the point where the symptom is no longer necessary—where the patient and family have "grown out" of the interaction patterns that fostered it, and have explored appropriate "alternatives" (Schwartz et al., 1985). However, the focus is not only interpersonal: considering bulimia as a rigid and extreme pattern of thinking, feeling and relating to others, with interconnections among many different systems (physiological, intrapersonal, familial, extrafamilial and sociocultural), Schwartz and co-workers are more individual-oriented when compared with the traditional structural family therapist. Family sessions are alternated by individual sessions, which are aimed at activating nonapparent "partial-selves" within the patient, so that she takes more direct control in significant relationships and in the direction of her own life. The authors believe that these alterations on an individual level will be facilitated when the patient's family of origin or marital relationship is also changing. The treatment, which is designed for an outpatient setting, goes through several stages, each of which contains different goals and techniques (Schwartz et al., 1985): (a) motivating the family and patient for differentiation, (b) guiding the differentiation, (c) targetting the symptom, and (d) inoculating the system against relapse.

Resistance and Motivation

Especially in the first phase of treatment, many therapists adopt a waiting attitude until the bulimic patient and/or significant others in her immediate social environment do really want to change and are ready to make a considerable effort for this purpose. This rather skeptical wait-and-see attitude is based upon the recurrent observation and experience of a strong resistance toward real change in the bulimic patient and her family. Some patients seem to have "incorporated" the bulimia as part of their lives while others appear to be attached to it in a love-hate relationship. Anyway, "most bulimics have grown intimate with the symptoms and the identity they signify, and have very mixed feelings about what the loss of the bulimia would imply— growing up, getting close to people, upsetting the family, and so on" (Schwartz et al., 1985, p. 293).

Beside, this restraining posture on the part of the therapist, one may also challenge the fear for change by introducing an *ordeal* (Haley, 1984; Madanes, 1981; Moley, 1983). The therapist first states to the patient and the family that he knows a strategy to solve the problems. It is, however, a very difficult one and, hence, he does not want to start therapy until he is convinced the patient really wants to change her life and give up her symptoms. One may even provoke the patient by asking her to consider carefully the consequences or dangers of improvement: giving up bingeing and vomiting might induce more severe emotional and relational problems, the family or spouse is not able to handle at this moment. So, in this early treatment phase the therapist does not give clear directives toward changing particular behaviors but prepares an ordeal, i.e., "a severe test," wherein, if possible, the husband or other family members are involved. This ordeal very often implies the paradoxical directive of prescribing the symptom, which at the same time dedramatizes the bulimic behavior by bringing it into the open in a preprogrammed way:

- In order to examine the relationship between anger, guilt and food, a bulimic patient was instructed to buy binge-food, keep it in the house and have a couple of planned experimental binges (Moley, 1983).
- Considering the wife's vomiting as "throwing away food," a couple was instructed to throw away the food three times a day instead of eating it, while the husband was asked to do the shopping of the food (Madanes, 1981).
- A bulimic wife was requested to be "completely, totally, without fail," honest in telling her husband each day about the times she would vomit for the next two weeks (Haley, 1984).

Once the patient and the family stand the ordeal and executed the directive, the therapist may again restrain them from changing. The family or couple is asked to discuss whether they are really ready to get over the problem, now that they have experienced a bit of what this could imply for the near future. The therapist further continues the treatment by regularly alternating between this restraining attitude and a direct move toward change. Moley (1983) uses the *Greek Chorus* technique we have discussed before: the patient is confronted with different positions of the team regarding the state of the problem; the therapist in the room takes an optimistic posture and states that the patient can move ahead, whereas the therapist(s) behind the one-way mirror warn(s) the patient about such a change and asks her to thoroughly consider the dangers of improvement.

Obtaining and Consolidating Change

Schwartz et al. (1985) state that they had more difficulty with those bulimics who began and closed therapy while still living in their parents' home. They emphasize that differentiation and launching from the family of origin are important steps in symptom control. Therefore the bulimic patient is encouraged to start living on her own. The launching often provokes a relapse into the symptoms on the part of the patient as well as a dramatic and emotional crisis within the family system. Here the therapist must be aware of the risk that the bulimic symptoms may even worsen once the patient lives on her own (without the drag of social control, the behavior can become ritualized in order to fill the emptiness of life). In order to avoid this risk but, at the same time, to promote separation from home, treatment in a day center may be a valuable alternative (Vandereycken & Meermann, 1984a). Another interesting possibility is to let the patient make this passage to independence through living for a while in another family (Jos Hendrickx from the Department of Child Psychiatry at the University of Utrecht, Holland, is experimenting with such a type of foster family care for bulimics). When the patient relapses into the symptoms, Schwartz et al. (1985) utilize some of the following symptom-specific interventions:

a. Stimulating the patient's awareness of the context and the sequences of thoughts, feelings or interactions with others that typically surround the symptoms, by using a diary.
b. Prescribing the patient to become depressed for a specific period of time each day or week to discover the issues in her life that are causing or maintaining the bulimic problems.
c. Redefining the bulimic episode as a helpful signal to the patient that a part of her is not being taken care of; she has to listen carefully to discover what that part might really want for her and search for alternative ways of acting on that intention that do not involve food.
d. Gradually giving permission and encouragement to the patient in order to try out some new behaviors without depriving herself of the binge-purge sequence.
e. Stimulating the patient to build up and maintain extrafamilial close relationships.

When the patient is differentiating and launching successfully from her family of origin, and is getting more control over the bulimic symptoms, the family therapist still needs to be available for a long period, especially at future points of crisis.

Conclusion

Although one can be impressed by the creative power of the uncommon strategic interventions, severe bulimia in our experience is not a single problem that can be challenged only by some hocus-pocus tricks. Many patients do relapse several times or, even when they obtain some control over their symptoms, many still have a distorted body image or a low self-esteem, and need therefore an intensive multidimensional treatment. Many actual forms of therapy for bulimia (mostly individual-oriented) do overemphasize the eating problems and the ultimate treatment goal of eliminating all bingeing and vomiting. Instead, it may be far more realistic "to break the sequence of behavior or thoughts involved in the syndrome, and thereby to give the patient more control over the symptom. This can be achieved by either changing the meaning of the bulimic behaviors and thoughts, or changing the interpersonal and/or intrapersonal interaction sequences that precede or follow the symptoms" (Schwartz et al., 1985, p. 300).

We do realize the fact that there still exists little experience among therapists about when and how family members or the broader social context need to be involved in the therapeutic work with bulimic patients. But we believe that a family-oriented approach, as in the case of anorexia nervosa, will become an essential component of any multimodal treatment that proves successful in severe bulimia.

GENERAL CONCLUSION

Looney et al. (1980, p. 507) cautioned that "a myopic focus on any single model can lead to the unfortunate situation in which treatment unit becomes a self-contained microcosm." This warning applies to the family therapy field in general as well as to its many different forms and schools. Fortunately, practitioners have again discovered that patients have families, but some are inclined to forget that patients have bodies too. Especially in the area of eating disorders, overenthusiastic family therapists seem to minimize or even completely overlook the devastating effects of starvation or binge-eating and vomiting. Some foster the naive conviction that by changing family interactions, a complex symptomatology as in the case of bulimia or anorexia nervosa will disappear all by itself. Or as Peggy Papp (1983, p. 88) points out: "There is a myth in our profession that if parents get together and free the child from the position of mediator, the child will automatically spring forth mature, well adjusted, and symptom free."

As we have underscored in the previous pages, all too often family therapists – including their great leaders – are lacking a sense of self-criticism. They abundantly describe their success stories, emphasizing the strength of family therapy, but seldom mention their failures, shortcomings and limitations. Most of them seem never to question the *ethics* of their profession. Whatever theoretical school one adheres to, each therapist has to examine time and again the ethical issues in choosing and executing a particular treatment format (Sider & Clements, 1982). In her brilliant autobiographical essay on anorexia nervosa, Sheila MacLeod (1981), sharply criticized certain (mainly structural) family therapists for their manipulative and ruthless styles and their ways of treating every family member, whether adult or not, "as a rather unintelligent child who can never hope to understand the mysteries of the hieratic profession whose skills are being utilized for the family's own good, and must therefore not be questioned" (p. 124). In order to speed up the treatment process, the family therapist may leave no stone unturned, no wound unprobed, according to MacLeod. Her criticism may be an overstatement, but others in more technical terms have warned that structural family therapists tend to overuse powerful tactics such as crisis induction "to push a family toward goals set by the therapist, rather than letting new patterns of family interaction evolve more naturally and with less intervention by the therapist" (Todd, 1985, p. 228). But the seemingly more elegant systemic-strategic approach sometimes underestimates the possibly dangerous condition of an emaciated family member. Would it be ethically justifiable to use paradoxical prescription for a life-threatening behavior?

Feelings of omnipotence inevitably make a therapist blind. A similar blindness as to the outside world may exist in family therapists who regard their special treatment room — including video cameras and one-way-mirror — as a laboratory where they can reshape individuals, families, if not even society itself. But many are narrow-minded while being only interested in a small slice of a *total ecosystem* (Keeney, 1984). They overemphasize the nuclear family and neglect the extended family and the larger peer and community networks (Todd, 1985). Viewed the increasing incidence of eating disorders, one might expect from the family approach at least some concrete guidelines for *prevention,* but they are, generally speaking, almost nonexistent (Vandereycken & Meermann, 1984b). We assume that this neglect is linked to the near absence of *research* by family therapists, as we mention repeatedly. This concerns both outcome and process investigation. Regarding the latter, few family therapists seem interested in the so-called nonspecific therapeutic factors. They usually focus on "new" and "powerful" techniques without proving their specificity. As Dare (1985) points out, there is a great need "to discover what a family therapist should best try to change if family therapy is to be helpful. At the moment the therapy is like a blunderbuss aimed at the most obvious and moving part.... The family therapist can only address available interventions toward what can be perceived. There is no way that this can be a refined treatment, even though video-taped demonstrations may appear both elegant and dramatic, and there may be developing evidence of useful effect. What is needed is that the family interactions, of the sort that can be tackled by family therapists, are assessed to see if they are relevant to the future course of the disturbance. Then the therapeutic efforts need to be researched to find out whether or not the changes they are intended to produce actually do occur, and to an extent required to modify the evolution of the anorexic patient's life. Then a useful paper on the family therapy of anorexia nervosa can be written. At the moment, all that can be written, are papers on family therapy" (p. 442). This chapter is an account of those papers. It is hoped that this book shows that treatment of eating disorders is not just a matter of techniques or methods, but is basically a question of attitude: a scientist-practitioner's view, from a biopsychosocial perspective, on a multidimensional problem which, among others, necessitates a constructive family-oriented approach.

REFERENCES*

Andersen, A.E. (1985), *Practical Comprehensive Treatment of Anorexia Nervosa and Bulimia*. Baltimore: Johns Hopkins University Press.

Andolfi, M. (1979), *Family Therapy: An Interactional Approach*. New York: Plenum Press.

Andolfi, M., Angelo, C., Menghi, P. & Nicolò-Corigliano, A.M. (1983), *Behind the Family Mask: Therapeutic Change in Rigid Family Systems*. New York: Brunner/Mazel.

Baker, L.C. & Pontious, M. (1984), Treating the health care family. *Family Systems Medicine*, 2:401-408.

Barnes, G.G. & Campbell, D. (1982), The impact of structural and strategic approaches on the supervising process. In: Whiffen, R. & Byng-Hall, J. (Eds.), *Family Therapy Supervision. Recent Developments in Practice*, London-New York: Academic Press-Grune & Stratton, pp. 137-150.

Barton, C., Alexander, J.F. & Sanders, J.D. (1985), Research in family therapy. In: L'Abate, L. (Ed.), *The Handbook of Family Psychology and Therapy*. Homewood (Ill.): Dorsey Press, pp. 1073-1106.

Benedetti, G. (1956a), Behandlung anorexischer Kinder durch Psychoanalyse der Mutter (Treatment of anorexic children through psychoanalysis of the mothers). *Helvetica Paediatrica Acta*, 11:539-561.

Benedetti, G. (1956b), Behandlung anorexischer Kleinkinder durch Psychotherapie der Mutter (Treatment of anorexic children through psychotherapy of the mothers). *Die Vorträge der 6. Lindauer Psychotherapiewoche*. Stuttgart: G. Thieme, pp. 159-171.

Benson, A. & Futterman, L. (1985), Psychotherapeutic partnering: An approach to the treatment of anorexia nervosa and bulimia. In: Emmett, S.W. (Ed.), *Theory and Treatment of Anorexia Nervosa and Bulimia*. New York: Brunner/Mazel, pp. 154-173.

Berlin, I.N., Boatman, M.J., Sheimo, S.L. & Szurek, S.A. (1951), Adolescent alternation of anorexia and obesity. *American Journal of Orthopsychiatry*, 21:387-419.

Blackwell, A. & Rollins, N. (1968), Treatment problems in adolescents with anorexia nervosa. Preliminary observations on the second phase. *Acta Paedopsychiatrica*, 35:294-301.

Blitzer, J.R., Rollins, M. & Blackwell, A. (1961), Children who starve themselves: Anorexia nervosa. *Psychosomatic Medicine*, 23:369-383.

Boscolo, L. & Cecchin, G. (1982), Training in systemic therapy at the Milan Centre. In: Whiffen, R. & Byng Hall, J. (Eds.), *Family Therapy Supervision: Recent Developments in Practice*. London-New York: Academic Press-Grune & Stratton, pp. 153-165.

Bruch, H. (1978), *The Golden Cage. The Enigma of Anorexia Nervosa*. Cambridge (Mass.): Harvard University Press.

Campbell, D. & Draper, R. (Eds.) (1985), *Applications of Systemic Family Therapy: The Milan Approach*. New York: Grune & Stratton.

Casper, R.C. (1983), On the emergence of bulimia nervosa as a syndrome: A historical view. *International Journal of Eating disorders*, 2(3):3-16.

Combrinck-Graham, L. (1985), Hospitalization as a therapeutic intervention in the family. In: Ziffer, R.L. (Ed.), *Adjunctive Techniques in Family Therapy*. New York: Grune & Stratton, pp. 99-124.

Compernolle, T. (1982), Adequate joint authority of parents: A crucial issue for the outcome of family therapy. In: Kaslow, F.W. (Ed.), *The International Book of Family Therapy*. New York: Brunner/Mazel, pp. 245-256.

---

* See also the bibliography at the end of this book.

Crisp, A.M. (1980), *Anorexia Nervosa: Let Me Be*. New York-London: Academic Press-Grune & Stratton.

Eiguer, A. (1983), *Un Divan pour la Famille: Du Modèle Groupal à la Thérapie Psychanalytique* (A Couch for the Family: From the Group Model to Psychoanalytic Therapy). Paris: Le Centurion.

Fishman, H.C. & Rosman, B.L. (1986), *Evolving Models for Family Change: A Volume in Honor of Salvador Minuchin*. New York: Guilford Press.

Frank, J.D. (1984), Therapeutic components of all psychotherapies. In: Meyers, J.M. (Ed.), *Cures by Psychotherapy. What Effects Change?* New York: Praeger

Frey, J. (1984), A family systems approach to illness maintaining behaviors in chronically ill adolescents. *Family Process,* 23:251-260.

Garfinkel, P.E. & Garner, D.M. (1982), *Anorexia Nervosa. A Multimensional Perspective*. New York: Brunner/Mazel.

Guidano, V.F. & Liotti, G. (1983), Eating disorders. In: Authors, *Cognitive Processes and Emotional Disorders. A Structural Approach to Psychotherapy*. New York: Guilford Press, pp. 276-306.

Gull, W.W. (1874), Anorexia nervosa (apepsia hysterica, anorexia hysterica). *Transactions of the Clinical Society of London,* 7:22-28. Reprinted in: Kaufman, M.R. & Heiman, M. (Eds.), *Evolution of Psychosomatic Concepts. Anorexia Nervosa: A Paradigm*. New York: International Universities Press, 1964, pp. 132-138. Also in: Andersen, A.E., *Practical Comprehensive Treatment of Anorexia Nervosa and Bulimia*. Baltimore: Johns Hopkins University Press, 1985, pp. 13-18.

Haley, J. (1980), *Leaving Home. The Therapy of Disturbed Young People*. New York: Mc.Graw Hill.

Haley, J. (1985), *Ordeal Therapy*. San Francisco: Jossey Bass.

Harbin, H.T. (1982), Family treatment of the psychiatric inpatient. In: Harbin, H.T. (Ed.), *The Psychiatric Hospital and the Family*. Jamaica (N.Y.): Spectrum Publications, pp. 3-26.

Hoffman, L. (1981), *Foundation of Family Therapy: A Conceptual Framework for Systems Change*. New York: Basic Books.

Hunter, D. (1985), On the boundary: Family therapy in a long-term inpatient setting. *Family Process,* 24:339-355.

Kascow, F.W. (1982), History of family therapy in the United States: A kaleidoscopic overview. In: Kaslow, F.W. (Ed.), *The International Book of Family Therapy*. New York: Brunner/Mazel, pp. 5-37.

Kaufman, M.R. & Heiman, M. (Eds.), (1964), *Evolution of Psychosomatic Concepts. Anorexia Nervosa: A Paradigm*. New York: International Universities Press.

Keeney, B.P. (1984), An ecological epistemology for therapy. In: O'Connor, W.A. & Lubin, B.L. (Es.), *Ecological Approaches to Clinical and Community Psychology*. New York: John Wiley, pp. 24-40.

Keeney, B.P. & Ross, J.M. (1985), *Mind in Therapy. Constructing Systemic Family Therapies*. New York: Basic Books.

Kwee, M.G.T. & Duivenvoorden, H.J., (1985), Multimodal residential therapy in two cases of anorexia nervosa (adult body weight phobia). In: Lazarus, A.A. (Ed.), *Casebook of Multimodal Therapy*. New York: Guilford Press, pp. 116-138.

Lasègue, E.C. (1873), De l'anorexie hystérique. *Archives Générales de Médecine,* 21:385-403. Reprinted in: Lasègue, E.C., *Etudes Médicales*. Paris: Asselin, 1884, pp. 45-63. English translation: On hysterical anorexia. *Medical Times and Gazette,* 1873, 2:265-266, 367-363. Reprinted in: Kaufman, M.R. & Heiman, M. (Eds.), *Evolution of Psychosomatic Concepts. Anorexia Nervosa: A Paradigm*. New York: International Universities Press, 1964, pp. 143-155. Also in: Andersen, A.E., *Practical Comprehensive Treatment of Anorexia Nervosa and Bulimia*. Baltimore: Johns Hopkins University Press, 1985, pp. 19-27.

Liebman, R. & Ziffer, R. (1985), Case consultation within a family systems network. In: Ziffer, R.L. (Ed.), *Adjunctive Techniques in Family Therapy*. New York: Grune & Stratton, pp. 181-207.

Looney, J.G., Blotcky, M.J., Carson, D.I. & Gossett, J.T. (1980), A family-systems model for in-
patient treatment of adolescents. *Adolescent Psychiatry,* 8:49-511.
MacLeod, S. (1981), *The Art of Starvation.* London-New York: Virago-Schocken Books.
Madanes, C. (1981), *Strategic Family Therapy.* San Francisco: Jossey Bass.
Minuchin, S. (1975), Structural family therapy. In: Arieti, S. (Ed.), *American Handbook of Psy-
chiatry (second edition). Volume II: Child and Adolescent Psychiatry, Sociocultural and Com-
munity Psychiatry.* New York: Basic Books, pp. 178-192.
Minuchin, S. & Fishman, H.C. (1981), *Family Therapy Techniques.* Cambridge (Mass.): Harvard
University Press.
Nichols, M. (1984), *Family Therapy: Concepts and Methods.* New York: Gardner Press.
Papp, P. (1980), The Greek chorus and other techniques of paradoxical therapy. *Family Process,*
19:45-57.
Papp, P. (1983), *The Process of Change.* New York/London: Guilford Press.
Piazza, E., Piazza, M. & Rollins, M. (1980), Anorexia nervosa: Controversial aspects of therapy.
Comprehensive Psychiatry, 21:177-189.
Pinsov, W.M. (1981), Family therapy process research. In: Gurman, A.S. & Kniskern, D.P. (Eds.),
Handbook of Family Therapy. New York: Brunner/Mazel, pp. 699-741.
Rollins, N. & Blackwell, A. (1968), The treatment of anorexia nervosa in children and adoles-
cents: Stage I. *Journal of Child Psychology and Psychiatry,* 9:81-91.
Rollins, N. & Piazza, E. (1981), Anorexia nervosa. A quantitative approach to follow-up. *Journal
of the American Academy of Child Psychiatry,* 20:167-183.
Seltzer, W. & Seltzer, M. (1983), Materials, myth and magic: A cultural approach to family ther-
apy. *Family Process,* 22:3-14.
Selvini Palazzoli, M. (1972), Racialism in the family. *Human Context,* 4:624-629.
Selvini Palazzoli, M. (1980), Why a long interval between sessions. In: Andolfi, M. & Zwerling,
I. (Eds.), *Dimensions of Family Therapy.* New York: Guilford Press,pp. 161-169.
Selvini Palazzoli, M., Boscolo, L., Cecchin, G. & Prata, G. (1974), The treatment of children
through brief therapy of their parents. *Family Process,* 13:429-442.
Selvini Palazzoli, M., Boscolo, L., Cecchin, G. & Prata, G. (1977), Family rituals: A powerful tool
in family therapy. *Family Process,* 16:445-453.
Selvini Palazzoli, M., Cecchin, G., Prata, G. & Boscolo, L. (1978), *Paradox and Counterparadox.*
New York: Jason Aronson (Original Italian edition published by Feltrinelli, Milan, 1975; French
translation published by ESF, Paris, 1978; German translation published by Klett-Cotta, Stutt-
gart, 1977; Dutch translation published by Samsom, Alphen a/d Rijn, 1979).
Selvini Palazzoli, M., Cecchin, G., Prata, G. & Boscolo, C. (1980), Hypothesizing-circularity-
neutrality: Three guidelines for the conductor of the session. *Family Process,* 19:3-12.
Sider, R.C. & Clements, C. (1982), Family or individual therapy: The ethics of modality choice.
American Journal of Psychiatry, 139:1455-1459.
Sperling, M (1950), Children's interpretation and reaction to the unconscious of their mothers.
International Journal of Psycho-Analysis, 31:36-41.
Sperling, M. (1978), Anorexia nervosa. In: Author, *Psychosomatic Disorders in Childhood.* New
York: Jason Aronson, pp. 129-173. Reprinted in: Wilson C.P. (Ed.), *Fear of Being Fat. The
Treatment of Anorexia Nervosa and Bulimia.* New York: Jason Aronson, 1983, pp. 51-82.
Stachowiak, J. & Briggs, S.L. (1984), Ecosystemic therapy: A treatment perspective. In: O'Con-
nor, W.A. & Lubin, B. (Eds.), *Ecological Approaches to Clinical and Community Psychology.*
New York: John Wiley, pp. 7-23.
Tomm, K. (1984), One perspective on the Milan systemic approach. Part I: Overview of develop-
ment, theory, and practice. Part II: Description of session format, interviewing style and in-
terventions. *Journal of Marital and Family Therapy,* 10:113-126, 253-272.
Vandereycken, W. & Meermann, R. (1984a), *Anorexia Nervosa. A Clinician's Guide to Treatment.*
Berlin-New York: Walter de Gruyter.
Vandereycken, W. & Meermann, R. (1984b), Anorexia nervosa: Is prevention possible? *Inter-
national Journal of Psychiatry in Medicine,* 14:191-205.

Weeks, G.R. & L'Abate, L. (1982), *Paradoxical Psychotherapy: Theory and Practice with Individuals, Couples and Families.* New York: Brunner/Mazel.

Wilson, G.T. (1985), *The Treatment of Bulimia Nervosa: A Cognitive-Behavioral Perspective.* Paper delivered at the 33rd Annual Convention of the American Psychological Association, Los Angeles, August 1985.

Winawer, H. (1983), The Heidelberg concept: An introduction to the work of Helm Stierlin and his associates. *Family Systems Medicine,* 1(4):36-40.

Wirsching, M. & Stierlin, H.(1985), Psychosomatics II. Treatment considerations. *Family Systems Medicine,* 3:281-290.

Chapter 12

A Family-Oriented Strategy in Outpatient Treatment*

Walter Vandereycken and Johan Vanderlinden

INTRODUCTION

The procedure utilized in our family-oriented strategy for outpatient treatment (like the pyramid model of family counseling presented in Chapter 14) is characterized by the sequential utilization of various treatment approaches following a hierarchy of interventions — from simple patient education and advice to a complex intensive treatment strategy. In this conceptual scheme, one can move from an initial level of problem difficulty, where perhaps only reassurance is required, to a final level of difficulty where intensive multimodal treatment is needed. Each level requires a different degree of therapist skill and competence. A close linkage between assessment and treatment is necessary in order to determine the (possibly changing) level of intervention needed.

As illustrated in Figure 1, the clinician's intervention may vary according to the "eye" ("I") level he chooses to approach the problem. With each patient, the physician has to start at the first level (problem identification or diagnosis) but whether or not he will become active at a higher level may depend on several factors. Among these, an important one relates to the physician himself, especially if the clinician involved is working in a private practice or in a setting with limited therapeutic possibilities or resources. Then he has to question his own position and whether he is the right person to treat this particular patient, recognizing the limits of his experience and/or his treatment potential. In general, when faced with an eating disorder patient, the physician (general practitioner, pediatrician) is advised to seek outside consultation with a psychiatrist or psychologist before starting a comprehensive treatment plan. Management of eat-

---

* Revision of a previously published article by the first author: "Outpatient management of anorexia nervosa" (*Pediatrician,* 1985, 12:118-125).

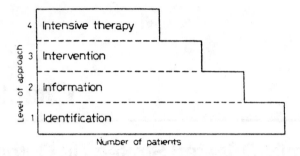

Figure 1. The four I or eye levels in problem management

ing disorders at the third and fourth levels (specific interventions or intensive treatment) might be too difficult unless the physician is both specially trained in psychotherapeutic methods and has had a good deal of experience.

IDENTIFICATION

The main aim of the identification phase is early detection with emphasis upon positive diagnosis and special attention for psychosocial assessment. *Early detection* is certainly the first and crucial step in secondary prevention because it enables early intervention which, is generally associated with good outcome (Vandereycken & Meermann, 1984b). But recognition of mild forms of anorexia nervosa or bulimia may be hampered by the patient who usually conceals the problem, and/or by the family who unwittingly colludes with this until the disorder becomes severe. The patient's indifference toward physical symptoms of starvation can mislead physicians, who are attuned to hearing complaints, into ignoring them (Casper, 1982). In fact, it is the contrast between the "abnormal" physical appearance (emaciation and symptoms of starvation) and the attitude of "normality" (reflected in professional, intellectual or athletic functioning) which must raise the suspicion of anorexia nervosa. All too often physicians tend to proceed in a "negative" diagnostic process which is primarily aimed at excluding somatic causes. Pursued by the nagging fear of missing something drummed into him as a medical student, a stream of differential diagnoses will run through the physician's mind. If he is not aware of the many physiological (metabolic and endocrinologic) abnormalities that may be associated with malnutrition, he will be tempted to ask for more and more extended technical investigations which only reveal more confusing abnormalities linked with an endless list of differential diagnoses! Such a diagnostic procedure would not only result in a series of unnecessary investigations but above all a delay before therapy can begin.

With some basic knowledge of the psychological peculiarities of anorexia nervosa and bulimia it should not be that difficult to reach a *positive diagnosis* based on the behavioral characteristics of the syndrome (as emphasized, for instance, in DSM-III). Instead of focusing on appetite or body weight, the physician should pay attention to the patient's attitude toward eating and body shape, and he will find that she expresses a pursuit of thinness or a weight phobia. When this positive diagnosis has been made, a limited number of technical investigations are necessary to document the physiological status of the patient. Usually a laboratory checkup (red and white blood count, electrolytes, liver parameters, total protein) and an electrocardiogram will suffice. The physician must realize then that the physiological abnormalities are signs of malnutrition and will usually return to the normal range with weight gain. Indeed, another pitfall is treating the physical sequelae of starvation instead of the starvation itself, e.g., prescribing sleeping medication for sleeplessness, laxatives for complaints of constipation, or hormones for amenorrhea (Casper, 1982).

Finally, the physician has to widen his medical diagnostic scope to a kind of *psychosocial assessment*. First of all, he will quickly learn that information from the patient's relatives (especially the parents) may tell much more than X-rays and endocrinologic tests. Furthermore, the family's perception of the problem may have important therapeutic implications. We already mentioned the patient's denial of illness (Vandereycken & Vanderlinden, 1983) as a crucial stumbling block. This implies that the attitude of the parents will influence the referral process. Especially in young adolescents, parental attitudes may serve as impediments to treatment (Andersen, 1985):

> *Denial or Recognition Failure:* The parents fail to recognize the seriousness of their child's eating disorder, e.g., because they admire her selfmastery, physical appearance/performances or intellectual productivity; the child's problem mirrors then a collusion with one or both parents.

> *Uncertainty or Confrontation Failure:* The parents do recognize the problem but assume a wait-and-see attitude because they fear that any intervention may only aggravate the problem or lead to disruptive family conflicts; often this attitude reflects the parents' lack of agreement on how to approach their child.

> *Impotence or Intervention Failure:* These parents want to solve the problem on their own; although they fail to handle it (mainly because of lack of joint authority) seeking professional help is viewed as an admission of their inadequacy or is felt as threatening because it might reveal other intrafamilial problems they prefer to keep concealed.

In each of these cases, self-protection or protection of the family is the main motive for the delay in seeking professional help or for the refusal of (some types of) treatment.

In recent years, the burgeoning popular and scientific interest in anorexia nervosa and bulimia has produced the risk of promoting the fashionable aspect or special attractiveness of this "modern" disease. This may lead to an overidentification both on the part of the family and the health care professionals. Both parties may be too easily alarmed when faced, for instance, with a child who sometimes refuses to eat. Anorexia nervosa means a lot more than periodic food refusal or a tendency to be slim, and periodic overeating is not necessarily a sign of bulimia. But in general, the physician more often encounters resistance on the part of the family. Besides those described above, it usually concerns parents who are alarmed by the weight loss or related signs of anorexia such as amenorrhea but who believe their child is the victim of a strange somatic illness. In fact, they are reluctant to face up to the psychological meanings of the eating disorder. Here, the general practitioner or the pediatrician has the advantage of being more easily accepted by the family than, for instance, a psychiatrist. He has to be careful, however, not to reinforce the parents' conceptualization of the "illness," e.g., by carrying out too many technical investigations before reaching a positive diagnosis as discussed earlier. The physician must use instead his authority toward the parents in a confrontational approach we describe later in this chapter.

INFORMATION

The physical examination of the patient is not merely a diagnostic observation procedure but the first step toward treatment if used as a means of confronting both the patient and the family with the seriousness and psychological nature of the disorder. The physician should inform the patient of the physical dangers of starvation, vomiting or laxative/diuretic abuse. Usually, parents welcome this injection of reality and authority, and experience considerable relief when the physician decides to intervene and, in effect, take over responsibility for the identified patient (Stern et al., 1981). Although it is essential to avoid a purely authoritarian role, the physician must win and sustain the confidence of both the patient and the parents in order that collaboration rather than contention becomes the basis and keynote of treatment. The patient should not leave after the first appointment with a feeling she has encountered an adversary, but rather someone who could turn into an ally. Therefore, the patient must be persuaded that treatment will be aimed at increasing rather than diminishing her own autonomy (Welbourne & Purgold, 1984).

Changing the patient's denial and resistance (in fact, fear of "imposed" change) into her being prepared to contemplate real change in herself is often a difficult task (Crisp, 1980). If the clinician tries to speak the anorexic's or bulimic's language, he may get in touch with the experiential world of the patient. "The aim is to convert the patient from someone exercising extreme resistance and denial to someone who can acknowledge 'the price she is paying' for her illness and move her from an egosyntonic position to that of a patient" (Kalucy, 1978, p. 200). The first thing to do then is to convince the patient and her family that they should participate in a treatment program. In doing this it is important to emphasize the *benefits of treatment* first of all for the patient herself. She can be told, for instance, that with treatment she can expect: (1) a decrease in the obsessive thoughts she has about food and body weight that interfere with her ability to concentrate on other matters; (2) a resumption of more normal eating patterns and hence that she will feel more comfortable when socializing with peers; (3) a relief from insomnia and depressive symptoms or mood swings and will feel less irritable; and (4) a restoration of her previous activity level, especially if she now feels she no longer has the energy to be active (Halmi, 1983).

An alliance can be established by addressing the patient's emotional isolation and unhappiness and by emphasizing that treatment is aimed at helping her resume a normal life. The patient must experience the physician's true concern for her future emotional and physical well-being for which a normal weight is a natural prerequisite (Casper, 1982). Moreover, it is only during weight restoration or after the patient has reached a normal body weight that she will reexperience the conflicts which led her to adopt an anorexic "solution." But the pitfall here is that the focus on weight gain may convey the message that the physician is not interested in the person of the patient but only in her body weight and physiology. "It is making a fundamentally anorexic mistake; it treats weight as a magical quality, allowing numbers on the dial to take over from reality. This is really the difficulty with all approaches to treatment which lay down rigid rules about weight gain" (Lawrence, 1984, p.76). One has to avoid the patient's body becoming the object of struggle and confrontation between herself and those who are trying to help her.

The *parents' support* is essential for the physician, and considerable time should be spent explaining the rationale and purpose of treatment in order to help ensure their continued cooperation. But in some cases, the parents must be first convinced of the seriousness of the disorder. The answer to the question of how to get the parents to comply with the diagnosis and/or the need for treatment will depend particularly on their conceptualization of the problem ("illness") and their attitude (fears, expectations) toward eventual treatment. Sometimes a direct confrontation with the severity of the condition must be deliberately exaggerated and dramatized as a kind of "horror" technique in order to frighten seemingly unconcerned parents (e.g., by quoting statistics on the mortality of anorexia nervosa). In the case of overanxious parents, the opposite must be done: clear factual information is given to reassure the parents or restore their confidence in their educational skills. The physician must be aware that most parents are inclined to feel guilty about their child's problem although this might be concealed behind a series of defense mechanisms as was described above. All too easily, the clinician may be tempted to act as a "superparent" who has to repair what the real parents have done wrong. Therefore, one has to avoid blaming directly or indirectly the parents for being the cause of the disorder (in anorexia nervosa the traditional scapegoat is the mother). A related mistake is to interpret each case of anorexia or bulimia as a sign of family pathology. Causal hypotheses related to a so-called typical anorexigenic family are still to be critically tested and, as yet, must be considered to be unproven generalizations (see Chapter 3).

A final remark concerns *lay literature* and *self-help organizations*. There is a bulk of recent popular literature on eating disorders: vulgarized scientific, general guidance or self-help, and (auto)biographic material (Vandereycken & Meermann, 1984a). This literature may be helpful both for patients and relatives to get a clearer picture of the disorder (e.g., its psychological nature associated with a complex disturbed physiology) and its treatment (e.g., the need for and the several forms of therapy). Reading such books may also have certain disadvantages:

- patients may learn new tricks (e.g., vomiting) in order to enlarge their abnormal behavior repertoire (Chiodo & Latimer, 1983);
- it may reinforce certain myths (e.g., the "disturbed" family);
- it risks inducing untoward effects deriving from the appealing image of a "fashionable" disease.

These risks also apply to self-help organizations* which, on the other hand, may provide an effective means of support, information and motivation for both patients and relatives. Many appear to be well-informed regarding the advice and guidance they offer, not in the least because they draw on the experiences of the patients and those living with them. Self-help groups complement professional treatment by serving as a bridge for people who are not quite ready to step into treatment or who are discouraged by their experiences therapy. Through supportive consciousness-raising experiences, these groups may help patients or parents become ready for or sustain the effort during treatment. Many organizations act as go-betweens in this respect and provide channels through which expert help can be sought.

INTERVENTION

We know little or nothing about the "natural" courses of anorexia nervosa and bulimia in their various forms and degrees of severity. When faced with early or mild forms of eating disorder, the question arises whether or not they represent transient stages of distress which may disappear completely without any therapeutic intervention. This means that in some cases *no treatment may be the prescription of choice* (Frances & Clarkin, 1981). The physician must question his "indispensability" and be aware that the greater the rescue fantasies he has, the greater the risk of ill-considered therapeutic activism. It is a basic principle that the patient herself can be or has to become the main agent of change.

---

* For a list of addresses in America and Europe see: Vandereycken and Meermann (1984a).

Moreover, the patient can turn to significant persons in her social milieu in order to get support or help. This implies that the physician, after the identification and information/confrontation process, may decide to give the patient the opportunity to reverse her problematic situation on her own. It is advisable then to schedule some follow-up appointments aimed at evaluating the patient's evolution. Remember, however, Gull's (1874) more than 100-year-old warning: "In the earlier and less severe stages, it is not unusual for the medical attendant to say, in reply to the anxious solicitude of the parents, 'Let her do as she likes: do not force food.' Formerly, I thought such advice admissable and proper, but larger experience has shown plainly the danger of allowing the starvation process to go on."

In a great number of anorexia nervosa patients specific therapeutic interventions are wanted or urgently needed. We prefer *a behaviorally oriented family approach* including a consistent and transparent strategy that:

- emphasizes the patient's responsibility for taking care of her own health;
- provides the parents with something concrete to do at home and thus decreases their anxiety and helplessness in dealing with an anorexic child;
- is aimed at avoiding self-defeating power struggles by neutralizing the problem of food refusal or threatening weight loss.

Such an approach is best characterized as "a collaborative effort directed and catalyzed by the therapist and carried out by the patient and her family in their daily lives. The therapist needs to be actively engaged in the process of treatment, at times being patient and understanding and, at times, being challenging and insistent" (Sargent & Liebman, 1984, p. 244). We will now describe briefly an outpatient strategy for anorexia nervosa which, according to our clinical experience, has a very favorable cost/benefit ratio (Vandereycken & Meermann, 1984a).

No causal explanations are given with regard to the anorexic problems following the axiom that we cannot change the past but can try to avoid repeating its unfruitful experiences. Two basic rules are explained: *the family has to restore its normal living pattern* and *the patient has to restore her health*. Weight restitution is the patient's own and primary responsibility, but her fear of losing control over eating and becoming overweight impedes cooperation. Therefore, assurance must be given, time and again, that the therapist will take care that the patient's weight will be restored to a normal age-appropriate level, i.e., fluctuating within reasonable minimum and maximum limits. A contract is made regarding minimal weight gain required (depending on the patient's physical condition, but usually a minimum of 500 g and a maximum of 3 kg a week, the latter limit selected in order to avoid overeating). If the patient does not meet this condition after a certain period (e.g., less than 1.5 kg after 3 weeks) consequences will follow with an increasing degree of severity (e.g., limitation of physical activity, interdiction on working or studying, hospitalization). All these consequences are decided upon, in agreement with the parents, before treatment starts. The patient has to eat in a separate room at the usual dinnertime, and she is free to eat what and how much she likes within this rule. However, she has access only to the same food the other family members are eating at the same time. Moreover, she is not allowed to eat in other rooms or at other times, to buy or hoard food, to interfere with cooking or with her mother's choice of menu. No family member is permitted to control her eating or to make comments about it; the same applies to her weight, which is only controlled by the therapist.

The rationale of this approach is twofold: (1) Anorexia nervosa patients have difficulty eating with others, and the more they are controlled, the less they eat; even if the other family members do not make any comments on her eating behavior while eating together, she will still feel nonverbal control on what is happening with her plate; therefore it is easier for her to start learning to eat normally again while being alone. (2) The family has to learn to resume normal mealtimes as a social event; this means that they have to return to their usual eating habits with no special menu (e.g., low-calorie diet) for one member and without controlling each other's eating behavior. Moreover, instead of talking about food or body shape, they have to resume normal dinner table talk so that dining may again become a pleasant family meeting. The patient may rejoin the family during mealtimes once she can eat properly for her age (but the therapist must be hesitant to allow this too soon).

It is the family's responsibility to see that these rules are respected and that eventual consequences of the contract will be carried out. We often explain here to the worried parents that, in order to prevent cardiovascular complications, it is far more important to be concerned about hyperactivity ("exhaustion of a weak body") than about the patient's eating behavior. "It is easier for you to achieve a decrease of her physical activity than an increase in her food intake." In this way we are deflecting attention onto a symptom which is less disruptive for family interactions. In other words, we ask the parents to be concerned in a constructive way. It would be an impossible and perhaps even an unhealthy task for parents (though many physicians appear to expect this from them) not to pay any attention whatsoever or to relinquish any concern. On the other hand, we ask the patient to report any interference of a family member with her eating or weight.

Such a *restructuring of the interactional nature of (non)eating within a family context* may soon have a great impact, especially if the parents are following the rules. Therefore, in the beginning, their cooperation is much more important than the patient's — who will usually try out the strictness of the contract by noncompliance or partial collaboration. If the parents do not comply, this can be used as a confrontation with the therapist's "growing evidence that there must be something wrong in this family." This might bring the parents closer to compliance or closer to the decision to hospitalize the patient. Indeed, although they help, some parents do not give up their own ineffective efforts to fatten the patient and they cannot admit having failed in this respect. Others sabotage the treatment or undermine the contract with the (unexpressed) intention or hope that the "expert" himself will fail too!

Crisis induction is a strategy aimed at bringing the parents to the point of admitting failure or impotence. The lunch session described by Minuchin et al. (1978) is partially directed toward the same purpose (see Chapter 11). The family is invited to have lunch with the therapist, who allows them to repeat their usual unsuccessful attempts to get the patient to eat. The therapist underlines their failure as strongly as possible and tries to get the parents to acknowledge that the patient has "won" again. Our contract system may be used in a similar sense. In a case where we feel that outpatient treatment is almost impossible for any chance of success, but the parents or the patients wish one last chance, we go along with their wish and design a time-limited (3-4 weeks) contract with strict rules as mentioned above. If they fail to reach the goal of a minimal weight gain within the prearranged time span, we label it as too difficult a condition to be treated on an outpatient basis. Usually the parents are more likely then to accept hospitalization or even to ask for it themselves. On the other hand, when the outpatient contract works, the changing family atmosphere and the patient's weight gain will reinforce the therapist's credibility to such an extent that he may shift the focus gradually from eating to interpersonal issues.

The further steps are usually centered around the particular *attachment-autonomy problems* in families with adolescent children. The aim is for the individual to achieve the next developmental step and for the family to allow this. We want to stress here that the so-called symptom-oriented approach we presented suffices in many cases to bring about all by itself a considerable reestablishment of a "normal" family functioning without engaging in specific family therapy. Whether the latter is really needed or not (or whether other interventions are wanted, e.g., individual psychotherapy) will depend upon the functional analysis of the anorexic symptoms and related intra- and interpersonal functioning during treatment. Therapy, even when focused on symptomatic behavior, is the best means for analyzing a problem and testing hypotheses with regard to the problem's etiology and, in particular, its maintaining factors. This is another reason for which we plead not to waste valuable time on complex diagnostic examinations, but rather to try out some therapeutic intervention as soon as possible. An early or final conclusion of this procedure can be that a more specialized intensive approach to treatment is necessary.

INTENSIVE THERAPY

An undetermined number of anorexia nervosa and bulimia patients need to induce and maintain significant changes in their life pattern. In many cases, this implies that several professionals are involved at the same time in the therapy of the patient and/or her family. Most common is the intentional splitting of different therapeutic functions, for instance, the physician takes care of the physical condition and the weight restoration, while a psychotherapist tries to get a grip on the patient's inner psychological and interactional experiences. Close contact must then exist among the therapists involved so that they are functioning as a unified team in order to avoid the danger of being played against one another. The discussion on the content and form of specialized and mostly inpatient treatment of eating disorder patients is treated elsewhere in detail (see e.g., Vandereycken & Meermann, 1984a). But what does concern the family physician is the *decision of hospitalization*.

With the exception of medical emergency indications the decision to hospitalize an anorexia nervosa or bulimia patient is usually based on a combination of criteria (Vandereycken, 1987):

1. *Medical criteria* which concern, in particular, a serious and potentially life-threatening deterioration of the patient's health:
   - severe acute or unremitting extreme weight loss (e.g., more than 30% below normal weight);
   - dangerous alterations in vital signs (postural hypotension, bradycardia, hypothermia) and electrolyte imbalance (hypokalemia);
   - intercurrent infection in a cachectic patient;
   - suicidal tendencies or attempts, and psychotic reactions.
2. *Psychosocial criteria* referring to a seriously disturbed life situation which may be, at the same time, cause and consequence of the eating disorder and thus create a vicious circle in which the patient is imprisoned:
   - marked family disturbance inaccessible to treatment;
   - abnormal social isolation with avoidance of interpersonal contacts or inability to engage in study or work.
3. *Psychotherapeutic criteria* especially in patients with a poorer prognosis (longer duration of illness, late onset of disease, occurrence of bulimia, vomiting or purging):
   - previous treatment failures, lack of motivation or even refusal to engage in outpatient therapy;
   - the need for an intensive psychotherapeutic milieu which can induce a change process that otherwise would take a long time to achieve.

The decision for hospitalization and its execution must be placed in a constructive therapeutic context instead of being the result of a power struggle the physician feels he is losing (Farley, 1985). In the latter case, referral for hospitalization disguises the clinician's counteraggression and frustrating helplessness: he is only interested in "winning" the battle by punishing the "stubborn" patient (or family) while keeping his own peace of mind. While admission to hospital might make the situation safe for a while, it may represent "a counterproductive retreat from confrontation with certain life difficulties and signify confirmation of sick role in the eyes of relatives who then dissociate themselves from active participation in therapy" (Morgan et al., 1983, p. 286). As Liebman et al. (1983) rightly stress, it is necessary to prevent the family from using hospitalization to reinforce the patient's role as the symptom-bearer for the family, as well as to prevent the parents from perceiving the admission as further acknowledgement of their personal failure as parents.

When there is no doubt about the need for hospitalization, the question arises of where the patient should be admitted. Some prefer a medical setting because it is less threatening and avoids the stigma of a mental hospital (Hodas et al., 1982). In our opinion (Vandereycken, 1986) this is only partially true. First of all, the family's attitude must be taken into account. For example, if the parents conceive the eating disorder as a somatic illness, this idea may be reinforced by a hospitalization in a purely medical setting. Moreover, we believe the major aim of the physician's work with anorexics or bulimics and their families is to help them over whatever treatment barrier exists. It is not so much a question of medical versus psychiatric hospitalization but rather of whether a particular hospital unit has sufficient experience with the treatment of eating disorders.

CONCLUSION

When faced with an anorexia nervosa or bulimia patient, the family physician plays an important role in the secondary prevention of the disorder. By making an early positive diagnosis he avoids the still too frequent situation that patients are burdened by too many technical examinations and that valuable time is wasted before treatment begins. According to the degree of complexity of the disorder as well as his own clinical experience and treatment potential, the physician must choose the appropriate level of outpatient management. It is a leading principle that outpatient therapy should be tried unless emergency situations force the hospitalization of the patient or unless there are solid reasons for preferring inpatient management. The physician is justified in attempting outpatient therapy on the condition that he regularly evaluates its costs and benefits both with respect to the patient and the family involved. The best guarantees for success are a constructive patient-family-therapist relationship and an explicit and consistent treatment plan based upon a multidimensional problem analysis.

REFERENCES

Andersen, A.E. (1985), *Practical Comprehensive Treatment of Anorexia Nervosa and Bulimia.* Baltimore: Johns Hopkins University Press.

Casper R.C. (1982), Treatment principles in anorexia nervosa. In: Feinstein, S.C. (Ed.), *Adolescent Psychiatry, Vol. X.* Chicago: University of Chicago Press, pp. 431-454.

Crisp, A.H. (1980), *Anorexia Nervosa—Let Me Be.* New York-London: Academic Press, Grune & Stratton.

Chiodo, J. & Latimer, P.R. (1983), Vomiting as a learned weight-control technique in bulimia. *Journal of Behavior Therapy and Experimental Psychiatry,* 14:131-135.

Farley, J.E. (1985), Preparing the family to make the decision about residential placement for an adolescent. *Hospital and Community Psychiatry,* 36:662-664.

Frances, A. & Clarkin, J.F. (1981), No treatment as the prescription of choice. *Archives of General Psychiatry,* 38:542-545.

Gull, W.W. (1874), Anorexia nervosa (apepsia hysterica, anorexia hysterica). *Transactions of the Clinical Society of London,* 7(1):22-28.

Halmi, K.A. (1983), Treatment of anorexia nervosa: A discussion. *Journal of Adolescent Health Care,* 4:47-50.

Hodas, G., Liebman, R. & Collins, M.J. (1982), Pediatric hospitalization in the treatment of anorexia nervosa. In: Harbin, H.T. (Ed.), *The Psychiatric Hospital and the Family.* Jamaica (N.Y.): Spectrum Publications, pp. 131 141.

Kalucy, R.S. (1978), An approach to the therapy of anorexia nervosa. *Journal of Adolescence,* 1:197-228.

Lawrence, M. (1984), *The Anorexic Experience.* London: The Women's Press.

Liebman, R., Sargent, J. & Silver, M. (1983), A family systems orientation to the treatment of anorexia nervosa. *Journal of the American Academy of Child Psychiatry,* 22:128-133.

Minuchin, S., Rosman, B. & Baker, L. (1978), *Psychosomatic Families. Anorexia Nervosa in Context.* Cambridge (Mass.): Harvard University Press.

Morgan, H.G., Purgold, J. & Welbourne, J. (1983), Management and outcome in anorexia nervosa. A standardized prognostic study. *British Journal of Psychiatry,* 43:282-287.

Sargent, J. & Liebman, R. (1984), Outpatient treatment of anorexia nervosa. *Psychiatric Clinics of North America,* 7:235-245.

Stern, S., Whitaker, C.A., Hagemann, N.J., Anderson, R.B. & Bargman, G.J. (1981), Anorexia nervosa: The hospital's role in family treatment. *Family Process,* 20:395-408.

Vandereycken, W. (1987), The management of patients with anorexia nervosa and bulimia. Basic principles and general guidelines. In: Beumont, P., Burrows, G. & Casper, R. (Eds.), *Handbook of Eating Disorders, Vol. I. Anorexia and Bulimia Nervosa.* Amsterdam: Elsevier/North Holland, pp. 235-253.

Vandereycken, W. & Meermann, R. (1984a), *Anorexia Nervosa. A Clinician's Guide to Treatment.* Berlin: Walter de Gruyter.

Vandereycken, W. & Meermann, R. (1984b), Anorexia nervosa: Is prevention possible? *International Journal of Psychiatry in Medicine,* 14:191-205.

Vandereycken, W. & Vanderlinden, J. (1983) Denial of illness and the use of self-reporting measures in anorexia nervosa patients. *International Journal of Eating Disorders,* 2(4):101-107.

Welbourne, J. & Purgold, J. (1984), *The Eating Sickness: Anorexia, Bulimia and the Myth of Suicide by Slimming.* Brighton: Harvester Press.

Chapter 13

The Family, the Hospitalized Patient, and the Therapeutic Team*

Walter Vandereycken, Johan Vanderlinden and Ellie Van Vreckem

INTRODUCTION

Once the decision of hospitalizing an eating disorder patient has been made and executed in a constructive way which makes the family co-responsible for the treatment (see Chapter 12 and 15), one must realize that the family is, to some extent, "hospitalized" too. This means that "the family as well as the patient have certain needs to which the entire treatment team must respond in order to have maximum therapeutic impact"(Stern et al., 1981, p. 396). By offering both family and patient a temporary "time-out" period (Hodas et al., 1982), the hospitalization breaks through a vicious circle of power struggles and dysfunctional interactions. But physical separation from the parents ("parentectomy") can assuage a crisis at home, and will not automatically change the family system nor alter the patient's relationships with psychic representations of the parents (Sours, 1980).

Intrafamilial conflicts or dysfunctional transactions may become externalized in the relationships between family members and treatment staff. The eating disorder may express the family's anxiety over developmental issues and possible splitting. Hospitalization can be threatening then for the family by fueling tension regarding issues of autonomy and dependence. Staff members may be viewed as "good" parents who are rescuing the "repressed" adolescent out of the hands of the "bad" parents. In other cases, the patient is scapegoated as the source of all problems in the family and hospitalization may reinforce that role which serves the protection of the family (e.g., denial of conflicts within the parents' marriage). Now the family feels relieved of a distressing responsibility

---

* Parts of this chapter are largely based upon excerpts from the book *Anorexia Nervosa. A Clinician's Guide to Treatment* (Berlin-New York, Walter de Gruyter, 1984) that Walter Vandereycken has written with Dr. Rolf Meermann from the University Psychiatric Hospital in Münster (F.R. Germany).

as long as the inpatient treatment staff focuses its expertise on the individual patient. Time and again, the therapeutic team has to find a sound balance between protection and confrontation (Harper, 1983). Since this is a complex but crucial matter, we will briefly highlight some peculiar issues of the triangular dynamics involved in the relationship between family, hospitalized patient, and treatment staff.

STRAIN ON THE FAMILY

Family reactions to the patient and hospital staff can be subdivided into three types of strategies used to control the treatment process (Krajewski & Harbin, 1982):

- The *overinvolved* family is enmeshed with both patient and treatment staff. This type of family may try to get more involvement in the decision making of the therapeutic team in order to obtain more control over the patient and to bring about a closer relationship between themselves and the patient.
- The *uninvolved* family, on the contrary, tries to control the treatment staff in order to increase the distance between themselves and their hospitalized family member (e.g., by opposing discharge from the hospital).
- The *pseudo-involved* family seemingly wants to be closely involved with the patient and the team. When pushed to change, however, their ambivalence and wish for increased separation emerge.

In our experience with hospitalized anorexics and bulimics, the first type of family reaction is the most common and the second rather scarce. Moreover, we encounter a fourth type, be it not so often, namely *normally involved* families. From the very beginning, we try to observe and to determine as soon as possible the type of family we are working with, and to understand the motivation and rationale of their attitude. Such observation must help us to have a better sense of what therapeutic strategies should be used and why.

The patient's and parents' usual responses to inpatient treatment appear to change according to a series of successive phases (Anyan & Schowalter, 1983; Seltzer, 1984; Stern et al., 1981). The major reactions are summarized in Table 1. In the beginning of the inpatient treatment ambivalence is high and the extent of the problem is minimized. This defensive reaction on the part of both patient and family then shifts to a more constructive working alliance with the staff. At the end of hospitalization, old or new problems may again put a strain on all parties involved.

Parents of anorexic or bulimic patients in residential treatment must cope with both the stress of the resultant separation and the burden of parenting a child now identified as severely disturbed or labeled as psychiatrically ill. Any shift of treatment focus, away from the individual patient and toward examina-

Table 1. The Patient's and Parents' Changing Attitudes During Hospitalization.

A. *Beginning phase*

The patient may:
- fear the separation from her family (e.g., expression of guilt feelings),
- postpone making real changes (e.g., no weight increase),
- test the integrity of the staff (e.g., splitting team members),
- manipulate the parents (e.g., insisting upon going home).

The parents may:
- feel guilty about what they have done wrong,
- experience frustration over the lack of tangible progress,
- criticize treatment procedures and test the authority of the team,
- doubt whether they have made the right decision about treatment.

B. *Middle phase*

The patient may:
- recognize the need to change the problem (e.g., weight gain),
- show a positive mood and openness (e.g., better contacts on the ward),
- be more accessible to confrontation (e.g., discussion of own feelings).

The parents may:
- feel confidence in the staff and support the treatment,
- shift their attention from weight to developmental issues,
- show greater willingness to discuss intrafamilial relationships.

C. *Final phase*

The patient may:
- deny the need for changes other than weight and eating,
- slow down the progress or relapse into the anorexia/bulimia,
- insist upon living on her own and becoming independent.

The parents may:
- be unduly optimistic about the patient's recovery,
- fear the responsibility for having the patient back home,
- stress the need for strict control over the patient's further evolution.

---

tion of family interactions, may prove threatening or psychologically painful for parents. Hence, it is no wonder that the treatment staff is faced with several negative parental reactions:

- *Ambivalence about the treatment:* parents may be skeptical about the appropriateness of a residential setting, especially with regard to a psychiatric unit or hospital. They may question their decision and fear negative consequences ("stigmatization"). Parents may criticize the treatment rationale or some therapeutic rules and interventions (e.g., restriction of visiting hours, the use of tube feeding or the lack of active "medical" intervention). They may doubt about the staff's competence and attempt to set one team member's comments or reactions against another's (particularly nurses are split into "good" or "bad").

- *Distress during treatment:* separation through hospitalization may arise an atmosphere of intrafamilial tension or even crisis in the parents' marriage (previously stabilized by the common concern about an "ill" child). Some parents may feel isolated or left alone, apparently convinced that problems encountered with their anorexic/bulimic child reflect unique and shameful family circumstances; they are particularly sensitive about being rejected and blamed as a scapegoat (the "bad" parents as cause of the illness).

In each particular case, one must remember that hospitalization itself may induce new problems or exacerbate existing ones: family alienation, fragmentation and isolation, but also enmeshment, overprotectiveness and noncompliance with the treatment program.

STRAIN ON THE STAFF

As a result of their personal characteristics, anorexic patients regularly place the whole team in situations of conflict. Their cachectic condition may evoke feelings of sympathy, worry, and willingness to help. But, on the other hand, the resistance to treatment (in fact a strong fear of changing), the lack of cooperation, the frustration caused by attempts at deception, and the patient's sometimes stubborn arrogance, may lead to anger and rejection. When staff members exhibit considerable counteranger, they in fact witness of the same frustrating helplessness the parents have experienced. Now the struggle over weight and eating is reproduced with the members of the treatment staff and results in the *re-enactment of intrafamilial conflicts within the hospital.* The anorexic's behavior and attitudes arouse, almost automatically, tendencies to counteract them, whether through (excessive) indulgence or covert aggression disguised as therapeutic pessimism, the use of coercive methods (e.g., tube feeding or complete seclusion) or the application of even newer therapeutic techniques. Driven into a corner, the therapist or team member is tempted to react with covertly aggressive displays of his authoritarian power or superior knowledge. But as such, he is building up the image of "omnipotent parent," an image the patients are determined to destroy.

On the other hand, there also exists a danger of overidentification with the patient, for instance with her success in gaining weight and in developing views that are congruent with one's own ideas. Then, the therapist is acting as many parents do: they wish to shape their child into a duplicate of their own ideals. Moreover, one must be aware that the patient is not just a pure victim of parenting failure, and one should beware of non-objective sentimentalization of the "poor" child and competitive criticism of the "bad" parents. It is helpful for the therapist to identify the family scapegoat without becoming drawn into the scapegoating process himself (Dally, 1977). Families have to be considered as treatment resources (Kuypers & Bebbington, 1985) instead of adversaries. All too often the treatment of eating disorder patients and their families is viewed as a continuing battle, whereas it is far more fruitful to look at the therapeutic process as a series of crises (Kalucy, 1978). In each crisis it is more constructive to analyze what kind of change the patient or the family is afraid of than to search for powerful tactics in order to tackle *resistance* — a term which by itself risks creating a confrontational atmosphere.

Many therapists are inclined to emphasize the family's resistance to treatment, its lack of cooperation or its tendency to deny the severity or significance of the problems. What is conceived of as a defensive fight of resistant patients/families on an *antitherapeutic battlefield,* may be created by the therapist's attitude itself. It seems to us that some types of treatment inevitably provoke antitherapeutic reactions on the part of the family. A treatment approach including parentectomy (strict isolation of the patient from her parents) might be the crucial factor in provoking negative reactions from the parents: they are officially blamed and in some way even punished, since the hospitalization seems to serve one main purpose, namely expelling the "pathogenic germs!" In a defensive therapeutic climate, the treatment staff, instead of questioning its own approach, may tend to suspect the family of being the cause of hindrances in the treatment. Then family therapy may risk becoming a too-easy response out of the staff's own frustration. Therefore, family therapy (for a discussion of when it is needed, see Chapter 15) must be incorporated in an overall treatment approach which witnesses the entire team's concern with the well-being of both patient and family.

The *cohesion of the therapeutic team* is the cornerstone of an effective in-patient treatment program. On many occasions, the team will have to face a "battle for structure," especially when their authority is tested by both patient and family. The team must "win" his battle, i.e., "establish the therapy situation as their domain, in which they decide what is therapeutic and what is not. This must be accomplished without humiliating the family or rendering them passive and submissive" (Stern et al., 1981, p. 401). The staff must resist becoming ensnared in the patient's or family's tendency to incorporate them into their way of life. Family members and the treatment team may get organized in a "too richly cross-joined system" in which the therapeutic subsystem has lost its effectiveness, is unable to maintain a meta-level from that of the family and is caught in a symmetrical game with the patient (Giacomo & Weissmark, 1985). Health care systems often share similarities with step families and especially new or inexperienced health care teams may resemble a "young family" in which the formation of new patterns is complicated by the preexistence of older and sometimes competing patterns of members from different families (Baker & Pontious, 1984). If the hospital staff wants to be a clear and constructive model of parenting, it must at least establish a firm but flexible inner structure allowing open communication without disguised subversion, and respectful negotiation without covert competition.

CONCLUSION

Hospitalization may have both constructive and disruptive effects on the patient and the family. It is important then not to start from a "defensive" point of view, suspecting that the family will somehow inevitably play an antitherapeutic role. If problems in the triangular relation between patient, family and staff do occur, the treatment team has first to question its own approach, especially whether or not they have disregarded or inadequately responded to the patient's and parents' ambivalence about treatment and their distress during hospitalization. One must try to avoid uncritically generalized assumptions as to the "pathological" nature of the family system, since many theories disguise in impressive neologisms a basic attitude of scapegoating toward the parents (especially the mothers: Calan et al., 1985).

Treatment of hospitalized eating disorder patients always involve the staff in the dynamics of the family process. The consistency of the therapeutic team as a whole is of decisive importance for the efficiency of an inpatient treatment program. Countertransference reactions on the part of the staff have to be recognized in time and worked out in mutual teamwork or by supervision in order to prevent splitting within the team, which inevitably means splitting of the triangle of patient-family-staff. Both the treatment team's cohesion and familiarity with eating disorder patients and their families are crucial with regard to treatment success. Whatever the concrete therapeutic approach, a congruence is needed among all parties involved. It is this congruence that will determine whether the patient and her family are allies or adversaries.

REFERENCES

Anyan, W.R. & Schowalter, J.E. (1983), A comprehensive approach to anorexia nervosa. *Journal of the American Academy of Child Psychiatry,* 22:122-127.

Baker, L.C. & Pontious, J.M. (1984), Treating the health care family. *Family Systems Medicine,* 2:401-408.

Calan, P.J. & Hall-McCorquodale, I. (1985), The scapegoating of mothers: A call for change. *American Journal of Orthopsychiatry,* 55:610-613.

Dally, P. (1977), Anorexia nervosa: Do we need a scapegoat? *Proceedings of the Royal Society of Medicine,* 70:470-474.

Giacomo, D. & Weissmark, M. (1985), An "overweight" anorectic family. *Journal of Strategic and Systemic Therapies,* 4(1):61-68.

Group for the Advancement of Psychiatry (1985), *The Family, the Patient, and the Psychiatric Hospital: Toward a New Model.* New York: Brunner/Mazel (GAP Report 117).

Harper, G. (1983), Varieties of parenting failure in anorexia nervosa: Protection and parentectomy, revisited. *Journal of the American Academy of Child Psychiatry,* 22:134-139.

Hodas, G., Liebman, R. & Collins, J. (1982), Pediatric hospitalization in the treatment of anorexia nervosa. In: Harbin, H.T. (Ed.), *The Psychiatric Hospital and the Family.* Jamaica (N.Y.): Spectrum Publications, pp. 131-141.

Kalucy, R.S. (1978), An approach to the therapy of anorexia nervosa. *Journal of Adolescence,* 1:197-228.

Krajewski, T. & Harbin, H.T. (1982), The family changes the hospital? In: Harbin, H.T. (Ed.), *The Psychiatric Hospital and the Family.* Jamaica (N.Y.): Spectrum Publications, pp. 143-154.

Kuipers, L. & Bebbington, P. (1985), Relatives as a resource in the management of functional illness. *British Journal of Psychiatry,* 147:465-470.

Seltzer, W.J. (1984), Treating anorexia nervosa in the somatic hospital: A multisystemic approach. *Family Systems Medicine,* 2:196-207.

Sours, J. (1980), *Starving to Death in a Sea of Objects. The Anorexia Nervosa Syndrome.* New York: Jason Aronson.

Stern, S., Whitaker, C.A., Hagemann, H.J., Anderson, R.B. & Bargman, G.J. (1981), Anorexia nervosa: The hospital's role in family treatment. *Family Process,* 20:395-408.

APPENDIX: Information Brochure For The Family

A member of your family or your partner has been admitted here* as a patient. We think it is important that you know our treatment principles. We also hope to obtain your cooperation.

General Treatment Principles

Problems with weight or eating patterns, known as anorexia nervosa or bulimia, are *psychosomatic illnesses.* Psychosomatic means there are concomitant physical and psychological features. The patient will be thoroughly screened for physical disturbances by the medical department. Psychological aspects are more difficult to assess. Experience has taught us that there is no clear, well-defined reason, somewhere in the past, but rather a multitude of different concurrent factors which have led to the actual situation. More important than "Why?" is the question: "How are we going to manage the problems with regard to the future?"

Experience has also taught us that disturbed eating patterns and weight abnormalities (especially weight loss) influence the patients' overall behavior, their feelings and thoughts, and their relationships toward others. Thus working on the consequences of their illness can be more important than worrying about the original causes. Talking does not help much as long as the weight and eating patterns are very disturbed. For this reason, priority is given to the *normalization of eating patterns and weight.* We hereby stress that the patient has to relearn to feed herself properly. It is a kind of reeducation program.

Restoring normal eating patterns and body weight is not sufficient. The patient also has to be able to fulfill a normal role in society: school, work, family, etc. Thus, the second aspect of treatment will be a training intent on *reintegrating the patient into society.* This means that problems centered around body image, sexuality, inferiority feelings, social inhibitions, etc. have to be treated. Different kinds of psychotherapy during and after the stay in the hospital will be used to this end.

All those therapy aims cannot be reached without *the active help of the family* (parents, partner, siblings). Usually in a longstanding illness like this the surrounding people have become overinvolved and nobody knows clearly what to do next. Many times well intended help becomes part of a vicious circle that ultimately only makes things worse. Many parents or partners develop guilt feel-

---

* Anorexia Nervosa Unit, University Psychiatric Center, Kortenberg (Belgium).

ings and wonder what went wrong. Instead of blaming someone or something, we prefer to search together for new solutions as a new approach is needed so as not to fall into the old trap again. The way you treat the patient on a visit or at home, after her discharge, is very important and full of consequences.

Concrete Details

Normalization of Eating Patterns and Weight
A written, detailed program has been given to the patient.* You can of course read it. In it we subdivide treatment into three phases. We need your help in enforcing the rules:
- At the beginning, visiting and other forms of contact (e.g., letters, telephone calls) are restricted. These restrictions are gradually lifted according to the patient's progress. If, however, the patient does not improve according to plan, further restrictions can be imposed. We need your help to hold the patient to those rules, so always contact the nursing staff before planning a visit.
- Do not disrupt the normal eating pattern in the hospital by bringing extra snacks or sweets. Do not bring any medication, including laxatives.
- Try avoiding topics such as food or weight. It is far more important to talk about other things.

Your Active Participation
- In addition to the general information offered here, we are of course always ready to answer additional queries. You can always telephone the psychiatrist or psychologist in charge. For concrete questions, such as visiting times, it is more efficient to contact the nursing staff directly.
- Twice monthly we have a special group for the parents and a separate group for the spouses of our patients. There you can exchange feelings, past experiences, frustrations, doubts, management problems or ask us for further information.
- It is also possible to have a personal meeting with the responsible psychiatrist or psychologist. You can ask for it or we will invite you and other members of the family for a separate family session.

Possible Problems

Many problems will arise during treatment. The main ones are:

---

* An example is reproduced in: Vandereycken, W. & Meermann, R., *Anorexia Nervosa. A Clinician's Guide to Treatment.* Berlin-New York, Walter de Gruyter, 1984, pp. 133-136.

- Separation from the family. This is hard on the patient and on you. The patient receives help from the other patients and staff to deal with feelings of being away from home in alien surroundings. The family, on the contrary, has to adapt on its own to a new situation missing one of its members. Therefore, we are always available for help; please do not hesitate to call!
- Later on, new problems arise: tensions, difficulties or conflicts will arise when the patient starts changing and is searching for a new role in the family. Especially difficult moments come when the patient, too afraid of change, blocks or even tries to avoid further treatment. These are frequent occurrences, so do not let it sap your determination to go through with the treatment.

Try to avoid on-the-spot decisons and get in touch with us first. This is of prime importance because the patient, who gets stuck, will try to manipulate you in any possible way.

Your patience and cooperation is a cornerstone of therapy we cannot do without.

Chapter 14

Parent Counseling: From Guidance to Treatment

Claire Perednia, Ellie Van Vreckem and Walter Vandereycken

INTRODUCTION

A whole evolution has taken place in the health care professionals' ideas about the role of parents in the development of an eating disorder and about their role in its treatment. As outlined in Chapter 11, for many decades parents were considered as pathogenic agents, having a noxious influence on the treatment of their anorexic child. As a logical consequence of this opinion, the therapist worked out a strategy to keep the parents at a "safe" distance from the patient. This strategy of so-called *"parentectomy"* was for a long time (and is sometimes still) conceived as the essential and most crucial therapeutic instrument. Such an attitude reflects a typical linear causal way of thinking in which the anorexia nervosa patient is just viewed as a pure victim of parenting failure. Hospitalization, then, is an act of rescuing that "poor" child which, at the same time, includes an indirect criticism of the "bad" parents.

This type of reasoning clearly shows that the therapist himself is drawn into the "scapegoat idea" (Dally, 1977). In anorexia nervosa, the traditional scapegoat is the mother who is blamed, often without any substantial evidence, by doctors, husbands, and even by patients themselves (Vandereycken & Meermann, 1984). In her book on psychotherapeutic abuse, Spitzer (1980) quotes the story of an anorexia nervosa mother who felt treated by a psychiatrist as if she was in a court-room playing both the role of the accused and the hostile witness: "Anything I said was pounced upon and questioned as though it had some hidden meaning, as if it contained some secret..." (p. 163). Her anorexic daughter was hospitalized and very soon the mother felt that the team overtly attempted to drive a wedge between herself and her daughter. This appeared to be coupled with an attempt to lay the blame for the anorexia upon the mother. This story illustrates many psychiatrists' attitude that family members, but espe-

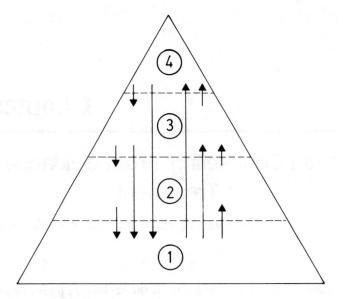

Figure 1.The "pyramid model" of parent counseling. (1 = guidance and educational counselng, 2 = family therapy, 3 = marital therapy, 4 = individual therapy.

cially parents, are the "enemy" fighting on an anti-therapeutic battlefield (Vandereycken & Meermann, 1984). The mother in Spitzer's chronicle is a vivid example of the conflicts many parents of anorexic patients face. They feel they have done everything for their children, "and yet there is that insidious poisoning which we all undergo, that somehow leaves me uneasy — a little, not exactly guilty, but rather responsible. Parents cannot avoid this sort of feeling. The psychiatrist would serve a much more useful role by attempting to allay this unwarranted guilt rather than exacerbating it" (Spitzer, 1980, p. 169).

Such a parent who has become a scapegoat or who feels guilty does not require treatment but is in particular need of understanding and reassurance (Dally, 1977). Hence, in our experience with the treatment of eating disorders, family therapy is not mandatory, but a *family-oriented* approach is! This means that we always try to work with the family in a constructive and collaborative way, following the principle that we have to meet the family's needs to the extent they "ask" for it and at the level they are "ready" to accept it (Vandereycken & Meermann, 1984).

This flexible attitude is represented in our *pyramid model* of parent counseling (see Figure 1) with different levels of approach; all parents are getting guidance and educational counseling (level 1); in several of them, a shift has to be made to family therapy (level 2), which in some parents ends up in marital therapy (level 3), while a few parents need individual psychotherapy (level 4).

We will first illustrate the model with the three cases we mentioned in Chapter 7 ("Case vignettes"). For the families we described, we have used three sources of information: the clinical impressions, the standardized interviews and the questionnaires.

Family A can be viewed as an example of the educational counseling approach; there is no apparent need for family therapy in order to restructure the system at home. The anorexia nervosa symptoms do not seem to be connected with marital or individual problems of the parents who seem satisfied with their marriage and have no special psychological complaints. The eating disorder appears to reflect some problems on the "educational" level: the parents are overprotective, especially mother who is too controlling in reaction to her youngest daughter leaving home. This would mean that the parents are on the threshold of a new developmental phase in the family life cycle. They are confronted with the "empty nest" phenomenon which requires a new equilibrium in their family as well as in their own marital relationship. Especially for this mother, who experienced a very close and warm atmosphere in her own family, such a confrontation can lead to some kind of crisis. Hence the basic approach in our counseling meetings is aimed at helping parents alter certain attitudes and preparing them for some changes in their family life.

In *family B* the anorexia nervosa problems obviously have a completely different meaning. From the family counseling meetings, it became clear that a very disturbing factor in this family is the exaggerated interference on the part of father's parents (especially of his mother). An extra difficulty is that the parents disagree about this matter and see it differently: father is not fully aware of the harmful influence of his mother upon his family and especially upon his wife. This reaction may be reinforced by his being absent from home very often for his job or his hobby. The situation is complicated by serious marital problems, experienced by both parents on a different level (for the mother it is an overall dissatisfaction, for father it particularly concerns the sexual relationship). Moreover, both parents admit a series of personal psychological complaints. It is obvious that the overinvolvement of the grandmother, together with the marital dissatisfaction, has become a chronic problem situation in this family, culminating in the anorexia nervosa problems of the daughter. According to the "first-things-first" principle, this issue is the main target to be tackled in family therapy sessions (level 2) sometimes even with the participation of the grandparents. The evolution of this family therapy will indicate if additional marital therapy (level 3) or parallel sessions of parent counseling (level 1) will be necessary.

In *family C,* the problems are even more complicated. With the exception of mother (who was reluctant to reveal personal opinions and feelings), all information sources indicate serious marital problems in this family, interwoven with individual problems, probably in both parents, but especially in the father, and serious parenting problems (rejection of the patient by both parents, a chaotic family life style etc.). First, this couple should come to a basic agreement about their positions both as parents and as partners. But the highly defensive attitude of both preclude the execution of the treatment plan, namely marital therapy (level 3) combined with parenting counseling sessions (level 1). In fact we had to limit our goal to the individualization process of the patient, completely separated from her parents.

Our pyramid model is based on a flexible and pragmatic viewpoint, each time "goods made to measure" in accordance with this family at this moment and in this situation. The first level consists of the more supportive, explorative or educational approach as to family management and problem solving skills. This type of counseling is meant for all the parents of our hospitalized patients and has two main goals: firstly building up a positive working alliance between the patient, the parents and the therapeutic team, and secondly, it also has a diagnostic function to see whether the family must be considered as a co-therapist or as a co-patient. In working with anorexia nervosa families, it is important to make a distinction between families in a kind of crisis situation and families with a more chronic (pathological) dysfunctioning. Characteristic for a crisis is the temporary character, caused by, for instance, the transition period of raising adolescent children or by the hospitalization itself. For these families parent counseling is the first step which stresses the role of the parents as educators and as co-therapists.

For those families, where the anorexia nervosa symptoms are an expression of a more chronic family dysfunctioning, the working strategy shifts from an educational to a more therapeutic level, i.e., from guidance to treatment. The parents (and other family members) are then considered as co-patients. This second level of family therapy, which focuses on the restructuring of the family system, is described extensively elsewhere in this book (see Chapters 15 and 16). When—from the work on the first or second level—it appears that marital and/or individual problems of one or both parents largely codetermine the eating problems, we shift to the next levels: marital therapy (level 3) and/or individual psychotherapy (level 4) for one or both parents.

This procedure is based on the principle: let us take the complaints of the parents "at face value," before engaging in active family intervention. Such an approach has two major advantages (van Engeland, 1976):

1. *Economic benefit:* Several parents can be used as mediators; they only lacked some knowledge and skills as educators. Why then problematize their partnership and ask them to talk about more as what they came for?
2. *Strategic benefit:* When the therapist has solid reasons to conclude that a "family problem" exists, he needs the parents' approval to act on this conclusion. Without the cooperation of the natural authorities in the family system (regardless how helpless the parents may be!), there is no real change possible. Some parents do not agree with the therapist's view. They do not want to question themselves, and sometimes this might be the end of therapy. But, by addressing them first in their role as mediators or co-

therapists, they may get the opportunity to experience that the problems are different from what they thought they were. Now, within a positive therapeutic climate, it is more likely that they will question themselves as individuals or marital partners, and hence become "co-patients" in the treatment process.

This is the basic philosophy of our work with parents. In the following part we will focus on the first (educational, supportive, explorative) level: family and parent counseling.

FAMILY COUNSELING

As Vandereycken and Meermann (1984) pointed out, we do not start working from the axiom that every family with an anorexia nervosa patient is — per definition — pathological and has to be "treated." That is the main reason why we offer all parents — from the beginning of the residential treatment — *family counseling sessions*. In these sessions — most often with, but sometimes also without the patient and/or the other children of the family — we address ourselves first and foremost to parents of a hospitalized child. This "family counseling" can eventually evolve to a kind of "parent counseling" — in principle without the patient or the other children — which stresses the role of the parents as educators, mediators or co-therapists.

The family counseling sessions have a double goal of working with the family in a positive atmosphere (the positive working alliance), and analyzing the presenting problem within the family context (the functional family analysis).

The Positive Working Alliance

The family counseling sessions are, in the first place, aimed at building a positive working alliance between the "therapist counselor" (representing the whole therapeutic team), the patient and the entire nuclear family. The implicit goal is to obtain an active participation from the family — especially from the parents — during the residential treatment. This is very important in order to avoid drop-outs during the inevitable crises occuring during treatment. For that purpose, these counseling sessions have an informative, a supportive and a motivational function.

The informative function consists of several aspects. One very important factor is the openness or high degree of transparency of our inpatient treatment program for both the patient and her family. We do this by making the initial interviews as freewheeling as possible, so that all kinds of topics and problems about our treatment program can be discussed. We give to all the parents an extensive information map with the general treatment principles. This brochure describes the eating disorder as a psychosomatic illness, i.e., the end-product of many somatic and psychic factors; the necessity of normalizing body weight and eating pattern; the goal of reintegrating the patient into society, and the need for active help on the part of the family (see Appendix of Chapter 13).

Another — sometimes very urgent — aspect of this informative function is to make the parents aware of the seriousness of the condition and the urge for treatment, they sometimes underestimate the somatic dangers of. For example, the malnutrition, emaciation or hypokalemia. Also, they often must be reminded of the psychological consequences of an increasing social and familial isolation, such as serious school retardation, loss of work, lack of social contacts, etc. Several parents often ask for more information about anorexia nervosa in the form of self-help literature (see also Chapter 12). Before simply suggesting some titles for lay people (examples: see Vandereycken & Meermann, 1984), it is important to know what type of information they are seeking and what the real motive is behind this request (e.g., alleviation of own guilt feelings). Moreover, we also offer the parents a redefinition of eating and weight problems into more workable concepts than their usually distorted idea of an illness.

The supportive function of the family counseling sessions is very important considering that a (psychiatric) hospitalization of a family member is an intrusive happening. The parents are often left with a lot of guilt feelings and/or a shocked self-confidence. They feel themselves culpable for the ongoing situation and ask themselves what they have done wrong in their child-rearing. They look upon the therapeutic team as a "super parent" who will take over the task in which they have failed. The hospitalization itself may have consequences toward the marital relationship of the parents. Either they find support from each other or the crisis reveals latent marital problems (e.g., parents blaming each other etc.).

Parents are sometimes ashamed to have a child that has been labeled as a "psychiatric" patient. They do not know whom to tell and how to deal with annoying or nasty questions of outsiders ("Such things would never happen in their families!"). Furthermore, most parents went through a lot of discouraging and painful experiences of unsuccessful contacts or treatments with different kinds of therapists. As a result, they feel more helpless toward the problems and lost the little self-confidence left. The family counselor must be aware of the danger that the parents might perceive an hospitalization as a further acknowledgement of their personal failure as parents. By a positive relabelling of the problems, we attempt to relieve their guilt feelings. We encourage them to verbalize these feelings of demoralization, ambivalence and criticism toward the therapeutic team and the treatment as a whole and call it their readiness to collaborate in a constructive way.

The most important support we can give them is to try to slowly demolish the myth of the completely powerless parent(s). We can do so by offering them a redefinition of the problems in such a way that they experience them as *within* their own reach, and not only as a matter for "experts."

Example: A couple of desperate parents stopped thinking how to take over the "power" in their family, once they learned how important it is to restore the normal dining schedule of the family.

We also stress our need to be supported and trusted by the parents. We make them aware of the importance of forming a united front, since without their help nobody can help their child. "Our central message is, our professional knowledge and your personal involvement should be blended into one powerful therapeutic fuel whose potential energy will be strong enough to induce the necessary change process if it is used in one and the same direction and for the same purpose" (Vandereycken and Meermann, 1984, p. 164). Whatever piece of information there is available can be helpful in this respect.

Example: A mother told us she found it strange that her daughter always smoked a cigarette outside the house and that she often drank a glass of water before eating. Investigating this further we discovered never mentioned and deep-seated compulsive rituals in her daughter's as well as in the family's life.

The motivational function of the family counseling sessions is another important aspect. Some parents are easily engaged in treatment because they experience some understanding and support from the therapist(s), especially when their guilt feelings are quickly relieved. But there are other parents whose motivation for participation and collaboration in treatment is a very difficult and delicate issue. Our experience is that in most of these cases confronting the parents directly and too early with their resistance usually has the opposite effect and should be avoided in order to get a foot in the door.

In eating disorders, there are sometimes indications of serious parenting failure, dating from before the admission, but sometimes also appearing during hospitalization. Harper (1983) mentions the following forms of parenting failure he encountered in anorexia nervosa families:

- provision of nocuous, dangerous (self-)medication;
- malignant denial of patient's life-threatening condition;
- persistent triangulation (e.g., by involving and manipulating the patient in divorce battles);
- subversion of treatment plans;
- parental desertion and depression;
- severe breakdown of the householding.

Special attention has to be given to families where the hospitalization of the eating disorder patient means that her role as a scapegoat — that mostly existed long before admission — is strengthened. This can result in a complete refusal of the parents to involve themselves into treatment ("she is sick, we are okay") in order to avoid a confrontation with their own (family, marital or individual) problems.

Example: While totally escaping in his job, a father persisted in refusing to join the counseling sessions, arguing that his daughter was just an egoist who already had received too much attention. In doing so, he reinforced the fusional relationship between her and his wive (with whom he covertly lived in discord) and hence doomed the treatment to failure.

On the other hand the family counselor must be aware of the pitfall of an — implicit or covert — identification with the victimized, "poor" patient. Such attitudes can create a power-struggle without any hope for a successful — even meaningful — cooperation with the parents. How can one expect that the "enemy" becomes an "ally?" Such a situation usually results in a failure, or premature termination of therapy. The family-counselor has to work, carefully and rather indirectly with the parents as allies instead of against them as adversaries. In these cases where symptomatology is very probably hiding serious problems (e.g., severe parental psychopathology or incest), he has to work with even more tact, patience and prudence.

The Functional Family Analysis

The second goal of the family counseling in sessions is a diagnostic one: "mapping" the eating disorder against the background of the family (dys)functioning in order to adapt the treatment to the real needs of the family. Firstly, it is important to distinguish the families that are in a kind of (temporary) crisis situation from those with a more basic (chronic) pathology. Not every family with an eating disorder patient is "disturbed." The need for family therapy stricto sensu will depend upon the functional analysis of the eating disorder within the interactional network of the family system. "We have to analyze if and in which way the individual's behavior is maintained by family interaction, and, conversely, if and how the symptomatology of the identified patient maintains a dysfunctioning family system" (Vandereycken & Meermann, 1984, p. 158). This can happen directly by inserting specific tasks in the interviews, and by observing the interactions (see Chapter 5) and also by means of specific questionnaires (see Chapter 6). A very useful analysis, however, is a rather indirect one, namely by observing the family's reactions during hospitalization: Does the family respect the therapeutic rules they agreed upon? How are the visits or week-ends at home? How does the patient's evolution relates with specific reactions from or toward the family? How does the family organize itself in the absence of the patient? A good functional analysis does not involve the problematic aspects alone: it is also important to see if the family uses the therapeutic situation to increase its possibilities of communication and problem-solving skills. This analysis, direct or indirect, will give — after some time — an indication whether the family has to be considered as a co-therapist (see Figure 1, level 1) or as a co-patient in general (level 2) or, more specifically, with respect to the parents' marriage (level 3) or regarding some individual parent's problems (level 4).

A common characteristic we saw in all eating disorder, especially anorexia nervosa families, is *the lack of adequate joint authority of the parents.* "Adequate" refers to the balance of control and autonomy proper for the age of the child. The parental authority needs to be rational in the sense that it should be flexible and in harmony with the child's level of development. "Joint" authority means that there must exist a basic agreement between the parents about child-rearing issues, that they function in concert and reinforce each other's requests and actions so that the child clearly knows what the expectations are (Vandereycken & Meermann, 1984, p. 153).

This lack of adequate joint authority of the parents and the resulting child-rearing problems, such as setting limits or establishing clear rules, can be of a primary or a secondary nature. When they are secondary, i.e., caused by an underlying dysfunctional family structure or by marital and/or individual problems of one or both parents, then we mostly shift to the next level(s) of our working model: family, marital or individual therapy respectively.

When we estimate theses child-rearing problems as primary—which means that there is no apparent need for specific therapy—the family counseling shifts its focus to parent counseling. We presume that the parents need some "education in education." We, thus, stay on the supportive, advisory-educational level but with more concrete attention for particular facets of parenting.

This strategy might also be indicated in working with parents who have a very strong resistance to therapy, although definitely needed. The parents, however, would refuse the proposition of any form of "therapy" ("there is nothing wrong with us") but they can more easily accept this kind of "educational" counseling that is less threatening. Through these sessions they get the opportunity to experience that their view on the problems needs to be changed and that more personal matters may be involved in it. In the meantime, the counselor may have gained their trust in order to now become their (marital or individual) therapist.

PARENT COUNSELING

In the parent counseling sessions, we address ourselves to the parents as a couple of educators who temporarily experience some problems in handling their adolescent child(ren). The eating problems are translated as an expression of a developmental crisis with which the parents as well as the patient have problems coping. The adolescent phase of children requires special problem-solving skills on the part of parents who are not trained for this task and, hence, may fail to a certain extent as many parents do. But certain shortcomings are understandable when one has no experience in a peculiar task.

Goals

The main goal of parent counseling is to teach the parents how to be co-therapists during the period of hospitalization. We underline the fact that the parents continue to be responsible for their child and that we can help them with our professional knowledge by giving them information and advice.

   Example: During the visiting-hours in the hospital, a couple observed that other patients usually had several friends who came visiting them. They now realized that their daughter had had too few contacts outside the family. We adviced them to invite more of their daughter's friends. Since they have four daughters, the parents always thought there were enough people in the house, thereby accentuating a rather fusional family atmosphere.

The anorexia/bulimia problems are very demanding to the competencies of the parents. A first step is to increase (or restore) their sense of competence and effectiveness by helping them acquire some new problem-solving or child-rearing skills, and enhance their identity and autonomy as parents of adolescent children. Adolescence itself is a critical moment in the family life cycle: an intersection between the increasing autonomy of the child and the decreasing control on the part of the parents (Compernolle, 1982). Finding the equilibrium point is a rather difficult issue for the patient as well as for the parents. As already stated, these families often show a lack of adequate joint parental authority. In some there is too much parental control and, therefore, creating some distance—some "private" space—is an important growth condition for the patient as well as for the parents.

   Example: Not infrequently, we have to advise parents not to open the letters nor read the diaries of their daughter, not to choose her clothes, to knock on the door before entering their children's room, etc.

In other families, the parental authority is too weak and must be reestablished. The parents have to learn to set up and consistently apply adequate, age-appropriate, rules.

   Example: In one family the parents were so indulgent that, in fact, the anorexic girl was governing the household (she did the shopping, cooking, cleaning etc.). Now that the daugher was hospitalized, we asked the parents to reintroduce the "old" family rules that existed before the anorexia started. The first week-ends that the daughter was allowed to stay at home were regarded as an experimental learning occasion to test it out.

We always emphasize the importance of a basic agreement between *both* parents about all these issues. They will need each other's help and support, especially in the difficult moments they will have to confront, such as, for example, manipulative attempts on the part of their child. Sometimes this can mean that one parent has to take more distance (usually the mother) while the other (usually the father) becomes more directly involved.

Example: We regularly ask the father to communicate to his daughter
the decisions taken in the parent counseling sessions.

Our experience shows us that such parent counseling sessions may reveal *hidden problems in the parents.* Some parents get completely stuck. They do not translate their good intentions and nice child-rearing ideas into every day practice. Or it can happen that their ambivalent attitude breaks the surface: "Help us, please, but do not ask us to change anything in our lives!" A wide range of obstacles can interfere with parenting. Interpersonal, marital or individual problems of one or both parent(s) can undermine their competency to fulfill their role as a parent. The emphasis must then (sometimes very gradually) be shifted to the therapeutic levels, where the parents are approached as "co-patients." Sometimes, it may be better to refer the parents to another therapist. Nevertheless, the impact of the parent counseling itself must not be underestimated. Several studies report the fact that the quality of parenting is influenced by the marital relationship. A remarkable finding is reported by Brody and Forehand (1985). They found that a parent training program for mothers (they did not include fathers in their study) had a positive influence on their marital relationship. The possibility that improvement of parenting may have a positive effect on the parents' marital relationship is worth studying.

Methods

As far as we know, there are not any parent training programs (PTP) specific for parents of adolescents with eating disorders and related developmental problems. Therefore, we inspired our practical work with the PTP for problem children which induced a popular self-help movement for parents (see e.g., Abidin, 1976; Becker, 1971; Miller, 1977; Patterson, 1975). Within an *experiential,* client-centered framework, Gordon's (1970, 1976) PTP teaches the parents some child-centered skills. Because older children are able to solve their own problems and have creative possibilities, the parents have to learn other ways of communicating with their child and other ways of constructive problem solving by active listening, giving I-messages and by using the no-loose method. Working in the same direction but from a social learning theory viewpoint, the *behavioral* PTP (Gordon & Davidson, 1981) supposes that child behavior can be influenced systematically. The parents learn to control or modify problematic child behaviors by training in the effective use of social learning principles, such as reinforcement, modeling, and punishment. In fact, many forms of PTP combine experiential and behavioral approaches, eventually adding other components such as the so-called "rational-emotive education" (Knaus, 1974).

Some useful aspects of these PTP for our work are:
1. *Teaching the parents to observe.* It is important in these families that the parents change their perception of the problems and "the patient:" They

are confronted not just with a "strangely sick" child but with a child who refuses to eat and, consequently, to grow up. For this purpose, we suggest that the parents:

- make a difference between an observation (what they see or hear) and an impression (what they think);
- take a distance from the situation by learning to react to what they really see and not on what they think to see;
- postpone their interpretation and not immediately react to the (problem) behavior.

The result often is that the parents feel much more comfortable in their role and that some misunderstandings — that caused much tensions in the past — can be avoided.

2. *Training the parents in the use of positive social reinforcements.* Giving constructive criticism and reinforcements are parenting skills that positively influence the parent-child relationship and, thus, also the child's development. "Constructive" means that the given criticism (appreciation) is concrete, motivated and that the non-verbal behavior fits with the verbal message.

3. *Helping the parents to learn the art of negotiation.* They first have to accept that in family life disagreements and conflicts are inevitable. This is an important issue in families with an anorexic daughter. The parents usually expect everything to be "perfect;" and have too high and unrealistic expectations of themselves as well as of their children. They also have to realize that these conflicts can be resolved in a way that is reciprocally satisfying and that this can be obtained by negotiation, which means that the adolescent is no longer under tutelage, but develops personal opinions.

An interesting and highly valuable method is the use of parent counseling groups, as will be described in Chapter 18.

CONCLUSION

The basic philosophy of our approach is: *to work with instead of against the family.* The model we presented is a flexible one offering guidance to all family members (family and parent counseling), family therapy to some of them, and marital or individual therapy to other parents. As does Andersen (1985), we can summarize the essential guidelines as follows:

- Do not assume dysfunction exists in the family just because there is an eating problem.
- Assume families have done their best, but are tired from stress and want help.
- Approach families in a non-blaming way and encourage their interest and investment in treatment.

As therapists we are, first and foremost, concerned with building a constructive and collaborative relationship with the family and especially with the
parents. We need their cooperation and at the very least they need our support
and understanding.

REFERENCES

Abidin, R. (1976), *Parenting Skills.* New York: Human Sciences Press.
Andersen, A.E. (1985), *Practical Comprehensive Treatment of Anorexia Nervosa and Bulimia.* Bal-
    timore: Johns Hopkins University Press.
Becker, W.C. (1971), *Parents are Teachers: A Child Management Program.* Champaign (Ill.): Re-
    search Press.
Brody, G.H. & Forehand, R. (1985), The efficacy of parent training with maritally distressed
    and nondistressed mothers: A multimethod assessment. *Behaviour Research and Therapy,*
    23:291-296.
Compernolle, T. (1982), Adequate joint authority of parents: A crucial issue for the outcome of
    family therapy. In: Kaslow, F.W. (Ed.), *The International Book of Family Therapy.* New York:
    Brunner/Mazel, pp. 245-256.
Dally, P. (1977), Anorexia nervosa: Do we need a scapegoat? *Proceedings of the Royal Society of
    Medicine,* 70:470-474.
Gordon, S.B. & Davidson, N. (1981), Behavioral parent training. In: Gurman, A.S. & Kniskern,
    D.P. (Eds.), *Handbook of Family Therapy.* New York: Brunner/Mazel, pp. 517-555.
Gordon, T. (1970), *Parent Effectiveness Training.* New York: Peter H. Wyden.
Gordon, T. (1976), *PET in Action: Inside PET Families, New Problems, Insights, and Solutions.*
    New York: Peter H. Wyden.
Harper, G. (1983), Varieties of parenting failure in anorexia nervosa: Protection and parentec-
    tomy, revisited. *Journal of the American Academy of Child Psychiatry,* 22:134-139.
Knaus, W. (1974), *Rational-Emotive Education.* New York: Institute for Rational Living.
Miller, W.H. (1977), *Systematic Parent Training.* Champaign (Ill.): Research Press.
Patterson, G.R. (1975), *Professional Guide for Families and Living with Children.* Champaign
    (Ill.): Research Press.
Schutze, G. (1980), *Anorexia Nervosa.* Bern-Stuttgart-Wien: Verlag Hans Kuber.
Spitzer, T. (1980), *Psychobattery: A Chronicle of Psychotherapeutic Abuse.* Clifton (N.J.): Humana
    Press.
Vandereycken, W. & Meermann, R. (1984), *Anorexia Nervosa. A Clinician's Guide to Treatment.*
    Berlin/New York: Walter de Gruyter.
van der Maas, J.J. (1985), Behandeling van ouders (Treatment of parents). *Kind en Adolescent,*
    6:219-226.
van Engeland, H. (1976), Gedragstherapie en gezinsinterventies (Behavior therapy and family in-
    terventions). *Tijdschrift voor Psychotherapie,* 2:132-141.

Chapter 15

Family Therapy Within the Psychiatric Hospital: Indications, Pitfalls and Specific Interventions

Johan Vanderlinden and Walter Vandereycken

INTRODUCTION

The vast majority of publications regarding family therapy deals with its use in an outpatient setting. For a long time, family therapy was considered as incompatible with a residential treatment program, since the latter focuses on the individual (the "symptom-bearer" or "designated patient"). But, as explained in Chapter 11, the "second generation" of family therapists has become more flexible in this respect, especially when faced with severe eating disorders. Indeed, there are times and conditions that hospitalization is the only possible course of action in some anorexics and bulimics (see Chapter 12). A specialized treatment center for eating disorders appears to be faced with a twofold trend (Vandereycken & Meermann, 1984): on the one hand it may see more and more cases in the early stage of the disorder, i.e., more referrals of patients with a good prognosis ("positive" selection); but, on the other hand, it may also see more and more treatment failures, especially those patients with long and intractable problems ("negative" selection). We, at our center, mostly encounter the second phenomenon: referral of older (married), severe, chronic or complicated cases, the majority of whom have been treated before (see Chapter 9).

For almost 20 years, our center has developed special interest in treating eating disorders (actually about 55 admissions per year), and the inpatient approach has been changed many times during this ongoing trial-and-error process (Vandereycken, 1985). In the last five years a standardized treatment program has been formed, which is:

● *time-limited,* with an average duration of three months (maximum stay is six months;) but intensive aftercare is provided;

● *multifaceted,* including group psychotherapy (two groups of eight patients each), a special behavioral contract (regarding weight and eating), occupational and art therapy (emphasizing free expression), and a specific psychomotor treatment (with e.g., body-image confrontation by means of video);

● *family-oriented,* including the flexible use of a variety of approaches, from educational guidance (see Chapter 14) to parent-counseling groups (see Chapter 18) and, finally, family therapy (the subject of this chapter).

In order to make the integration of family therapy in the residential program as effective as possible, the family therapist should have a *central position* within the team (see also Harbin, 1982; Sargent, Liebman & Silver, 1985; Seltzer, 1984). In our unit the principal therapist coordinates several functions or tasks: he meets the family during the first interview at admission; at the same time he is involved in the inpatient group psychotherapy; he will be responsible for the aftercare program; and, finally, he will accomplish the role of family therapist where indicated. This central and coordinating position contrasts considerably with the strong division of therapeutic functions so common in residential treatment centers or psychotherapeutic communities. Although centralization of different functions within one therapist definitely demands a great amount of knowledge and therapeutic skills, it has in our experience some important and specific benefits (Vandereycken et al., 1986):

● It avoids the patient's almost notorious game of playing off therapists against each other (splitting the team).

● It enhances consistent action and avoids endless discussions among therapists.

● Information from different angles (referring context, individual, group, family or partner) is gathered in a more efficient and integrated way, which helps the planning and realization of treatment strategy.

● Centralization often brings about some extra motivation on behalf of the family therapist.

● It is reassuring for the patient's relatives to know that there is one person they can call upon.

However, the introduction and integration of family therapy within an inpatient treatment is not always welcomed with great enthusiasm but can often provoke a highly resistant attitude on the part of the ward staff. This was not the case in our unit, since the introduction of the family-oriented approach was carefully planned and gradually tried out, with close attention for developing a working alliance with all team members. If one is surrounded by a skeptical and resistant team, Treacher (1984) describes several practical guidelines for the beginning family therapist, to avoid this resistance and make the family approach work. First, the family therapist has to analyze and understand the structure of the hospital and form a working alliance with the entire ward staff. Second, when the initial strategies of the family therapist prove successful, it is then possible to move toward deepening the family-orientated approach, so that ward policy concerning, for instance, admission and discharge, can be changed. However, for the family therapy approach to be influential at all, it must avoid taking up a messianic position.

Our family approach may be characterized as *directive family therapy* (Lange & van der Hart, 1983), i.e., pragmatic, eclectic and flexible, using structural, strategic and behavioral elements. The main focus is on the here-and-now situation, aiming at stimulating change in the actual problems that are presented by the family. We do not always find it necessary that all family members should be present at the therapy sessions, although we invite the whole nuclear family at least for the first interview. Depending on the analysis of the family functioning and its evolution during treatment, we may decide to work with the whole family or meet only with separate subsystems (parents, children, with or without the patient). At all times we try to adjust our family therapeutic approach to the special needs and growing capacities of that particular family, together with the patients' developmental status. This pragmatic approach necessitates a flexible attitude on the part of the therapist, and a continuous assessment and functional analysis of the anorexic or bulimic symptoms against the background of the family system. We have to analyze repeatedly if and in which way the individual's behavior is maintained by family interaction and, conversely, if and how the eating disorder maintains a dysfunctional family system. Questions such as "What function does this symptom serve in this family?" or "What gain is achieved through it?" are sometimes difficult to answer until some therapeutic intervention has occurred. Therefore, treatment itself is the best way to test and reformulate clinical hypotheses about the nature and function of a particular eating disorder. Ultimately, such a functional analysis is completed at the end of a successful therapy (Vandereycken & Meermann, 1984).

INDICATIONS AND CONTRAINDICATIONS

The question of whether family therapy is indicated or not in the case of an hospitalized patient is for many family therapists an irrelevant question. From a rigid systems perspective, they strongly believe that an eating disorder, just as any other symptomatic behavior, always has a special function within the family (or broader social system). Hence, the system is the "patient" and family therapy is always the treatment of choice. We, on the contrary, do not think that family therapy is mandatory, but a family-oriented approach is. "The difference lies, of course, in the word 'therapy,' which somehow presupposes that something is wrong in the family and has to be changed then. We prefer to work 'with' the family in a constructive and collaborative way: we need their cooperation and they need at least our support and understanding. Functional problem analysis during the treatment of the 'identified patient' will reveal in which way the eating disorder is interwoven with family (dys)functioning, and to what extent and at which level interventions in the family system are necessary and possible" (Vandereycken & Meermann, 1984, p. 165).

Based on a detailed functional analysis and clinical assessment of the eating disorder within the family system, we sometimes find *no family dysfunctioning*. This finding has also been noticed by Andersen (1985), who states that 12% of the families with an eating disorder sample seemed to provide enough support so that the patient was nurtured, and enough separateness so that the patient could grow! Hence, in those families where the functional analysis does not reveal any major interactional (marital) problems or hidden conflicts within the family system, which further shows the existence of clear intergenerational boundaries (also in relation to the parents' family of origin), family therapy will not be necessary. Here, we like to stress the advantage of working in a hospital setting which enables the therapist to experience the impact patients may have on those surrounding them. Each therapist and nurse working with anorexics or bulimics in a residential treatment program knows the difficulties of living with such patients far much better than an outpatient family therapist who only meets the family in his office during a relatively brief period of time. What we like to underscore is that the eating disorder itself may have a disruptive effect on the social system the patient is living in. "In our experience, it is a mistake to start from the axion that every anorexic's family is somehow 'disturbed' and must, therefore, be 'treated.' True, every family we saw was in one sense or another 'dysfunctional' at the moment of referral or admission to the hospital. But which family would not be in some kind of crisis when being faced with a severely starving family member? Which parents would not be upset when they are searching for professional help fearing that their child is in a medically dangerous condition? In other words, a family *crisis* is not necessarily a sign of family *pathology*" (Vandereycken & Meermann, 1984, p. 158). Hence, a so-called symptomatic or individual-oriented treatment (hospitalization) may sometimes suffice to bring about all by itself a reestablishment of a normal family atmosphere.

On the other hand, the functional analysis may reveal *serious problems* such as high conflict (avoidance), disorganization and unhealthy cohesion in the family system, sometimes reflected by severely disturbed or psychopathological behavior in one or more other family members.

> *Example:* Olivia, an 18-year-old girl, was admitted to our hospital because of an extremely therapy-resistant anorexia nervosa complicated with binge eating episodes, vomiting and abuse of laxatives. The family consisted of two other girls (17 and 21 years old) and one boy (22 years old), who all appeared to have serious eating problems. Both parents were at the moment living together, but they struggled for more than 15

years with serious marital problems and they had already separated several times in the past. All these years, both parents misused their children by involving them in their ongoing fights, for instance, by forcing them into coalitions with one parent against the other.

In recent years, we have seen more of these severely disturbed families; not commonly there even exist incestuous relationships between father and daughter(s), which mostly are hushed up with dogged determination or only brought into the open during the final phase of the treatment. The question with regard to these families is not merely whether some family therapeutic intervention is indicated — there is no doubt about it — but in which form, for instance whether it is meaningful to see all family members together and at what moment in the treatment this should be done.

Moreover in many of these very disturbed families we often decide at the beginning of the treatment to work toward a definite separation between (at least) the patient and the parents. Therefore, we may work only with the separate subsystems (i.e., children and parents apart). Then, the major focus will be on decreasing the chaotic family atmosphere. The hospitalization serves the final goal of separating the patient from the family in order to promote and stimulate individuation, usually combined with marital therapy for the parents.

As mentioned in Chapter 11, other clinicians also warn the inexperienced family therapist and stress the need for careful assessment and treatment planning in the following situations (see e.g., Liebman, Sargent & Silver, 1983):

- patients with a long history of eating disorder and a significant delay in psychosocial development;
- single-parent families or broken homes (see Chapter 17);
- families in which one or both parents display severe psychopathology;
- families in which previous family therapeutic attempts have failed.

But still many questions concerning (contra)indications for family therapy in hospitalized eating disorder patients remain unanswered. At the moment, we do not have clear-cut and research-based criteria for the use of family therapy in general or for the application of specific strategies or techniques in particular. We do not know what sort of interventions from the therapist results in what sort of responses in the family and the patient. We even believe that the so-called nonspecific therapeutic factors (Frank, 1984) — such as creation of hope, constitution of a warm working alliance, redefinition of the probem as a resolvable one — are very important elements in the family approach, as also underlined by Yager and Strober (1985).

Although there seems to exist general agreement about the usefulness if not preference of family therapy in fairly young patients who still live in intact families, there are divergent and opposing opinions about whether family therapy is indicated in bulimics and in older chronic or married patients. In our experience with older and chronic cases of anorexia nervosa and bulimia, the family approach is very often a crucial element in the treatment process (see Chapter

16). The fact that adult patients are married or have already lived for several years away from their family of origin can be very misleading. They seem to have reached a certain independence but a great deal of these so-called grown-up women still have strong emotional ties with their family of origin. The eating disorder appears to be at once cause and consequence of a strong attachment to their family of origin (Vanderlinden & Vandereycken, 1984).

In sum, although many questions remain unanswered because of lack of research in this area, it is our experience that a family-oriented approach is mandatory in an inpatient treatment program for eating disorders. The indication for specific family therapy, however, must be based on careful (re)assessment of the eating disorder within the context of the family system.

SPECIFIC STRATEGIES AND SPECIAL TECHNIQUES

In our experience, the therapy process during inpatient treatment passes through several stages, each of them necessitating specific clinical strategies and interventions. These phases are offered only as a flexible framework for the clinician, rather than as absolutely necessary steps to pass through with each family. Though this framework and its related treatment strategies do also apply to bulimic patients and their families, this population requires additional interventions, which will be described separately.

Beginning Phase: Preparing the Family System for Change

Effective family therapy for anorexia nervosa and bulimia in an inpatient setting begins with *contacting the family or spouse before admission.* The presence of important family members during the first interview has become a basic rule. If possible, we request that everyone living with the patient – at least both parents – must attend the first interview. This procedure is aimed at underlining the importance of the family's co-responsibility and cooperation. We will not admit a patient without the family's (parents', spouse's) explicit willingness to support the treatment. This commitment, in our experience, can be crucial for avoiding a premature termination of treatment (Vandereycken & Meermann, 1984). Otherwise the risk that the patient might create a power struggle between the team and the family over some aspects of the inpatient treatment program would be much greater (Stern et al., 1981). Hence, the first contact with the family can be decisive in determining the success of the hospital phase of treatment (Treacher, 1984).

The most important goal of the first meeting is *to constitute a warm working alliance* with all family members. For this purpose, we start the conversation by asking all family members to introduce themselves (age, profession, hobbies, etc.). We thus emphasize that we are not only interested in the identified patient, but in the whole family as well. We try to listen carefully to their questions and

Table 1: An Outline for the Beginning Phase

- Contact the family or spouse before admission.
- Constitute a warm working alliance with all family members.
- Listen carefully to the family's feelings of guilt, anxiety, despair, shame, anger,...and provide support.
- Approach the family members in a positive way and compliment them upon their (over)involvement with the patient.
- Consider the eating disorder patient as entrance to the family system.
- Neutralize the symptoms of the eating disorder.
- Redefine the family system as co-therapist and engage the family in major therapeutic decisions.
- Assess several levels (behavioral, experiential, cognitive) of the entire family and its various subsystems (parents, children and separate family members), including the grandparents' position (the transgenerational per spective).
- When the initial functional analysis reveals that the eating disorder might have a special function within the family system, develop an appropriate hypothesis.

provide an answer when possible. We give information about the inpatient treatment program (see also the brochure in the Appendix of Chapter 13). We further stress the importance of their collaborations without which we are as helpless as they were before. We deliberately avoid labeling the family sessions as family "therapy" in order not to enhance the resistance of family members who might otherwise feel accused and blamed for being the cause of the problem.

The family therapist needs to realize that for many families this might be the first time they have sat down together to discuss the problem directly and overtly. This interview is therefore usually anxiety-laden and requires great skill of the therapist (Harbin, 1982). Hence, the family members, especially the parents, must be given the opportunity *to talk about their feelings* of guilt, anxiety, shame, anger, helplessness, and so forth, while the therapist provides corresponding support. We tell them that the question of "who is right or wrong and who is guilty" does not matter. What matters is whether or not they are ready to cooperate in a joint effort to solve these problems here and now. We try to create a positive, nonjudgmental atmosphere and pay special attention to stopping any attempts by one family member to blame another.

Only after every family member has introduced himself/herself, we ask the family to explain in detail for what problem they expect our help. We are attentive to giving every member the opportunity to expound one's own view. Special attention is also paid to what has been tried out in the past to solve the eating problems. This analysis can give clues to the family therapist about which strategy might be appropriate.

Example: The functional analysis of the eating problems of Jane (18 years old) revealed that during the last weeks both parents had been discussing, sometimes for several hours, with their daughter the dangers of not eating, and how she was ruining her life. All day long, mother listened to her daughter's ideas about food, her fears of becoming overweight and her complaints of stomachache. This attitude resulted only in both parents becoming overstrained, while Jane continued to lose weight.

In this case, we *compliment the family,* in particular both parents, *for their involvement,* care, patience and endless efforts they employed in dealing with their anorexic daughter (the step toward the hospital is not a sign of defeat but of genuine concern). We advise them to talk no longer about food and weight, since they all have learned now that this was just not a good strategy to challenge the eating problems. This advice has become a general rule in our treatment program, and the hospitalization often helps to *neutralize the symptoms,* although most parents during the first weeks after admission keep on being extremely preoccupied with their daughter's weight.

We try to *involve the family in all major therapeutic decisions,* starting with the decision of hospitalization. Therefore we force the parents to deliberate and agree on our proposal to hospitalize their daughter (the decision to hospitalize an eating disorder patient can be based on several criteria: see Chapter 12).

This decision-making process offers the therapist important information about the communication and problem-solving skills of the family, the intergenerational boundaries and the like.

> *Example:* In the case of Marilyn (a 16-year-old student who displayed a severe and long-lasting anorexia nervosa) both parents started to argue about our proposal to hospitalize their daughter. Marilyn's brother replied, very upset, that he was not planning to visit his sister in a mental hospital. The parents could not come to an agreement and asked for some time to reflect. Two days later, Marilyn herself phoned us to make practical arrangements for hospitalization. Only after both grandparents from mother's side had given their approval to our proposal did the parents no longer disagree with each other about the recommended hospitalization for Marilyn.

The next important step is *the functional analysis of the eating disorder within the family system,* aimed at formulating an appropriate hypothesis (see Figure 1). One must be aware that such a functional analysis is not confined to the first meeting. Assessment and reassessment must be a continuous activity during the whole treatment process. When gathering information, it is helpful to keep the following questions in mind (Papp, 1983):

1. What function does the symptom serve in stabilizing the family?
2. How does the family function in stabilizing the symptom?
3. What is the central theme around which the problem is organized?
4. What will be the consequences of change?
5. What is the therapeutic dilemma?

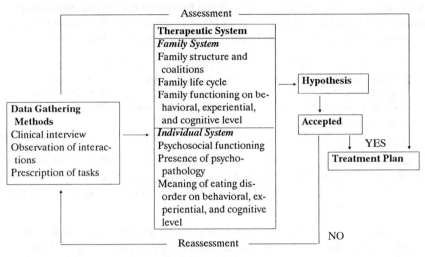

Figure 1: Different Steps in the Functional Analysis.

While doing this, we consider the *identified patient as entrance to the family system*. One has to realize the enormous power connected to the function of the "scapegoat," who very often controls all family interactions. Therefore, we ask all family members how they behave with regard to the eating problem, for instance, what happens before, during and after mealtime (the *behavioral* level).

Example:

Therapist: "Who calls everyone for dinner?"

Mother: "I do."

Therapist: "What do you say to your daughter?"

Mother: "Nothing special, I just ask her to come and sit down at the table."

Therapist: "What do you do, when she refuses to eat?"

Father: "We ask her, at the beginning very kindly, to eat just one bite and then another one."

Therapist: "But who asks this?"

Mother: "Mostly I do. Is this so important?"

We ask the family how they feel about this life-threatening problem and how they express their feelings to one another (the *experiential* level). Feelings in these family systems are often repressed, and the parents are even reluctant to show their daughter how helpless they feel regarding the eating problem. We encourage the different family members to express the way they experience

things at home. Not seldom, we see parents becoming depressed during hospitalization, meanwhile inducing feelings of guilt indirectly ("you are leaving us"),
when their daughter likes to be in the hospital or is making clear improvement.

Example: In one family, mother displayed a conversion reaction — she
lost her voice and could not speak for several days — at the moment her
daughter informed her of the good news that she was menstruating
again after three years. The daughter reacted with confusion and became quite tense.

The family therapist must also know how each one perceives the problem and
reacts to each other's perception (the *cognitive* level). An historical perspective
of the extended family, including the parents' family of origin — the transgenerational perspective (see Chapter 17) — can often help the therapist to obtain a
clear understanding of the family's belief system (White, 1983).

Example: During the first interview a father became very silent and
tense when we asked him about his relationship with his family of origin.
After a while, his wife answered with fear in her voice that her husband
had cut off all contact with his family, after their second daughter — actually 23 years old and showing an extreme form of anorexia nervosa —
was born. The grandparents, in particular grandfather, had expected to
have a grandson, and were very disappointed with the birth of a second
granddaughter; they even refused to visit the newborn. Father was
deeply hurt by this rejection and reproached himself for not having a
son. Thus, the functional analysis revealed that his belief, "my daughter
should have been a son," played an important role in the development
of the anorexia nervosa.

Apart from the family system, we have to pay special attention to *the individual life cycle,* the personal process of development and psychosocial
functioning of the patient and the other family members. We think that many
family therapists have intentionally sought to bypass the individual level in order
to deal directly with interactions on the family level. In our experience with
severe cases of eating disorders, one must be aware of the sometimes considerable retardation in the patients' personal development because of their regression into the symptoms (see also Papp, 1983). Moreover, the anorexia or bulimia
may create considerable psychobiological deterioration that must be dealt with
(e.g., restoration of normal weight and healthy eating patterns). The presence
of psychopathology in other family members needs to be detected, since this information can give clues to the therapist regardless of whether sessions with all
family members are indicated.

The family therapist must collect all this information in order to answer the
pivotal question: if and how the symptomatology of the identified patient is interwoven with a dysfunctional family system (Vandereycken & Meermann,
1984). When the functional analysis indeed reveals that the eating disorder has

a special function within the family system, the family therapist must *develop an hypothesis wherein he connects the eating disorder with the family system.* Moreover, our goal is to clearly relabel the eating problem as a *resolvable* family problem.

> *Example:* In Mary's family, the functional analysis revealed that her bulimia was functioning as the homeostatic regulator of every family transaction: the eating problems served as lightning-conductor for severe marital problems between her parents, whom she also protected against feelings of pain and sadness in the confrontation with Mary's brother and sister, who were both reaching adolescence and launching. Finally, Mary herself (a 22-year-old university student) still had extremely strong emotional ties with her parents and could not manage or was afraid to develop an intimate relationship with someone outside the family. She called the bulimia her "one and only friend." In this family, hospitalization was labeled as a first and necessary step to promote the separation-individuation process of Mary and to give both parents the possibility of facing their marital problems, together with their ambivalent feelings toward the launching of the other children.

An appropriate relabeling of the problem, however, is a difficult task when family therapy takes place within a residential setting. Treacher (1984) even states that "reframing psychiatrically-presented problems is an art in itself. Reframing forms an essential phase of the first interview in hospital because it helps to arrest the processes which underpin the move to hospitalize the patient."

Middle Phase: Conducting the Family System Toward Individuation

Challenging Resistance
The shift to the middle phase of treatment may begin as soon as the end of after the first interview, but can also take several weeks. Families with an eating disorder patient often display a strong need to label the eating disorder as caused by a "strange" physical illness, as is often evidenced by the parents' doctor shopping (Yager & Strober, 1985). Others consider their daughter as a victim of our weight-obsessed society. In general they put the cause of the problem outside the family's or parent's responsibility (see Chapter 7): it was the general practitioner who overlooked or mistreated the anorexia nervosa; it was problems at school or just a too-heavy weight which caused the eating problems. Anorexic and bulimic families are indeed experts at displacing responsibility and initiative onto others, while appearing to comply with external demands. But ultimately, such passive compliance produces no real change (Stern et al., 1981).

Most families hope that the treatment staff will take over all responsibility concerning their daughter as soon as she is hospitalized. In the beginning phase

Table 2: An Outline for Challenging Resistance

- Offer a systemic hypothesis, wherein the symptom is connected with the family's functioning.
- Alternate between active provocation and restraining from change.
- Increase the stress level by encouraging conflict and disagreement.
- Promote direct and open communication and negotiation.
- Challenge family structure, coalition patterns and implicit beliefs about the patient's illness.
- Encourage and teach the family to formulate clear, realistic and pragmatic goals.
- Observe and listen carefully to the family in order to reassess and redefine the hypothesis and change the treatment plan when indicated.

the family's major concern is how the weight and eating behavior are evolving. As such, in many cases families continue avoiding confrontation with hidden interactional conflicts.

Now the offering of a *hypothesis wherein the therapist connects the eating disorder with the family's functioning* must have top priority, although this step should be carefully planned. When redefining the eating disorder, it is important to use the family's own words, to speak its own language. Attentive listening and observing is then crucial, since most families give several clues, often expressed on a metaphoric level, which can be employed for effective relabeling of the eating disorder.

Examples:

- A mother said, "When I am together with my daughter, we always fight and argue. Our relationship is really 'suffocating,' both for myself and my daughter." In this family the anorexia was relabeled as a sign of the suffocating relationship between mother and daughter. Consequently, the treatment goal would be to change this relationship by introducing more distance between mother and daughter so that they both could start "breathing" again.
- Another mother said, "Our family is just like a warm nest, where everyone can find security and love." In this case the family therapist redefined the anorexia as an indirect message from the daughter to her family that the time was ripe for flying out of the warm nest. Preparing the family and the daughter for this important step was formulated as the most important treatment goal.

We further alternate our therapeutic attitude *between active provocation,* stimulating the family system toward change (the "direct" approach), while *at times we restrain the family from change* (the "indirect" approach). We usually start trying to break through the resistance to change both in the family system and the patient, with a direct and active provocation of the family system. Here again, we use the eating disorder or the identified patient as entrance to the family system. If the family controls the therapeutic system through the identified patient, the therapist, too, must try to control the therapeutic system using the same channel (Andolfi et al., 1983). That is why we first try to challenge the family's belief system about the eating disorder. In families that tend to deny the dangers of a bulimic or anorexic condition, the decision to hospitalize the patient often functions as an initial, direct provocation of the family's belief system.

> *Example:* In order to confront the patient and her family with the gravity of the emaciation, we sometimes put the patient in a wheel-chair and forbid her any physical activity on the ward, while visits are strictly limited in order not to exhaust her.

Once the family and the patient have realized the seriousness of the eating disorder, we further *dismantle the function of the symptoms and of the identified patient.* Our goal is to destabilize the dysfunctioning family equilibrium by inducing a crisis.

> *Example:*
>
> *Therapist:* "And how old does your daughter appear? I mean, when you observe her way of living and thinking, is she really behaving as a 22-year-old grown-up woman? She doesn't work, she's extremely dependent on her family, she has no friends — "
>
> *Mother:* "When I was 22 years old, I was already married and...pregnant."
>
> *Therapist:* "But look at her, she's behaving like a pitiful 12-year-old girl!"
>
> *Patient (furious):* "I want to live my own life. But how can I when my mother thinks she must take care of everything for me...It is she who treats me like a child!"

It is useful to bear in mind that "resistance" in these cases often means anxiety for (imposed) change! The family therapist must be aware that many patients are afraid to give up their symptoms and that most parents become anxious or depressed when confronted with the growing up of their daughter. Hence, to challenge the ambivalence and resistance toward change, the therapist may confront the family with the consequences of giving up the symptoms and then even *restrain the family from change.* Meanwhile, we invite them to think about a future without eating problems.

> *Example:*
>
> *Therapist:* "Can you imagine your life without bingeing and vomiting? Would giving up your eating pattern change your life?"

Patient: "It's very hard to imagine my life without bulimia. I am used to living this way for many years, I suppose. Well, I'll have to start working again."

Therapist: "Yeah, find a job, and what else?"

Mother: "Maybe, she'll go out and meet a boy..."

Therapist: "But you just mentioned that both your parents are thinking and worrying about you 24 hours a day. What are they going to do as soon as you starts to improve? Actually, all of you are very close to each other, but what will happen in the future? I am just wondering, at the moment, whether it's not too dangerous for all family members that you give up your symptoms. I mean, it could break up, for example, the closeness among all of you."

At other times, in order to *increase the stress level in the family,* we push the family toward dealing with hidden conflicts, especially in those families which are experts in avoiding or detouring overt conflict.

Example:

Mother: "I don't agree with my husband. In my opinion he's too strict with the children."

Therapist: "Do you often quarrel with your husband about the way to handle your daughter?"

Mother: "Oh no, I hate conflicts and discussions."

Father: "I think we don't quarrel more than other parents do. Usually I get along quite well with my wife. In the best families, there always exists some disagreement."

Therapist: "Marilyn, how do your parents get along? What's your point of view on this issue?"

Marilyn: "I don't know."

Therapist: "Do you think they have a happy marriage?"

Enactment sequences at this stage of therapy offer the therapist the opportunity to uncover hidden conflicts, intergenerational coalitions and often marital schisms (Frey, 1984). Whatever the conflict is about, our goal is to *support and strenghten the parental unity, and thus restructuring intergenerational boundaries.*

The family therapist must recreate a private psychological space for the parents as partners before marital problems can be handled in separate sessions. Meanwhile, the family therapist *promotes direct and open communication* and *teaches the family to negotiate.* At this time in the treatment process, the patient still remains on the ward 24 hours a day. Family therapy sessions are planned to discuss and negotiate about the frequency of visits, the schedule of visiting hours, the problems and tensions which arise during the visits in the hospital. Most families at this stage are still preoccupied with the evolution of their daughter's weight curve, but we teach them to look at it in a different way. The tensions, for instance, that they experience during the visits are very often expressed by fluctuations in the patient's weight (Harper, 1983).

Example:

Therapist (showing the weight curve): "How can you explain that these weight fluctuations always happen before or after the weekend visits?"

Mother: "Oh, that doesn't mean anything; it might just happen by accident."

Patient: "I don't know. I was not aware of the relationship between visits and weight fluctuations. The only thing I know is that as soon as I see my parents, I get nervous."

Therapist: "Do you know what makes you nervous?"

Patient: "I think — sorry, dad, for saying this — it's my father. I don't know what to tell him when he visits me. It's so strange, at home he's seldom there and now he is paying too much attention to me...I feel annoyed."

Anorexic and bulimic patients very often have irrational beliefs and perceptions about themselves (i.e., about their body, about nutrition and weight, about performances and achievements, etc.) as well as about their family and the outside world. They often perceive their family as the only place where they can survive, while the outside world is judged as dangerous and threatening. In our experience, these irrational beliefs are produced, maintained or reinforced by the family members themselves who sometimes seem to give hypnotic-like suggestions to the patient (Ritterman, 1983). For example, some parents encourage their daughter to start dieting, and siblings may admire her determination, thus focusing her attention even more strongly on her body. In other cases, mothers regularly complain, usually in an indirect way, about all the bad sexual experiences they had with their husbands, thereby giving the message that "men and sex just ain't no good." The therapist must try to *detect and challenge irrational and implicit family beliefs,* including specific values, traditions, customs, prescriptions for specific roles, and rules and attitudes concerning relationships and the expression of emotion (White, 1983).

Example: When discussing the weekend visits, the family and Rosaline (a 17-year-old anorexic) agree that nobody outside the family will be invited to the hospital. There exists a strong belief that Rosaline is not ready yet for confrontation with the outside world and the peer group, and needs to be protected by the parents. Hence we see that the family script is brought into the hospital, thus disconnecting the patient from the outside world.

Mother: "I think Rosaline is still too emaciated and too sick to receive visitors; it will upset her, and she will lose still more weight."

Therapist (toward father): "What do you think about your wife's concern? Do you agree that visits from friends should be forbidden at the moment?"

Father: "I don't agree at all."

Therapist (surprised): "You don't agree?! Why don't you then start arguing with your wife?"

Father: "O, arguing always ends in needless, quarreling, and I hate quarrels."

Therapist: "So, you're doing your best to avoid disputes as much as possible. Are quarrels so dangerous?"

Father: "Well, it's better to surrender in time than to lose everything in a fight."

Therapist: "'Everything' could mean your marriage?"

Father: "Yeah, maybe…"

Once the therapist has overcome the family's initial resistance to change and once the interactional relabeling of the eating disorder is accepted, we will *encourage the family and the patient to formulate clear, realistic and concrete goals.* These goals must fit the family's life cycle and the stage of the therapeutic process the patient is in.

Example: In Jane's family, the anorexia was relabeled as an indirect message and signal of being too close with one another. The main goal of family therapy was defined as loosening the tight relationships in order to facilitate everyone's growth. At this stage in the treatment process, Jane was still hospitalized. The parents decided to visit her only very briefly, thus giving her the opportunity to meet other young people and friends. For the very first time in her life she was also free to buy new clothes, without the companionship and influence of her mother, who used to make the choice in Jane's place.

In general, since we are dealing mostly with late adolescents (18 to 25 years old), treatment goals are usually centered around the separation-individuation process of the patient, the launching from the family system. The family therapist will try to promote the development of autonomy and increase the independence both in the patient and the other family members. When married patients are concerned, the same basic goal (successful launching from the family of origin) very often deserves priority, before marital problems can be dealt with (see Chapter 17). In younger patients increasing parental effectiveness or strengthening the parental coalition, especially around executive functioning, will be the primary goal.

Consolidating Change

Once the family's initial resistance has been transformed into a collaborative attitude, the family therapist has to further consolidate change in the family system. Ideally this consolidating of change should start already in the middle phase of our inpatient treatment program (i.e., after about four weeks). However, some very rigid families will need much more time before resistance toward change can be challenged successfully. In these cases, alteration of the family's scenario will only start to emerge at the end of the inpatient treatment (i.e., after about three months) or even later during the aftercare program.

At this stage in our treatment program, the patient will be gaining weight steadily and, consequently, obtaining more autonomy and responsibility. The patient is obliged, for instance, to spend, every week, one afternoon, one evening and the whole weekend outside the hospital, but not necessarily at home. Weekends can offer the best opportunity to provoke some interactional conflicts between the parents and the hospitalized patient, especially when everything seems "suspiciously quiet" both at home and in the hospital (Vandereycken & Meermann, 1984).

Meanwhile, once the initial resistance starts to decrease, the family and the patient pass through a period of crisis and instability, which is necessary to break through the pathologic homeostasis of the family system (Andolfi et al., 1983). Since the old family scenario, e.g., protecting the patient against the outside world or the avoidance of conflicts, can no longer be employed, the family feels insecure and will need the *encouragement of the whole treatment staff to explore, experiment and learn new and more independent behaviors, feelings and thoughts.* At this point, the therapists are functioning as (re)educators. The patient will be invited to plan in detail the free moments outside the hospital (in particular the weekends), make practical arrangements when needed and discuss her intentions in the family sessions. Especially in bulimia patients, this careful planning of leisure activities is extremely important, since bulimics often fly back into the symptoms as soon as they are confronted with empty moments and unexpected situations.

At this stage, common questions asked by most parents are: What do we have to cook when our daughter returns home for the weekend? How should we react when she refuses to eat or starts bingeing? Do we have to control her and give special attention? Can she go out with friends or would she be better off staying at home? All these questions can be used as input *to promote conflict resolution and direct communication* between the hospitalized patient and her parents. Intrafamilial conflicts often occur during weekends at home. But this

Table 3: An Outline for Consolidating Change

- Encourage the family members toward exploration, experimentation and learning of new independent behaviors, feelings and thoughts.
- Strengthen appropriate coalitions.
- Reinforce age-appropriate behavior, e.g., contact with peers and launching from the family of origin.
- Further encourage conflict resolution and direct communication.
- When resistance toward change emerges, again use active provocation or restrain the family from change.
- Plan marital and/or individual therapy when indicated.
- Predict relapse, after discharge.
- Constantly, reassess and reevaluate the formulated goals.

may be a time for the patient and family to try new approaches to solving their problems, with the hospital in the background (Harbin, 1982).

Homework tasks are also given, aimed at *strengthening appropriate coalitions.* The patient can be given the task to spend the weekend outside the family of origin and plan some activities with friends. Or we will encourage a temporal coalition between the father and his daughter and advise them to do some leisure activity together. The purpose is to disconnect the mother-daughter coalition on the one hand, and to give the daughter the opportunity to change her perception of her father, on the other. Next we often encourage both parents to plan some leisure activities together and ask them to prepare themselves for a life without an eating disorder patient. All these tasks are designed to restructure the family system, to make intergenerational boundaries clear.

Meanwhile we try *to reinforce age-appropriate behavior* in the patient. She must abandon the role of identified patient and begin to assume the role of a "normal" adolescent or grown-up female. Family sessions are focus now on the discharge of the patient from the hospital, together with a careful planning of future activities. We always make it a condition for discharge that the patient applies for a job or returns to school or previous work. The risk of relapse into the symptoms will be much greater if no meaningful activity during the day is provided, particularly in bulimics.

A great number of our patients have the intention to leave their family and start living on their own (approximately 30% are indeed launching from the family one year after discharge: see Chapter 9). An intermediate step toward successful launching from the family may be the introduction of partial hospitalization (day treatment) at this stage in our therapeutic treatment: five or three days a week (from 9 a.m. to 5 p.m.) in the hospital while the patient rents a small flat or room not too far from the hospital.

The discharge from the hospital and planning of future-oriented activities, together with the separation of the patient from the hospital and/or family, always causes anxiety, both in the patient and the family system. At this time in the treatment, the patient becomes in touch again with her inner feelings, for instance, of guilt, sadness, ineffectiveness, and "her feeling of being excluded from the world of peers" (Sargent et al., 1985). Meanwhile, the parents may be confronted with the pain of the separation of their daughter, and/or will be concerned with their own marital relationship. Some parents also fear to take over again the responsibility for their daughter (in case of younger adolescents). Hence the issue of discharge often results in a temporal recurrence of the eating problems, while old resistance toward change can reemerge, or other family members may display problem behaviors or try to sabotage therapeutic gains (Frey, 1984).

Example:

- At the time the anorexic daughter (23 years old) rented a flat for herself — a decision that was overtly agreed upon by both parents in the family session — mother wrote a letter to her still-hospitalized daughter, saying that she was lying sick in bed, afraid she might have a heart disease. This letter provoked intense feelings of guilt and fear in the patient, together with a considerable drop of her weight curve.
- At the end of her inpatient treatment, Regina, a 32-year-old married woman (admitted in our hospital for a severe anorexia nervosa with bingeing episodes and vomiting), started to discuss directly and openly the communication and sexual problems with her husband. After this session the so-called always-quiet husband became very anxious and insisted on stopping the marital sessions, shouting to his wife that "we can handle our marital problems ourselves and don't need any professional help." Regina was furious and said she was thinking about a divorce if her husband refused to collaborate in the marital sessions. This situation escalated to a suicidal attempt by the husband and provoked a relapse of Regina's anorexic symptoms as well as a premature termination of treatment.

When resistance or ambivalence toward change reenters into the therapeutic scene, we will try once more to *alternate* our therapeutic attempts *between provocation and restraining from change.* At this stage in our therapeutic approach, especially in difficult and chonic cases, we introduce a strategy, based on Peggy Papp's (1980, 1983) technique of the "Greek Chorus" (see Chapter 11). When practicing the Greek Chorus in an inpatient treatment, we often try to make a therapeutic triangle between the family, the family therapist and the therapeutic team. In general, the therapeutic team functions as protagonist, thus encouraging the patient and the family toward change, while the family therapist restrains the family from change. The family therapist even states that change will cause many more problems and tensions in the family system; and next he advises the family to learn to live with a chronic eating disorder patient. These opposite attitudes and messages often provoke confusion and crisis in the family system and may further destabilize the dysfunctional family equilibrium.

Example: Suzy, an 18-year-old student with a very therapy-resistant anorexia nervosa, was showing almost no progress after three months of hospitalization. To challenge the patient's and the family's resistance toward change, the family therapist gave the following message: "Now, after three months of hospitalization, I've learned that you're right, Suzy, in your decision not to change. You have convinced me that relinquishing your eating problems not only would be a very difficult task, but would probably also cause too many other problems and tensions that your family just can't handle at this moment. First, your parents will have to face their marital problems. Then, your mother may become depressed when confronted with her grown-up girl leaving her. And, finally, you Suzy, you're just not ready yet to manage all the consequences of giving up your anorexic symptoms. That's why I think we should change the therapeutic goal and start helping all of you to live with someone who suffers from a chronic eating disorder. I know that my colleagues in the therapeutic team won't agree with this, since they still believe in your capacity to grow and change. But personally, I think you're better off to stay like this." The parents were clearly confused and Suzy angrily stated that she would prove to me in the next weeks that she "was not such a hopeless chronic case"!

In some very therapy-resistant family systems, the therapeutic team and the family therapist may decide to give only one and the same message, i.e., that solving the eating problems will be an impossible task in our special treatment program. Meanwhile, the family has to make a choice between referring the patient to another residential unit where further treatment will take at least one year or just accept that they have a daughter with a chronic eating disorder. However, one must be very careful when giving such paradoxical messages (see also Todd, 1985). Some families may indeed accept this pessimistic point of view and may even become more depressed and cut off all contact with the therapeutic team.

When the first signs of improvement appear, the family and the patient — and, not uncommonly, the therapeutic team — may display an euphoric state of mind, thus believing that "the ugly corner has been turned." At this stage in the treatment process, the family therapist will *predict a relapse* in order to undermine overoptimistic reactions in the family and to maintain control over the symptoms (Weeks & L'Abate, 1979). Most families, indeed, will pass through a period of crisis when the patient is discharged from the hospital. Hence, anticipation of a relapse works disenchanting and reduces both the therapeutic team's and the family's feelings of frustration and failure once they are inevitably faced again with new or old problems (Frey, 1984).

In the final phase of inpatient treatment, as the patient's symptoms are improving, some parents become increasingly aware of individual and marital concerns, and they must be given the opportunity to deal with these affairs in *separate marital sessions.* As mentioned earlier (see Introduction), we recommend that all these different therapeutic tasks (family therapy, marital therapy, group or individual therapy) are carried out by the same therapist. At this point of therapy, the parents may experience feelings of alienation to one another, they may feel insecure toward their future roles as marital partners, without the presence of the children. Parents can become depressed or anxious when confronted with the growing separation and individuation of their daughter. Intergenerational issues, i.e., problems with their own parents, may (re)appear (see Chapter 16). For example, some parents now realize their long-lasting emotional dependency or the presence of strong loyalty feelings toward their own parents and family of origin. Lack of resolution of these problems may lead to recurrence of the eating disorder patient's symptoms or to the development of symptoms in another family member (Sargent et al., 1985). One of the most important tasks of the family therapist, at this point, is to support the parents' marital dyad, while promoting open communication between both spouses. At the same time, the therapist must be very attentive that the parents no longer involve the patient or other children in their marital conflicts and, if they continue to do so, he must intervene and stop these interactions as soon as possible.

In our inpatient treatment program, patients have directive group therapy (Vandereycken et al., 1986) in which they deal with their individual problems. As part of the aftercare program, we encourage the patients to further explore their individual problems after discharge from the hospital, preferably during the *directive group therapy sessions on an outpatient basis.* Issues that often must be dealt with in these group sessions are: the patient's fear of separating from her family and gainning more autonomy and responsibility; feelings of dissatisfaction or confusion with her "new" body and sexual identity; feelings of ineffectiveness in communicating and interacting with peers or family members; concerns about how to date a boyfriend and start a sexual relationship etc. A significant remission of the presenting symptoms, together with a clear improvement in interaction and self-experience of the patient, forms the basis for discharge from the hospital. Therefore, *reassessment and reevaluation of the formulated treatment goals are needed.* At the very end of the inpatient treatment we usually plan a session with all family members to evaluate what has been accomplished and what still has to be done. Just as with the decision to admit the patient, we now discuss and negotiate whether or not the patient and the family are ready for discharge. The final decisive meeting often functions as a kind of farewell ritual (Van der Hart, 1983), at least with respect to leave-taking from the hospital.

Final Phase: Ensuring the Long-Term Result

Generally speaking, the final phase in our treatment program should start immediately after the patient's discharge from the hospital. However, in a great number of families, the middle phase of our treatment will continue after dis-

Table 4: An Outline for the Final Phase

- Plan intensive aftercare and long-term follow-up.
- Gradually decrease contact with the patient and the family.
- Be available for the patient and the family for an extended period.
- When every therapeutic attempt has failed, teach the family to live with a chronic eating disorder patient and/or refuse further treatment.

charge for several months before the final phase is reached. Several elements in the final phase of family treatment require our special attention (see Table 4).

Clearly, a planned discharge is crucial, since there are very real dangers of relapse as the identified patient leaves the hospital and/or returns home (Treacher, 1984). In our experience, *the providing of an intensive follow-up treatment* is the cornerstone of a successful treatment outcome over the long run. Therefore, we try to motivate patients to join our outpatient group therapy, as mentioned earlier. Meanwhile, we provide therapy sessions for the whole family or marital therapy for the parents, when indicated. Married patients or those who are living together with a boyfriend will be encouraged to attend separate marital therapy sessions. Once more, we recommend that all the major therapeutic tasks are executed by one and the same therapist so that the aftercare program is closely linked to the inpatient approach. Ideally, the outpatient treatment should be carried out by the same therapeutic team involved in the inpatient treatment. The primary therapist during hospitalization should then be also the outpatient therapist. If the patient/family has to be referred to another outpatient therapist, the latter must be involved in the final stage of the hospitalization. This means, at least, that he must have met his future clients before discharge from the hospital and he must agree on the general treatment approach used thus far by the hospital staff, and take an active part in the aftercare planning (Vandereycken & Meermann, 1984).

The splitting of the separate subsystems after discharge — i.e., parents versus children or patient — has several purposes: first, it may further strengthen clear intergenerational boundaries and, second, it underlines the necessity of giving all responsibility concerning eating behavior and weight to the patient. Therefore, we make a clear contract with every patient as to the maintenance of a normal body weight and healthy eating pattern (see Vandereycken & Meermann, 1984).

At this final stage in our treatment program, *the frequency of contacts with the family must decrease.* In the first weeks after discharge we meet the family regularly to evaluate the reintegration of the patient (in case of younger adolescents) or the evolution of her separation from the family (in older patients). The contacts with the family then gradually decrease as soon as we think that they no longer need the support and guidance of the therapist and that they can handle their problems and conflicts all by themselves. However, in our experience, the *therapist should be available for the family over an extended period of time.* Clinical experience has taught us that improvement rarely happens suddenly in the treatment of severe and chronic patients whose evolution often shows periodic remissions and relapses. It is, therefore, naive to expect a spectacular change or "recovery" after only a couple of months.

Many family therapists have a strong belief that once they have changed the family structure and destabilized the system's equilibrium, or have strengthened appropriate coalitions and intergenerational boundaries, or once the anorexic or bulimic daughter starts living on her own, improvement on all (biopsychosocial) levels will follow automaticly. Therapists who focus only on the interactions in the family neglect the considerable developmental retardation which exists in eating disorder patients. Once they have given up their symptoms, many patients go through a period of "loss of identity." They often feel empty or insecure and have to start a completely new life. Therefore, they will need the support and guidance of the therapist over a long period. We recommend an aftercare of at least one year and planning of follow-up sessions for up to five years after admission (in our center, an independent assessor rates the patient's evolution at fixed and regular points of time, namely after 6 months, 1 year, 2 years and 5 years according to a standardized procedure). Planning such a long-term follow-up also conveys to these families the continuing availability of the therapist (Frey, 1984).

The therapeutic strategy and outcome have to be evaluated constantly. But, *when every therapeutic attempt has failed* and when the treatment team, after careful consideration, does not believe anymore that improvement is still possible, we recommend *the family learn to live with a chronic eating disorder patient and, consequently, we refuse further treatment.* If the patient and the family do not make any effort to change, if they put most of their energy into criticizing and undermining the therapeutic strategy, termination is probably appropriate (Stern et al., 1981). But any experienced therapist also knows that in some cases repeated hospitalizations are inevitable and that a readmission is sometimes the best means to shake up a family that was waiting for the magical treatment or entertaining the hope that the eating disorder "will just go away."

Additional Interventions in Bulimics

Although bulimic patients and their families pass through similar stages in the treatment process, some additional interventions and techniques have proven, in our clinical experience, to be very useful (see Table 5). Bulimic families tend to deny very strongly the presence of bulimic behaviors (bingeing, vomiting, laxative abuse etc.). Family members, in particular the parents, seem to be blind to the repeated disappearance of food supplies in the kitchen and refrigerator. They even seem to lose their olfactory sense, since they do not notice the

Table 5: Additional Interventions in Bulimia

- Bringing the eating problems into the open.
- Dealing with the ambivalence toward change.
- Engaging the family or spouse as co-therapist.
- Encouraging contact outside the family of origin.
- Promoting the launching from the family.
- Attacking the bulimic identity.
- Detection, (re)experiencing and/or relabeling of underlying emotional problems.
- Providing support and encouragement by means of a long-lasting follow-up.

sour smell of the vomitus in the toilet. And, even when they discover or know about these things, they avoid communicating or discussing these strange observations with other family members. They act as if they have dissociated these observations from their conscious mind, or are keeping the bulimia secret from the others.

Example: Dorothy (actually 26 years old) was already bingeing and vomiting for more than four years. All this time, mother, who had noticed from the beginning the sour smell in the toilet, supposed that her husband was vomiting because of his liver disease. Surprisingly enough, she never asked her husband if he was indeed vomiting. Father, on the contrary, had never observed or smelled anything unusual!

As distinct from anorexia nervosa patients, who mostly experience great difficulty in hiding their abnormal eating and weight from the other family members and the outside world, a great deal of the bulimics still have a normal weight and display normal eating habits in the presence of other family members.

Hence, the seriousness of the bulimic symptoms is largely underestimated or even completely neglected by the family. In the beginning phase of the treatment, it is therefore of crucial importance that the therapist tries to *bring the eating problems and the related psychobiological deterioration into the open.* Next, the family may be asked to calculate the sum of money their daughter is wasting every week! Both the family and the patient must be aware of the gravity of the eating problems in order to motivate and encourage the family in challenging the eating and related problems. In our experience, most bulimics experience great relief at the moment they can openly discuss their eating problems with the other family members. In our treatment approach, all bulimic patients are given a brochure, aiming at informing them in detail about all the risks and dangers of vomiting, bingeing and laxative abuse, together with several guidelines and concrete steps to achieve control over the eating symptoms (principles of stimulus control and self-management comparable with the approach used in cases of addiction).

Although resistance or ambivalence toward change exists in almost every family system entering the treatment room, particularly in bulimics and their families the therapist must be very sensitive to their ambivalence regarding any of the changes the therapist might advocate (Schwartz et al., 1985). Most of these families, once they realize the seriousness of the bulimia, present the family therapist a list of clearly defined problems (mostly eating behaviors) and they often have a request for help. They often state that they are ready to cooperate and follow any directive or task the therapist may give. Here exists a great danger or possible pitfall for the therapist who might feel himself forced or seduced to offer immediately a concrete treatment plan, without taking into account the possible resistances in view of the considerable consequences of change. In our experience, whenever we immediately offered some practical guidelines and strategies to challenge bulimic eating patterns, most families were only trying to convince us that we just did not give the right directive. Hence, to avoid this possible pitfall in the early stage, we never start our therapeutic attempt by offering a well-defined treatment plan. We first try to *mirror the family's attitude toward change,* thus demonstrating a skeptical or ambivalent attitude whether or not they "are ready for real change." Next, we ask the family and the identified patient to consider all possible (negative) consequences, of the disappearance of the symptoms or related problems. Possible consequences of changing may be that the patient is no longer the "weak, vulnerable" child close to her mother. The eating problem is no hindrance anymore for developing relationships outside the family, applying for a job or dating a boy.

Once the therapist has a clear view of the family's ambivalence, he may start by engaging other family members (or the spouse) as *co-therapists.* Although it is a general rule in our treatment approach to give all responsibility concerning food, eating behavior and weight to the bulimic patient, one can ask how much the family may tolerate. Especially in those bulimics still living in their family or with their spouse, we often encourage the family or spouse to *set limits* as to the bulimic eating patterns.

Examples:

- The family may decide to lock the kitchen or other places wherein the food is supplied.
- All binges must be paid for by the patient.
- The patient may still binge, but only on one type of food, in one particular place and only once a day (e.g., between 6 and 7 p.m.).
- Vomiting in the bathroom or toilet is forbidden; the patient must use a special bucket and clean it all by herself.

In the case of bulimics, hospitalization can be used as a first step of reducing the patient's dependence on her family, and breaking her isolation together with the addiction-like vicious circle of bingeing and vomiting. Bulimics, generally speaking, develop very quickly a strong bond with the hospital milieu and treatment staff. Moreover, most bulimics even stop bingeing and vomiting from the very first day of admission in the hospital (because of the structured milieu and the presence of social control). Here the danger exists that the patient may ensconce herself in the protection and safety of the hospital environment. In our treatment program, the bulimic patient, therefore, is forced after three weeks of hospitalization to spend two afternoons and the weekend outside the hospital. In the meantime, we encourage her to plan clearly and structure these moments in detail, in such a way that she will have the opportunity to develop contacts and relationships outside the hospital and family milieu.

Some families, at this point, may be prepard for the *launching* of their daughter. In others, the therapist may decide to force the patient to leave the family and start living on her own. We often label the launching as a basic condition for further therapeutic treatment. During the first months after the separation from the family, most bulimics tend to relapse into the old symptoms and pass through a tumultuous period (see also Schwartz et al., 1985). The family therapist must therefore carefully plan the disengagement of the family. Next, he must prepare both patient and family for a possible relapse into the symptoms (we even predict it), since otherwise both parties may use this as an excuse for returning home again.

Bulimics often perceive themselves as incompetent, weak, inferior, abnormal and so forth, when they compare themselves with others. But, on the other hand, they appear to be hypercritical and demand perfection. These *irrational beliefs* and expectations may be challenged by means of a cognitive-oriented therapeutic procedure in individual and/or group therapeutic sessions (see e.g., Fairburn, 1984; Vandereycken et al., 1986). But, since we are systematically involving the family in our treatment, we established that these unrealistic beliefs are often reinforced by (in)direct messages from the other family members. Parents often perceive their bulimic daughter — already long before the onset of the bulimia — as "different from the other children," as "not so intelligent but having other capacities," or as "a strange, special child from her birth on." Surprisingly enough, besides the creation of this identity of a "peculiar, vulnerable" child, most parents have very high expectations of their daughter (perfectionism and achievement are the hidden key words in their education). Now, the patient is caught between conflicting messages and, as long as the parents perceive her as weak, they will further try to protect her. The family therapist must, therefore, challenge these conflicting perceptions and expectations (both in the patient and in the family system) and undermine the "bulimic identity" whenever possible.

In many cases the bulimia conceals *unresolved conflicts of a highly emotional nature*. At the time of referral to our unit, a great number of our bulimic patients and families may still be suffering from traumatic experiences which have been repressed or dissociated from the conscious mind. Not uncommonly, we established that unusual traumatic events had taken place in the parents' family of origin. The therapist must try to detect such traumatic events and provide special means to help working through these painful experiences.

Examples:

- In a few cases, the bulimic patient appeared to mourn silently for the loss of a parent.
- In some families we found out that the grandparents had suffered a lot during the Second World War.
- In other cases, the bulimic patient was traumatized by an incestuous relationship or by a sexual assault (e.g., rape).
- Another patient was severely burned as a child due to an accident in the absence of her mother.

In the severe and chronic cases we are faced with, patients often relapse during the treatment process into the bulimic symptoms. Especially at these moments they may again feel depressed and overwhelmed by self-depreciating thoughts (sometimes even suicidal tendencies). Next they may isolate themselves completely from the outside world and decide to give up therapy. Most families will react with despair, thus believing that nothing will ever stop their daughter from bingeing and vomiting. Hence, the family therapist must provide support and encouragement over an extended period to both patient and family. A long lasting follow-up is therefore recommended. In our outpatient group therapy for bulimics we immediately contact the patient (or her family) when she is absent from the session. In our experience, bulimic patients often test the patience and perseverance of those surrounding them — including the therapist — and often require direct encouragement to continue the often-frustrating trial-and-error process of finding a way out of the repetitive patterns they are imprisoned in.

CONCLUSION

Currently, the importance and effectiveness of incorporating family therapy within the psychiatric hospital in the treatment of eating disorders can only be estimated by means of clinical experience (see also Chapter 9). Nevertheless, we hope that the present chapter may stimulate others in contacting, joining and introducing family members and/or important others into the treatment process. Since anorexia nervosa and bulimia are recognized as multidetermined syndromes, a flexible, multimodal and eclectic approach (using structural, strategic and behavioral elements) is needed for successful challenging of the eating disorder within the family system.

The outline and description of the several stages in our family therapeutic approach during hospitalization have been very schematic. However, we would like to warn the inexperienced clinician against carrying out our therapeutic strategies literally, like recipes in a cookbook. Ideally, both patients and families should evolve from one stage to another, but in our clinical experience this is rather exceptional. Moreover, they fluctuate from one stage to another and many families may even fall back into a previous stage, or break off their therapeutic engagement before the final stage has been reached.

Hence, family work with eating disorder patients, be it in an inpatient or outpatient setting, is most challenging for the family therapist and all team members whose skills and personal involvement will be tested, sometimes to the extreme.

REFERENCES

Andersen, A.E. (1985), *Practical Comprehensive Treatment of Anorexia Nervosa and Bulimia.* Baltimore: Johns Hopkins University Press.

Andolfi, M., Angelo, C., Menghi, P. & Nicolò-Corigliano, A.M. (1983), *Behind the Family Mask. Therapeutic Change in Rigid Family Systems.* New York: Brunner/Mazel.

Fairburn, C.G. (1985), Cognitive-behavioral treatment for bulimia. In: Garner, D.M. & Garfinkel, P.E. (Eds.), *Handbook of Psychotherapy for Anorexia Nervosa and Bulimia.* New York: Guilford Press, pp. 160-192.

Frank, J.D. (1984), Therapeutic components of all psychotherapies. In: Meyers, J.M. (Eds.), *Cures by Psychotherapy. What Effects Change?* New York: Praeger Special Studies.

Frey, J. (1984), A family systems approach to illness-maintaining behaviors in chronically ill adolescents. *Family Process,* 23:251-260.

Harbin, M.T. (1982), Family treatment of the psychiatric inpatient. In: Harbin, M.T. (Ed.), *The Psychiatric Hospital and the Family.* Jamaica (N.Y.): Spectrum Publications, pp. 3-25.

Harper, G. (1983), Varieties of parenting failure in anorexia nervosa: Protection and parentectomy, revisited. *Journal of the American Academy of Child Psychiatry,* 22:134-139.

Lange, A. & Van der Hart, 0. (1983), *Directive Family Therapy.* New York: Brunner/Mazel.

Liebman, R., Sargent, J. & Silver, M. (1983), A family systems orientation to the treatment of anorexia nervosa. *Journal of the American Academy of Child Psychiatry,* 22:128-133.

Papp, P. (1980), The Greek Chorus and other techniques of paradoxical therapy. *Family Process,* 19:45-58.

Papp, P. (1983), *The Process of Change.* New York: Guildford Press, pp. 46-56.

Ritterman, M. (1983), *Using Hypnosis in Family Therapy.* San Francisco-London: Jossey Bass.

Sargent, J., Liebman, R. & Silver, M. (1985), Family therapy for anorexia nervosa. In: Garner, D.M. & Garfinkel, P.E. (Eds.), *Handbook of Psychotherapy for Anorexia and Bulimia.* New York: Guilford Press, pp. 257-279.

Seltzer, W. (1984), Treating anorexia nervosa in the somatic hospital: A multisystemic appraoch. *Family Systems Medicine,* 2:195-207.

Stern, S., Whitaker, C., Hagemann, M.J., Anderson, R.B. & Bargman, G.J. (1981), Anorexia nervosa: The hospital's role in family treatment. *Family Process,* 20:395-408.

Todd, T.C. (1985), Anorexia nervosa and bulimia: Expanding the structural model. In: Mirkin, M.P. & Koman, S.L. (Eds.), *Handbook of Adolescents and Family Therapy.* New York: Gardner Press, pp. 223-243.

Treacher, A. (1974), Family therapy in mental hospitals. In: Treacher, A. & Carpenter, J. (Eds.), *Using Family Therapy.* Oxford: Blackwell, pp. 166-188.

Vandereycken, W. (1985), Inpatient treatment of anorexia nervosa: Some research-guided changes. *Journal of Psychiatric Research,* 19:413-422.

Vandereycken, W. & Meermann, R. (1984), *Anorexia Nervosa. A Clinician's Guide to Treatment.* Berlin-New York: Walter de Gruyter.

Vandereycken, W., Vanderlinden, J. & Van Werde, D. (1986), Directive group therapy for patients with anorexia nervosa and bulimia. In: Larocca, F.E.F. (Ed.), *Eating Disorders: Effective Care and Treatment.* St.Louis: Ishiyaku EuroAmerica, pp. 53-69.

Van der hart, O. (1983), *Rituals in Psychotherapy. Transition and Continuity.* New York: Irvington.

Vanderlinden, J. & Vandereycken, W. (1984), Directive family therapy in adult patients with severe or chronic anorexia nervosa. *International Journal of Family Psychiatry,* 5:267-280.

Weeks, G. & L'Abate, L. (1979), A complication of paradoxical methods. *American Journal of Family Therapy,* 7:61-77.

White, M. (1983), Anorexia nervosa: A transgenerational system perspective. *Family Process,* 22:255-275.

Yager, J. & Strober, M. (1985), Family aspects in eating disorders. In: Hales, R.E. & Frances, A.J. (Eds.), *Psychiatry Update, Annual Review. Volume 4.* Washington, D.C.: American Psychiatric Press, pp. 481-502.

APPENDIX: CASE PRESENTATION—A FAMILY OF ANGELS

INTRODUCTION

The family we have present is one of those complex and challenging cases we are regularly faced with in our inpatient program. Besides many moments of frustration, desperation and sometimes even anger, we were overcome at other times with feelings of admiration and astonishment during the therapeutic work with this family. We have chosen this difficult case because it demonstrates the step-by-step process or trial-and-error procedure of putting concepts and methods into practice. It further illustrates how much patience and perseverance on the part of the family therapist is sometimes needed before change clearly starts to occur. Meanwhile, we hope that this case history demonstrates the importance of therapeutic work with the family when the therapist is confronted with an eating disorder patient, without neglecting the ongoing interchange and mutual influence of individual and familial factors.

The family consulted us regarding the eating problem of their 19-year-old daughter Helen, who displayed a typical anorexia nervosa, with significant weight loss (39 kg for 170 cm), hyperactivity, amenorrhea, vomiting and a distorted, implacable attitude toward weight and food. "Here's a family of angels," father ironically remarked when we met for the first time. Already during the first interview the family clearly showed some of the well-known interaction characteristics to such an extent that they looked like a caricature of a text book case: a high degree of cohesion and enmeshment, an extreme triangulation (a strong coalition between mother and daughter against father) and an unusual absence of clear intergenerational boundaries.

The family consisted of both parents, two sons and one daughter (the identified patient). Father, a 48-year-old industrial engineer, looked much older than his age, as though he had suffered a lot in his life. Outside his work and family environment, he avoided contact with other people as much as possible. He further attached much importance to the traditional Catholic rules and values. He had refused sexual intercourse with his wife for several years "to punish her for a moral lapse," i.e., an extramarital relationship she had five years before. "At this moment," he said, "I am still suffering every day from the misstep of my wife," and he still maintained the feeling that he was a "cuckold." His wife, a 42-year-old housewife who regularly showed mood fluctuations, was bowed down with worries and feelings of guilt, because of her "misstep." When having conflicts with her husband, she always took refuge, whether in the relationship with her daughter or in the (ab)use of alcohol and medication. Peter, the eldest son (22 years old) ran away from home three years ago, after a serious conflict with his father about his being homosexual, and he never returned home. Nobody in the family has since received any communication from Peter. At one point, a family member might believe he was just missing, at another point he would be judged as deceased. Meanwhile, mother had traveled to Rome, Paris, London and Amsterdam in search of her son, but returned each time without any result. The younger son, Alfred (16 years old), was in continuous rebellion against his father, while having a close relationship with his mother.

PREPARING THE FAMILY SYSTEM FOR CHANGE

The First Interview

Six months before admission to our hospital, mother and daughter made a bet as to who could lose as many kilograms as possible during a one-week holiday. Helen lost four kilograms and won the stake (ten dollars) but she could not stop dieting. She even started vomiting and became strikingly hyperactive. At the time of referral to our hospital, Helen had lost 19 kg: she looked completely exhausted and avoided all eye contact. Even during this first interview, father started to criticize and to blame his wife for being too mild and lenient with their daughter. Meanwhile, both mother and daughter could not help laughing: mother even reported with some pride about their bet and the onset of the anorexia nervosa. Alfred, the younger brother, refused to sit down and walked crisscross through the therapy room.

The constitution of a working alliance with each family member separately was extremely difficult: when we invited one member to expound his or her view regarding the eating problems, he or she was immediately interrupted by another family member. When we were enjoining mother, for instance, father promptly intervened and cut off the conversation, because he felt he was being blamed for causing the problem. After only a few minutes, we decided to use and impose our leadership and authority as much as possible. Otherwise, this first interview would have ended in a complete chaos.

Finally the family, the patient and the therapist agreed upon the hospitalization of Helen. This decision was based on the following considerations: first, we

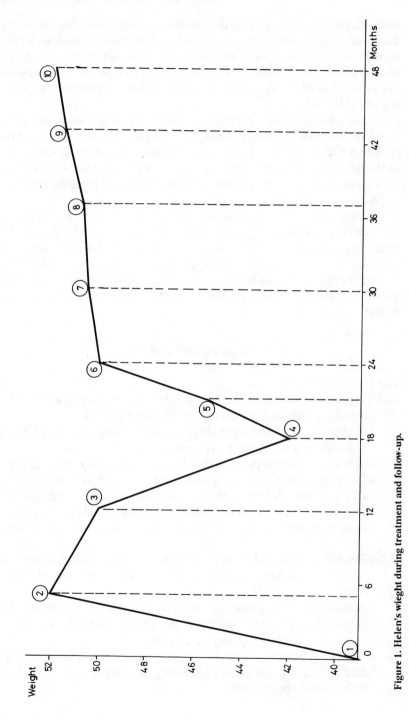

Figure 1. Helen's wieght during treatment and follow-up.

were worried about the serious deterioration of Helen's health, caused by the acute and extreme weight loss during the past few weeks. Second, we were confronted with a markedly dysfunctional and sometimes chaotic family atmosphere including an explosive relationship between the parents and a striking social isolation of all family members. Third, previous outpatient therapeutic attempts had failed.

On the other hand, we realized the possible pitfall of our therapeutic proposal: the fact that this family immediately agreed upon the decision of hospitalization could also be understood as a means of expelling the scapegoat out of the family system. We therefore explained to the parents the importance of their collaboration and participation in the therapeutic program and decided to plan one family session per week.

The family therapist was trying to involve Helen's family—and in particular both parents—as much as possible in the inpatient treatment. The family was sent home with several homework assignments: they had to fill in some self-report questionnaires and were asked to reflect upon how they could help promoting change in Helen's condition. In the meantime Helen stayed at our inpatient unit and, since she happened to have artistic talents, she was instructed to make a drawing of her family.

Assessment of the Family System

The Family Structure

After the first meeting we could summarize our impressions as follows:
- Helen sat close to her mother, between both parents.
- Mother and daughter were always looking at one another, while father addressed himself directly to the therapist.
- Helen was dominating the family life by means of her anorexia nervosa.
- The communication was characterized by a typical pattern: therapist asks question—father or mother responds—discussion between father and mother starts—father begins to shout—mother, daughter and younger brother laugh—conversation stops—therapist asks question—etc.
- The family clearly demonstrated a highly enmeshed structure with a particularly strong coalition between mother and children against father.
- Although there existed high conflict and tension within the family (especially between the parents), the family was trying to avoid confrontation with these conflicts at all costs.
- The eating disorder seemed to protect the parents against marital discord (threat of separation) by inducing an overprotective attitude from both of them toward Helen.

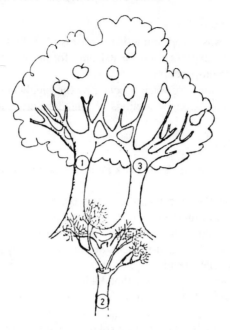

Figure 2. Helen's first sketch of her family. (1 = Father; 2 = Helen; 3 = Mother)

We were amazed by Helen's sketch of her family (see Figure 2), who clearly demonstrated the dysfunctional family hierarchy and lack of intergenerational boundaries, and thus strongly confirmed our first impressions and assumptions. Helen drew herself as a tree which functioned as a buffer between father and mother, while all her roots were connected with those of her mother. In her experience, both brothers were nonexistent.

A more detailed functional analysis of the family system further revealed the following findings.

The Behavioral Level:

- With regard to the anorexia nervosa, father and mother both displayed opposite behaviors. Mother reacted with gentleness and patience, father with strictness, severity and, next, overt anger: he threw plates and food on the floor and in a particular instance even refused to eat as long as his daughter refused to do.
- Separate interviews with the spouses gave evidence of the supposed existence of serious marital conflicts over many years. Once mother had informed her husband about her extramarital affair, regular escalating disputes with physical violence arose, often in presence of the children, who were used as arbitrators in the parents' battle. Father had refused sexual intercourse ever since.

The Experiential Level:
- This family was programmed to repress all feelings as much as possible, or to express them in extreme forms of acting-out (e.g., aggression between parents).
- On the other hand, we were touched by the highly emotional family atmosphere, dominated by feelings of guilt, anxiety, sadness, anger and helplessness.

The Cognitive Level:
- In this family, achievement, work and perfectionism were highly appreciated values.
- There existed a strong belief that the children must be protected by their parents and must obey in every situation without protest.
- Sexual relationships in adolescents were judged as being caused by a lack of discipline and self-respect. Sexuality was only accepted within a loyal marital relationship.
- All family members believed that Helen was suffering from a somatic disease; they further perceived her as a helpless girl who had been vulnerable and weak from the time of her birth.

In order to have a clear understanding of this cognitive level, we also gathered information concerning each parent's family of origin, since this is where the attitudes, perceptions and beliefs originated.

Therapist: "Can you give me some information about your family of origin? Are your parents—Helen's grandparents—still alive?"

Father: "Well, my father is now 85 years old, while my mother died during the Second World War in a bombardment (...). My father has always been a very dominating person."

Mother: "Oh yes, my husband still consults on every decision with his father (...)."

Therapist (toward mother): "And how is your family?"

Mother: "Well, both my parents are still alive. Our family, too, suffered a lot but after the second world war. My father was arrested and put into prison for several years because of collaboration with the Germans. This has provoked, and it still does nowadays, high tension and chronic conflicts between my parents (...)."

Therapist: "And how do you relate to them today?"

Mother: "Oh, my mother has always been a meddlesome women. She has always interfered in our family life; today she still tells me what is right or wrong (...)."

Hence, information about the extended family revealed that both parents had grown up in families traumatized by the Second World War. The traumatic events in both families provoked strong emotional ties among the family members, together with a marked distance set up against the dangerous outside world, as a means of survival and to protect the family system. Moreover, both parents still showed an intense emotional attachment toward their family of origin, and hence, were still strongly influenced by their parents' values and belief systems. This might explain why this family was experiencing so much trouble and pain in the confrontation with the separation-individuation process of the children.

Assessment of the Individual System

Besides a detailed analysis of the family life cycle, one should also give special attention to the individual life cycle of each family member. In this family, everyone showed maladaptive and even psychopathological behavior. Mother had serious mood fluctuations, and often felt very depressed. For many years she consulted several psychiatrists and regularly abused alcohol and tranquillizers. Father was very distrustful, sensitive and suspicious as to the outside world. He clearly displayed a paranoid attitude, with frequent aggressive outbursts toward his wife and children, which not uncommonly escalated into physical violence. Peter, the eldest son, had run away from home at the age of 19 years, after a severe conflict with his father, who could not accept the homosexual orientation of his son. This emotional cutoff (Bowen, 1978) appeared to be the only way for him to gain independence and autonomy from his parents. Helen, the identified patient developed a serious anorexia nervosa and was extremely socially isolated. She had no contacts with peers outside the family and experienced her brothers as nonexistent. Psychological assessment further revealed a serious developmental retardation (e.g., infantile and immature behavior), the presence of a marked depressed and anxious state of mind as well as a weak ego-functioning, although she was very intelligent and artistic. Helen's general behavior resembled a borderline personality disorder. Alfred, her youngest brother, had chronic conflicts with peers at school; at home he was struggling with his father. He could not manage to develop a solid relationship outside his family of origin. During the family therapy sessions, he always looked very strained and displayed a rather hyperkinetic behavior.

Conclusion

The functional analysis and assessment of both the family and individual systems clearly showed that the eating disorder of Helen had, indeed, a special function within the family. We were confronted with severe marital discord and the presence of quite abnormal behavior in both the parents and the children.

This analysis immediately raised some serious therapeutic questions. Is family therapy in this particular family indicated, and are they ready to handle the consequences of real change at this moment? Should we first focus on the marital problems or give priority the restoration of intergenerational boundaries? Or should we decide to meet the family only on a supportive basis, while silently disconnecting and separating the patient from her family?

CONDUCTING THE FAMILY SYSTEM TOWARD INDIVIDUATION

Challenging the Resistance to Change

As mentioned earlier, we were astonished by the clarity and accuracy of Helen's sketch (see Figure 2) of her family of origin. This "portrait" was in high contrast with her verbal description, which presented a normal family without special problems. We decided to use Helen's sketch as input into the family system to test the family's resistance toward change and to prepare a redefinition of the eating disorder in connection with the family's functioning. Before the family session, we asked Helen if she agreed with our proposal to discuss her sketch of her family. She at first hesitated and then whispered, "Okay." This session took place about two weeks after her admission to the hospital.

> *Therapist:* "As you know, we asked your daughter to make a drawing of the family and bring it to this session." (Helen shows the sketch to her parents.)

> *Father:* "She has much creativeness and imagination, but what the hell has she done with her life!?"

> *Therapist:* "Ask her, she sits next to you."

> *Father:* "What does this beautiful drawing mean?" (Helen does not respond.)

> *Mother:* "Please, Helen, give some explanation, this might help curing you, sweetheart." (Helen still does not answer. We decide to increase the stress level by means of active provocation, while using Helen as entrance to the family system.)

> *Therapist:* "Your 'sweetheart' has lost her tongue. How old is she?"

> *Father:* "She's 19 years now, and I order her to immediately give the information we've asked for."

> *Mother:* "Don't be so hard, daddy. You see (toward therapist), my husband never has patience." (Father and mother start quarreling and then Helen suddenly intervenes.)

> *Helen* (showing with her finger on the drawing): "This is my father and this is my mother."

Mother: "And you are just standing in the middle between your parents?"

Helen: "Yeah!"

The discussion then following aroused a highly strained and emotionally atmosphere, and the session ended in a quick-tempered dispute between both parents, who advised each other of being the cause of the problem. Again we had to take up an authoritarian attitude to stop the parents' fight and explain to them that no one was to blame. The only question that mattered was how Helen could "develop her own roots and grow up as a young tree," apart from her own family. The hospital environment was relabeled as a "temporal guest family" for Helen.

Challenging the Family Structure and Belief System

After this session, it became clear to us that restoring clear intergenerational boundaries deserved top priority. As long as Helen was functioning both as buffer and go-between between father and mother, she would have extreme difficulty reaching autonomy and independence. For this reason we decided to focus in the next family sessions on strengthening the parental coalition and creating an unanimous attitude in the parental dyad with regard to their daughter. Although both parents were struggling for many years with serious marital conflicts, we tried to emphasize the importance of parental collaboration and joint authority. For this purpose we planned several separate sessions with the parents.

Therapist: "In our last meeting, you (= parents) told us about your serious marital problems. But do you think you can put these aside for a while, and try to find a compromise concerning your attitude toward Helen. In our experience, this might be crucial for a successful solution of your daughter's problem."

Mother: "My husband and I never agreed upon the education of our children. He's a very severe man (she laughs) and I know I am too weak, let's say, a bad or failing mother." (Father grumbles.)

Therapist: "What matters now is if both of your are ready to discuss, negotiate and agree upon one common attitude with respect to your daughter. Later on we'll offer you the possibility of handling your marital problems."

Both parents agreed upon our proposal and finally made the following arrangements:

- Their own visits to the hospital would be limited to a frequency of once a week (i.e., Sunday afternoon 2-5 p.m.) so that Helen during the visiting hours would have the chance to meet other people from outside the family and thus break through her social isolation.

- During visits, conversations about food and weight were forbidden; whenever this issue would arise, the parents should interrupt the conversation immediately.
- The parents were ordered not to discuss their marital conflicts in the presence of Helen, nor to inform her regarding any marital disputes at home.
- The parents were encouraged to talk instead about future plans regarding their daughter, and to stop "psychoanalyzing" Helen's condition as well as their own pasts.

It soon turned out that we had been much too optimistic and had underestimated both the rigidity of the dysfunctional family structure and the severity of the marital schism. Despite all our encouragement to make explicit arrangements, the old family scenario was repeated already during the first visit in the hospital, i.e., severe disputes between both parents took place in the presence of Helen, who was indirectly blamed for having caused the marital tensions. In the next session both parents accused each other of breaking the arrangement made with the therapist.

Though Helen had already stayed five weeks in our inpatent unit, she still tended to isolate herself most of the time from her fellow patients. In the group psychotherapy, she said she was feeling very guilty for being the cause of the marital tensions between her parents. One month later, at the time her parents started to discuss the issue of separation, Helen began to mutilate herself: she burned her arms with cigarettes and cut herself with a knife. This self-mutilation was interpreted, on the one hand, as an ultimate maneuver to play the "sick" child and thus reunite her parents, and, on the other hand, as an expression of her ambivalence toward separation from her family.

When confronted with the self-mutilation of their daughter, the parents were deeply shocked and finally awakened. Now they realized the importance of a marked and clear boundary between their marital relationship and their daughter's life. From this moment on, the parents started to increase little by little their collaboration and endorsement of our treatment. Notwithstanding all this, the old family scenario would return on several other occasions during the further course of the treatment process.

Besides the restructuring of clear intergenerational boundaries between parents and daughter, we also centered our therapeutic attempts on challenging the cognitive belief system of both patient and family. One of the most striking beliefs in this family system was the absolute conviction that children must be protected by their parents against the dangers of the outside world. This family was completely isolated and even alienated from the normal social network outside the family. The "emotional cutoff" of Peter and the anorexia nervosa of Helen could be understood as the fear of the family system for the launching and autonomy of the children. At the same time, these extreme reactions (running away and self-starvation) might be seen as signals — cries for help — that something in this family system absolutely needed to change.

Again, we used Helen's drawing (Figure 2) in challenging the family's belief system, together with the relabeling of the eating disorder as a psychological problem of growth and gaining more autonomy, having considerable consequences for both patient and parents. This relabeling, often expressed on an indirect metaphorical level, had to be repeated again and again during treatment.

> *Therapist:* "Do you know what happens with little trees in the wood that don't receive any sunlight, standing in the dark, overshadowed by their big neighbors?"
>
> *Mother:* "They will probably dry out and never grow up to become adult trees."
>
> *Father:* "Yes, but look at our daughter — that girl needs care and protection. You can't compare a tree with a starving girl!"
>
> *Therapist:* "What happened with both of you when you were around the age of 19 years? How did your own parents react at that time? Did they protect you as much as you intend to do now with Helen?"
>
> *Father:* "At that time, my mother had just died. I was the oldest son next to my father. I worked night and day, struggling to survive."
>
> *Therapist:* "You had a lot of responsibilities, although your father was a severe man. I guess that's the only way to grow up, just take up your own responsibility..."
>
> *Mother:* "Well, when our daughter decides to grow up and become a young woman, we'll have to find a way to dig out this little tree and put it somewhere else."

Until the discharge of Helen from our hospital, the exploration of how one could find a way "to dig out this little, overshadowed tree and plant it somewhere else," became the main topic in our family sessions.

At this point in treatment the self-mutilation of Helen suddenly stopped. She became more involved on the ward and even started to discuss and explore, although hesitatingly, some future plans. However, three more months of intensive inpatient treatment were needed before she reached her target weight (52 kg), and before both parents and daughter agreed upon a realistic plan for the future. Meanwhile, one of the most important tasks on the part of the family therapist was to provide support and encouragement for Helen's parents. On several occasions, we had to assure them over and over again that Helen no longer needed their protection and that nobody was to blame for the past. The more the parents were distancing themselves from the care and concern for their daughter, the more their marital conflicts escalated bringing the theme of separation or divorce into the open.

Preparing the Discharge from the Hospital

In the last phase of inpatient treatment, Helen returned home for the weekend. The discussion and detailed preparation for the first weekends outside the hospital was of crucial importance, since we were expecting that the separation from the inpatient treatment milieu would probably provoke high tension, insecurity and anxiety, both in the patient and in the parents. The latter were clearly overoptimistic and appeared to expect that after discharge from the hospital all eating and other psychological problems in their daughter would disappear at once. Father was even silently hoping "that the harmony in his marriage may return spontaneously as soon as the daughter returns home!" We therefore confronted the family with the transition and adaptation problems they could expect and even predicted an extremely difficult time for all family members, with the possibility of a relapse into the anorexia.

Helen's own idea of studying at a boarding school, hence living apart from the family during the week, was strongly sustained by the family therapist and the other team members. The parents, in particular father, reacted with disapproval. Father felt rejected by his daughter and even stated that "his daughter was just not ready for this." After many hours of discussion, the parents finally agreed upon their daughter's proposal, but still remained very skeptical. The implicit message sent to Helen was that "she still needed the protection of her parents."

Three weeks before Helen's discharge from the hospital, a totally unexpected event occurred. Peter, the oldest son, who had already been missing for more than two and a half years — one family member even thought he was deceased — suddenly phoned his mother and asked if he might come home on holiday to visit his family. He further informed his mother that he was all right and lived as a guest of a family in another country. Since then, the "prodigal son" has re-established regular contacts with his family up to the present, though he has continued to live his own life far away from home. Before discharge from the hospital, careful reassessment of the family and individual system was needed in order to reformulate appropriate therapeutic goals when indicated.

Reassessment of the family system: Alterations in the family structure and boundaries between the subsystems at the end of the inpatient treatment (i.e., after five months), were again clearly demonstrated by a drawing Helen made during her last week in the hospital (see Figure 3). Once again, we decided to use this information as input in the family session. Helen's picture showed that a weak boundary between the subsystems had been constructed. She stated that, although she was no longer experiencing herself as being locked between both parents, this disentangling process made her very anxious at certain moments.

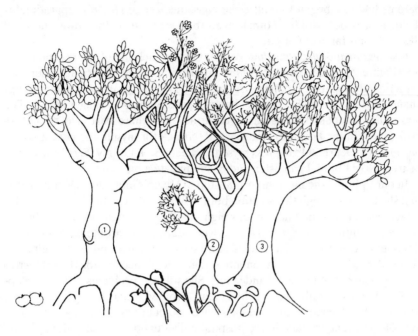

Figure 3. Helen's sketch of her family made during her last week of hospitalization. (1 = Father; 2 = Helen; 3 = Mother).

Since she was trying to make more distance between herself and her parents — particularly from her mother — and to become more independent, she felt "as if she had no roots anymore." On the other hand, the sketch showed she clearly idealized her parents' unity and togetherness. Though the parents had realized the importance of a common consistent but nonprotective attitude toward their daughter, their marital relationship got worse and they were considering a divorce. They agreed upon our proposal to start a fortnightly marital therapy while we also planned one outpatient family session per month.

The behavioral, experiential and cognitive level: As mentioned earlier, both parents no longer displayed opposing behaviors with regard to their daughter. They now realized that Helen's weight and eating behavior was her own responsibility. Escalating disputes, accompanied by physical violence between them on the part of parents, no longer occurred. Nevertheless, they were still at certain points trying to involve their children as coalition partners in their ongoing marital conflicts. At the end of hospitalization, the parents no longer felt guilty for having caused the anorexia nervosa. On the other hand, they were still experiencing great difficulty in expressing their feelings toward each other directly. Next, they no longer perceived their daughter as a helpless, weak and dependent girl who needed parental care and protection. Meanwhile, the parents had just begun to realize the consequences of Helen's separation-in-dividuation process for their own lives and became aware of their own emotional ties with their family of origin.

Reassessment of the individual system: On the backside of her second drawing (Figure 3), Helen explained how she perceived and experienced her own evolution during the inpatient treatment: "The situation in our family has changed a lot. This makes me feel happy, because it was no longer livable. The atmosphere is not so suffocating anymore, although there exists a lot of sadness now. Here (in the hospital), I've learned to think for myself and not for someone else. I've learned to express myself and hence a lot of my fears have disappeared. Now I think I can listen and communicate a bit."

In our opinion, the most important step in Helen's individual evolution, was that she broke through the isolation both in her symptoms and in her social interactions. She reached her target weight of 52 kg (see number 2 in Figure 1), stopped vomiting, and her menses returned during the last month of inpatient treatment. Although she had gained more self-confidence and felt herself more cheerful, she was fearful of autonomy and independence outside the protective environment of both hospital and family. She still had problems with the acceptance of her sexually mature body and avoided relationships with boys. Moreover, Helen still showed ambivalence and conflicting expectations about her role as young woman: in the hospital individuality and self-differentiation had been emphasized, while loyalty toward her family of origin was still highly valued by her parents. Hence, overviewing Helen's evolution, we had expected that the steps toward autonomy and separation from her family would certainly be very stressful. We therefore advised her to join our fortnightly outpatient group therapy for anorexia nervosa patients.

CONSOLIDATING CHANGE

During the first seven months after Helen's discharge from the hospital, family life was suspiciously quiet and stable. Helen integrated herself at the boarding school without any special difficulties. She was gradually making contact with peers and said that she was gaining more self-confidence. At this time, our most important task was to encourage Helen toward exploration, experimentation and the learning of new behavior. She completely changed both her wardrobe and outlook: she even started to experiment with makeup and went out for dancing. At the same time, very slowly, Helen's weight was decreasing, which we interpreted as an indirect signal that some problems still remained untouched.

The parents, when faced with the idea of an eventual divorce, flew into each other's arms and were living for some time in a "honeymoon" state of mind. The more we tried to confront them with their denial of the marital conflicts, the more they claimed that they now "live in harmony for ever." We therefore stopped our attempts of direct provocation of the marital system and we adopted a wait-and-see attitude of careful listening and observing.

The Relapse into the Symptoms

Seven months after discharge from the hospital, Helen's weight suddenly began to drop quickly (see numbers 3 and 4 in Figure 1). She displayed hyperactive behavior (e.g., studying) and again became obsessed by food, calories and weight while her menses ceased. Not surprisingly, we did ascertain at about the same time that the parental conflicts and disputes had returned. Helen still had difficulty escaping from her traditional role as mediator between her parents. Once again the question of divorce and separation arose. Although we expected this crisis to come out, there was some hesitation in our reaction to it. According to the arrangements of the outpatient therapeutic contract concerning Helen's weight, she had to be readmitted to the hospital as soon as her weight dropped below 46 kg (i.e., 6 kg below target weight). Nevertheless, we decided, by mutual arrangement with Helen and the parents, to refrain from proceeding with these arrangements and abandon the consideration of readmission for the time being. This decision was based on the following considerations:

- Helen's physical health was still in good condition; the vomiting had never returned.
- As contrasted with the highly resistant attitude at the beginning of treatment, the family was now clearly aware of the psychological meaning of Helen's weight loss.
- Although she was relapsing into the anorexic symptoms, Helen had built up a certain degree of autonomy and independence from her parents; she had some good and solid relationships outside the family, and at school she was behaving quite normally (besides a strong tendency to reduce her food intake).
- We also feared that a rehospitalization of Helen would elicit a conflict-detouring process, and thus help both parents to flee from their chronic conflicts.

We asked Helen to fix a minimum weight, under which outpatient therapy no longer would be possible and rehospitalization would be unavoidable. She herself determined a threshold of 42 kg as absolute minimum. Hence, we were further delegating the responsibility toward Helen and thus modeled for the parents the trust and belief in their daughter's capacities of change and growth.

Separation of the Parents

With regard to the marital schism, we decided to change our therapeutic strategy. At this time, instead of directly confronting the parents by means of active provocation and supporting their proposal to separate, we now restrained them from negotiating an eventual divorce.

> *Therapist:* "Now, at last, I'm convinced of the fact that you better stay together, because the separation will probably cause too much pain and sadness, which neither of you can handle at the moment. I guess the best thing to do now is just try to accept and live with these conflicts for the time being."

> *Father:* "Oh no, I'm no longer afraid to leave my wife and children and the house I have lived in for more than twenty years. I just can't stand this situation one minute longer. I'll search for an appartment to live on my own from now on."

> *Mother:* "I must admit that our planning to separate makes me very sad and frightens me. But for all of us, I believe it's the only solution to survive. Otherwise we'll be fighting till the end of our lives. And now I realize how unhappy we all feel."

> *Therapist:* "Yes, I know, but do you think you can handle the consequences of the separation at this moment. I mean, the loneliness, the reactions from your parents and colleagues. In fact, it looks as if your fights resulted in making a strong bond between both of you."

Quite astonishingly, our therapeutic strategy turned out to be successful this time insofar as that both parents no longer hesitated about their decision to separate and started to negotiate practical arrangements. Although we remained skeptical, we agreed upon the parents' demand for help in this painful and exhausting negotiating process. Father proposed to leave the house, and he rented a small flat. Eighteen months after Helen's hospitalization and more than one year after her discharge from the hospital, father moved away from his wife and family and the separation was put into practice. The parents decided to meet once a week for two hours to discuss practical arrangements (e.g., expenses, attitude toward the children etc.). From then on we switched over to individual sessions for each of the spouses. Father, in particular, felt very depressed and tended to set himself apart completely. He became even more isolated than he had been before: he started to drink and was risked developing a serious alcohol problem. The only person he regularly met with was his own father. During the first months after the separation, mother, who lived together with Alfred (the youngest son), felt greatly relieved. Later on, she had to fight against her loneliness and had great difficulty with the increasing independence of both Helen and Alfred.

The Individuation of Helen

Once the children were informed of their parents' decision to separate and live apart, Helen's weight started to increase. During the week, she was still stay-

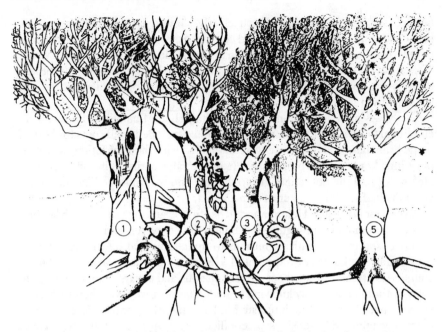

Figure 4. Helen's sketch of her family made two years after the beginning of treatment.
(1 = Father; 2 = Helen; 3 = Mother; 4 = Alfre; 5 = Peter).

ing at the boarding school and during the weekends she alternately stayed with her mother or with her father, but this made her confused. She therefore decided to leave the boarding school and to live on her own. To make the execution of her plan possible, she applied for a weekend job and rented a small flat in a neighboring city not far from her parents (see number 5 in Figure 1). At the time Helen's menses returned (see number 6 in Figure 1), her mother suddenly phoned us and asked for an appointment as soon as possible. Although Helen's weight kept on increasing, mother said that she was fearing a relapse into the anorexic symptoms! A detailed exploration of her fear revealed an alcohol problem in mother together with periodic binge eating. She further stated that now that her daughter had a boyfriend, the distance between mother and daughter would even become greater.

Helen indeed reported that, at the time her menses returned, she had fallen in love with a boy. In the outpatient group therapy, she explored her feelings of uncertainty and inferiority toward her boyfriend. She even believed that she "was just not good enough" to enjoy the pleasure of this relationship, since her father continuously repeated that she "first had to finish her studies before dating a boy." These unrealistic beliefs were challenged and questioned during the group therapy sessions, and we explained to her the way both parents were trying unconsciously to make her feel guilty. Once again we asked Helen to make another drawing about how she was actually experiencing her life and family relations (see Figure 4). The sketch clearly showed that Helen's scope has broadened: she made a beautiful and colorful drawing, wherein she also placed her two brothers, Peter and Alfred. On the backside of her sketch Helen wrote: "I tried out two different solutions: first I planned to grow higher than the others, but this was too difficult; next I decided to search another place in the soil, wherein my tree may become solidly rooted."

Two years after admission to our hospital, Helen finally had loosened the emotional ties with her mother and, next, had developed solid roots for herself. Some branches of Helen's tree were entangled with those of father, who went on writing her letters on moral issues (e.g., the value of discipline and virginity). Helen stopped the outpatient group therapy and we continued having irregular individual sessions on her demand.

Several months later, Helen reported her first sexual experience with her boyfriend (see number 7 in Figure 1). Though she enjoyed it and was sexually responsive, she reacted with vaginismus to the attempts at having sexual intercourse, and she felt very disappointed. Helen said that as soon as sexual intercourse was attempted, she became very anxious and always felt the urge to run away, without consciously knowing or understanding why. We therefore asked her whether she would be interested in learning self-hypnosis in order to explore any underlying tensions or conflicts regarding her vaginismus. Helen agreed to our proposal and we introduced the hypnoanalytic technique of the "affect bridge" (Watkins, 1971). The exploration under hypnosis of Helen's anxiety revealed several repressed traumatic incestuous sexual experiences with her father at the age of six and seven years. The conscious awareness of these traumatic events helped Helen to deal successfully with her vaginismus (see number 8 in Figure 1). She further evolved toward being an independent, fullblown and attractive young woman.

FOLLOW-UP

Approximately three years were needed before the consolidation of change in this family was actualized. The family system was no longer ruled or guided by rigid, homeostatic forces which hampered the transition from one phase to another in the family life cycle. As Helen's colorful family sketch clearly demonstrated, the family was now a continuously evolving system governed by morphogenetic forces, which were introducing change, flexibility and growth but also instability into the family system. We therefore decided to decrease our contact with both Helen and the parents. We were convinced that now at last Helen and the other family members could further evolve all by themselves. Indeed, both parents stated that they no longer needed our help and asked to stop the individual sessions. Helen was still requesting help and support, but only once every two months.

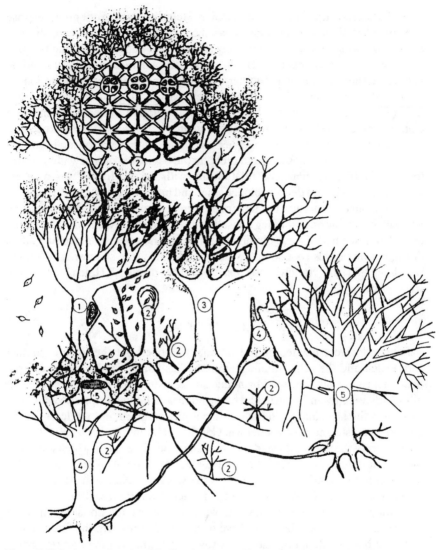

Figure 5. Helen's "very last sketch" of her family. (1 = Father; 2 = Helen; 3 = Mother; 4 = Alfred; 5 = Peter).

During the following twelve months (see numbers 8 to 10 in Figure 1), Helen further stabilized her weight. She studied during the week and worked during the weekend. On several occasions, her father wrote her a letter condemning his daughter for her "unrespectable and vulgar" behavior. Father phoned us twice with the message that he was worried about his daughter's sexual behavior. Helen, indeed, was experimenting with dating boys, but finally became seriously engaged with the expectation of marrying her boyfriend.

At the last individual therapeutic session, Helen brought to our great surprise "her very last sketch of her family," as she stated (Figure 5). Again, she had drawn a growing family, wherein many changes had happened during the previous two years. With regard to Helen, some part of her trunk was still standing between father and mother. But her own trunk and branches were no longer entangled with those of her father – Helen was no longer influenced by her father's messages. Moreover, her trunk had developed a shape resembling a club or cudget, so she was finally armed against her parents' interference into her personal life. In the meantime, her roots had continued growing in several directions, while sowing seeds and creating the beginning of a new life in more fertile soil. In particular, the relationship with her boyfriend was now experienced as solid and deep-rooted. Father and mother were now clearly differentiated from one another, but father lost a great number of his leaves, while he was still distancing and isolating himself from the outside world. Mother, on the other hand, seemed to have obtained a stable position. Alfred's tree had fallen down, but one of his roots created a new and stable tree somewhere else. He was doing all right, "following the example of his brother," Helen told us with some pride.

CONCLUSION

Four years were needed before we finally stopped our therapeutic contact with Helen and the other family members. This family was no longer imprisoned in a rigid isolation ruled by homeostatic, change-inhibiting forces. Flexibility, individuality and growth had replaced the old family script. After all, flexibility was the key concept in the treatment process itself, not the least for the family therapist. One may wonder what kind of interventions or specific strategy on the part of the therapists made these changes possible and in which way these interventions have influenced the family system. We first of all presume that the nonspecific therapeutic factors such as the working alliance, trust, hope and belief in one's own approach have been of crucial importance. Others may state that "time heals all wounds." Indeed, we cannot prove the possible impact of our therapeutic work. Maybe we have been a guide for a trip the family could or would have made all by itself. Anyway, it was a fascinating and rewarding trip...

REFERENCES

Bowen, M. (1978), *Family Therapy in Clinical Practice.* New York: Jason Aronson.
Watkins, S. (1971), The affect bridge: A hypnoanalytic technique. *International Journal of Clinical and Experimental Hypnosis,* 19:21-27.

Chapter 16

The Family Therapist Faced with Chronic Cases, Broken-Home Situations, and Transgenerational Issues

Johan Vanderlinden, Claire Perednia and Walter Vandereycken

INTRODUCTION

The literature on the use of family therapy in eating disorders deals mostly with young patients who live in an intact nuclear family. Since there is a lot written about such cases (see Bibliography on Family Aspects of Eating Disorders in this volume) and since we are usually faced with far more complicated cases, we would like to highlight some topics which are generally overlooked in the current literature. In a specialized treatment center such as ours, the majority of patients referred show a long history of eating disorder for which several treatments, including family therapy, have usually been tried out in vain

Instead of looking at chronicity in a pessimistic way, we try to consider it as a special challenge to our treatment potential. Although we too fail in several cases, some extraordinary and unexpected results have reinforced our attempts at approaching these cases as if everything could still change regardless of what has happened before. We adopt the same stance with all our patients, but we have learned to set limits, too, and to accept failures as well: they constitute the best feedback for our work and the most powerful antidote against the illusion of omnipotence. Specially challenging are single-parent families and broken-home situations, because the "normal" family structure here is already basically disrupted, regardless of the existence of eating disorder itself. In these and many other cases we have realized the sometimes enormous influence from the outside on the nuclear family, especially from the grandparents. Therefore, we also pay specific attention to transgenerational issues which may be of particular significance in the treatment of eating disorder patients.

CHRONIC CASES*

Treatment of severe eating disorders necessitates, as is noted repeatedly throughout this book, an intensive and multidimensional approach. Outpatient family therapy will certainly be the treatment of choice in young nervosa patients. But in recent years, we have been confronted with a growing number of patients presenting a severe form or a chronic course of anorexia nervosa and/or bulimia, including previous treatment failures and even more deteriorating behavior (vomiting, purging, kleptomania, self-mutilation, and suicidal tendencies). Here, experience has taught us that, in most cases, admission into a hospital, which provides a specialized treatment setting for eating disorders, becomes unavoidable in order to break through the vicious circle in which these patients are caught.

However, hospitalization does not exclude the necessity as well as the possibility of involving the patient's natural milieu in the treatment, i.e., taking the family influences into consideration. Especially in older and in severe cases of eating disorders, the family approach did become a crucial element in the treatment process, since a great deal of these so-called grown-up women still have extremely strong emotional ties with their family of origin, as this chapter demonstrates.

Case Reports

Case 1

Julia is 33 years old. She is married to Marc, a 36-year-old hairdresser. They have two girls (age 6 and 9). From the beginning of their marriage — 10 years ago — Julia has been developing a severe and chronic form of anorexia nervosa, with hyperactivity, extreme loss of weight (33 kg for 1m66), binge eating and vomiting, excessive use of laxatives, and a strong preoccupation with food and a thin body ideal as the most important features. Before her admission at our unit she had been hospitalized several times in both general and psychiatric hospitals. Hence, Julia has spent a considerable time in various hospitals, separated from her husband and two children. Tube feeding, psychotropic drugs and a sometimes strict isolation from the outside world were the most important therapies she had received in the past. Julia was referred to our unit to give her "a last chance," but at that point no one believed that anyone or anything could ever stop her starving.

We asked the referring physician if the patient could attend the first interview in companionship of her husband and both children. They were all present

---

* Parts of this section are based upon excerpts of a previously published article by Johan Vanderlinden and Walter Vandereycken: "Directive family therapy in adult patients with severe or chronic anorexia nervosa" (*International Journal of Family Psychiatry*, 1984, 5:267-280).

at the intake interview, but also was Julia's mother. Before starting the interview, we asked Julia and her husband whether they agreed with the presence of
the mother during the intake. The fact that they did not object was, in our view,
a symptom of a lack of intergenerational boundaries. It was Julia's mother who
answered almost all of our questions. She motivated Julia — her "little
daughter" — for accepting admission at our hospital. Julia herself looked physically exhausted and played the pitiful patient. Julia's husband and two children
tried to avoid all our questions.

During the first interview, it became clear that Julia started dieting shortly
after her marriage. And since then, marital conflicts have existed up to the present. Julia's husband became an alcoholic. But strikingly enough, the anorexic
symptomatology appeared to have also a meaning with respect to Julia's family
of origin. The marriage of her parents was characterized by endless conflicts,
and Julia's father appeared to be an alcoholic too. On the basis of this information, we formulated the following hypothesis: Julia was sacrificing her own
health to hide the conflicts both in her own family and in her family of origin;
because of an overinvolvement with her family of origin (especially with her
mother), she presented a very low level of self-differentiation and had never become a grown-up woman.

Julia stayed in our hospital for about five months. During the first weeks, the
medical team had to fight for her life, because although she was dangerously
emaciated she refused to eat and opposed every treatment. She seemed to be
stuck in a negativistic attitude and a stubborn refusal to cooperate. Therefore
she did not attend the normal group therapeutic activities. In the beginning, we
planned one family session every week to gather more information and to discuss the visits. After a while we decided to work only with the couple, because
marital tensions became more apparent. We explained our working hypothesis
to them and stated that both of them were afraid to be confronted with their
marital conflicts. But, we said, this could be the only way of dealing with it and
maybe they should go on living as they had done the last ten years. Shortly after
this session — Julia was in the hospital three months without any considerable
change — the husband suddenly phoned us, telling us very self-confidently that
he had made the decision to divorce.

This message almost had the effect of an exploding time bomb within the
marital relationship and provoked an intense emotional crisis in both the patient
and her husband. The equilibrium of the marital system was fundamentally disturbed. This severe crisis was the first and most important step in the therapy,
leading to a striking change in Julia's behavior. Indeed, once she realized and
discussed with her husband the consequences of an eventual divorce, she started
very slowly to eat again, and engaged herself in the therapeutic program. Now
the overinvolvement (enmeshment) between Julia and her mother became very
clear. The husband refused further cooperation and we switched to a therapy
involving the family of origin. Julia's father, however, refused to collaborate, so

we had to work with Julia and her mother. The central theme in these meetings was the preparation of a "new life" for Julia as a divorced woman.

After five months of hospitalization, she was discharged from the hospital and weighted 48 kg. We carried out an aftercare program for two years: about 25 sessions with Julia and her mother. The divorce and the separation from her children — they lived with their father — made Julie depressed for a long period. It was the first time that we saw her express some genuine feelings. After about 15 months, Julia started a part-time job as librarian. After her discharge from the hospital (about four years ago) she never fell back into her anorexic symptoms and her weight remained well controlled within a normal range (about 45 kg). These days, she lives on her own, and at the age of 37 she became a full-blown woman.

Not all our patients are doing so successfully. Many relapse in their anorexic or bulimic symptoms and sometimes rehospitalization is necessary. We will illustrate this in the following case example.

Case 2

Margareth, an attractive 37-year-old woman, married to a 43-year- old computer-programmer was admitted to our hospital with a severe anorexia nervosa symptomatology: daily vomiting, considerable hyperactivity, a strong preoccupation with food, amenorrhea for two years, 20% loss of weight. She also displayed obsessive-compulsive behavior, such as washing her hands and brushing her teeth about 25 times a day. The anorexic symptoms started about two years before, after a period of depression but without any clear precipitating event. Margareth seemed to have, however, some problems with her two adolescent daughters (13 and 17 years of age). The fact that they became more and more involved in social contacts (peer relations and activities) outside the family life was a change she had difficulties accepting. This separation-individuation process of the children would confront the parents with their marital relationship, in particular with their communication and sexual problems.

We assumed that the anorexic symptomatology of Margareth served as a regulator of the family homeostasis, i.e., as a protector against a possible family crisis. First we decided to work with the entire family (while Margareth was hospitalized) and to focus on the adaptation problems between the adolescent girls and their parents. We tried to strengthen the coalition between the parents and to make clear boundaries between them and the children. But the longer we worked with the entire family, the more the marital conflicts became apparent and, therefore, we decided that marital therapy was needed.

After five months of total hospitalization, with very slow progress, we shifted to partial hospitalization (five days a week in day treatment on the same unit). Now the spouses had to spend more time together and were forced to face their marital problems. The harder they tried to communicate and solve these problems, the more they became aware of the alienation and distance between themselves. This process ended up in a deep marital crisis: both of them formulated—very carefully—the desire for a temporary separation.

Meanwhile, Margareth was discharged after five months of total hospitalization and two months partial hospitalization. Weight gain (from 45 kg to 55 kg) and normalization of eating habits came only very slowly and required a great effort. During the aftercare, which consisted of marital therapy and directive group therapy for anorexic and bulimic patients, both spouses became very anxious. Facing the possibility of a definitive separation, they were stuck in a marital crisis. Margareth relapsed into her anorexic symptoms: she flew into hyperactivity, dieting and vomiting, and lost weight again very quickly. Her husband refused to collaborate any further in the marital therapy as long as his wife did not regain weight.

Following the agreements in the outpatient treatment contract, Margareth was readmitted at our day hospital only four months after discharge. In the beginning, she was very negativistic, refused to cooperate and convinced almost all the team members that she was "a hopeless case." After about two weeks, we decided to change our therapeutic strategy: instead of pushing, encouraging or stimulating her in order to induce change directly, we had chosen to follow an indirect strategy. The following message was given to the couple: "After all these months of intensive psychotherapy, almost every team member is convinced at last that solving your eating problems will be a very difficult task and will need much more time than we thought in the beginning. We think also that the eating pathology has a very important meaning within your relationship and that maybe it is much better to remain anorexic than to face a marital crisis and, eventually, divorce. So, we believe that both of you cannot benefit anymore from our special treatment program. That's why we are thinking about stopping this approach and, "if you wish", referring Margareth to another residential unit, namely the psychotherapeutic community, where further treatment will take at least one year." The couple's answer was very direct and clear: we will prove to you in the next weeks that your approach is the best therapy for both of us and that the team's opinion is wrong. Nevertheless, we remained skeptical and decided to give them a "last chance." After this session, Margareth showed a considerable improvement, both in her anorexic behavior and in the relationship with her husband. Both spouses were trying to convince the team that Margareth was not a hopeless case and that recovery was still possible.

After discharge from the day hospital, Margareth attended outpatient marital and group therapy for about one and a half years. Meanwhile, our therapeutic strategy was still characterized by an indirect approach, and every improvement had to challenge a somehow skeptical attitude on the part of the therapist. But the couple kept on proving to us that things can really change! Today, Margareth is three years out of the hospital and has not had further treatment (on her request) for more than six months. She has developed an active social life but, though the marital relationship has improved considerably, she believes that, in fact, her husband is the wrong man for her. She realized this particularly when her eldest daughter married, a difficult moment Margareth could overcome without relapsing into anorexia. Nevertheless, she still has difficulties with food and weight, and may vomit at moments of great tension.

Treatment Considerations

The previous case examples illustrate some of the principles in our therapeutic approach (for a detailed description of the different treatment phases, basic strategies and interventions see Chapter 15). However, the therapeutic work with severe and chronic eating disorders is often quite demanding and frustrating, in particular for the therapist. Hence, it may be useful to reconsider some basic principles and possible pitfalls in the treatment of chronic eating disorders. Generally speaking, one may state that the longer the duration of the eating disorder, the more the patient and those surrounding her (family, husband, relatives etc.) are able to adapt to living with someone who displays a chronic anorexia nervosa or bulimia. Hence, in these families there usually exists a highly rigid structure together with a strong resistance or ambivalence toward change. Besides these characteristics, previous treatment failures may further discourage both the family and the therapists to such an extent that change in the patient and family is the last thing one expects. The conviction that the patient is intractable, regardless type or intensity of treatment, undermines some basic conditions for therapy, especially the nonspecific factors (creation of hope, establishment of a working alliance, relabeling of the problem as resolvable etc.). We therefore try to convince ourselves, especially in the beginning phase of treatment, that change and growth in this particular patient is still possible. On the other hand, we have been confronted several times with dramatic and spectacular changes in patients who were labeled as incurable because of the chronicity of their symptoms and because previous therapeutic attempts had failed. Hospitalization in our specialized unit is often interpreted by the family as "the therapy of the last chance." Such an attitude may lead to tapping new sources of energy and growth, both in the patient, the family and the therapeutic system. We further try to explain to the patient and the family "that everything has a price" and that a real change will demand a high price that must be paid by everyone living with the patient around whose illness the whole family life has been organized. During the entire treatment process, we continually repeat this message and encourage the patient and family to reflect upon the consequences of change and whether or not they want to pay such high price for change and growth.

Some family therapists (e.g., the Milan School) recommend a paradoxical therapeutic approach, especially when chronic cases and rigid family systems are concerned. Although such paradoxical attitude (e.g., "it is better for you to stay ill") may have considerable impact (see Hsu & Lieberman, 1982) its effect is unpredictable and, therefore, not without serious risks (e.g., a feeling of being abandoned by the therapist may evoke suicidal tendencies). For this reason, we prefer to start with a direct approach (active provocation). Later on in the therapeutic process, when a direct attempt has failed to promote any change, we switch to an indirect approach such as the "Greek Chorus" technique (see Chapters 11 and 15). On the other hand, when faced with chronic eating disorder patients, one must always be very attentive to detect those patients who start treatment with one ultimate goal: to convince themselves and the family that they are incurable and will never be able to change. These patients often start the therapy with suspicious but great enthusiasm, seducing the therapist to intervene immediately with an active therapeutic strategy. However, it soon turns out that they intended to sabotage all therapeutic arrangements and may often provoke an extremely negative therapeutic atmosphere (which can have a devastating influence in a group treatment setting). In these cases, the therapist has to question his position in such a pseudo- or, better, anti-therapy situation and perhaps may refuse to give further treatment when the patient keeps on sabotaging every therapeutic attempt. Indeed, some of these patients tend to reconcile themselves even more with the anorexic or bulimic identity, when they passed "the most specialized" treatment for eating disorders without any improvement! Not uncommonly, one may discover these chronic patients as active leaders in self-help organizations where they give one and the same message: "Once anorexic, forever anorexic."

But, finally, the therapist must accept and respect his and the patient's own limitations because some patients have "the right to stay ill" (Hall, 1982).

BROKEN-HOME SITUATIONS

Characteristics

Generally speaking, one may state that there has been a dramatic growth in the number of broken-home situations and single-parent families in the last decade. Currently, the incidence of broken homes in families with an eating disorder patient varies considerably among the reported studies, probably because of sociocultural influences (see Chapter 3).

We are regularly faced with two major types of single-parent families: (1) because of the divorce of the parents (who usually are still emotionally involved with one another, although they are legally separated), and (2) because of the death of one parent (leaving the other usually overinvolved with the children)

In our experience, these families have two characteristics in common: first, the non-custodial or absent parent (divorced or deceased) often continues to play a significant role in the life of the family (see Morawetz & Walker, 1984); second, the eating disorder patient often functions as a link or go-between between the custodial parent and the absent (divorced) parent or she must replace (in practice or symbolically) the deceased parent.

Example: Since the sudden death of her mother four years ago, Suzy (an attractive 22-year-old young woman) has developed an extreme bulimia nervosa with dayly bingeing, vomiting and laxative abuse. The functional analysis revealed that no one in the family (father, three daughters and one son) ever talked about their feelings concerning the loss and death of mother. Suzy, on the other hand, told us that almost every day she silently weeped for the loss of her mother, whose grave she frequently visited with fresh flowers. The bulimia was interpreted as an expression or sign of the family's repressed feelings or unfinished mourning process concerning the loss of mother.

The functional analysis of a single-parent family system may further reveal (Morawetz & Walker, 1984) that:

- The identified patient functions as the embodiment of the absent parent; this often happens in families who are suddenly confronted with the death of one of the parents or with an emotionally unresolved divorce.
- The identified patient replaces the deceased or absent parent and has to play a parental role; in these families we often found confusion or a complete lack of intergenerational boundaries.
- The family has run wild and has become chaotic, displaying a complete absence of hierarchic boundaries and executive functions within the family system on the one hand, and an extreme, rigid boundary against the outside world on the other.
- All guilt concerning the loss of the deceased or absent parent is projected upon the identified patient who becomes the scapegoat and is indirectly blamed for having caused the loss of the marital partner.
- The reentry on the social scene of the single parent with the hope of engaging in a new relationship provokes a lot of fear and strain, mostly neglected and/or projected upon the identified patient.
- The single parent becomes dependent again on his/her family of origin, a situation which again may awaken separation-individuation issues and/or conflicts between dependency needs and autonomy wishes.

In single-parent families and broken-home situations, the eating disorder often reflects the impossibility of the youngster and the family overcoming a crisis and for them to make the transition to the next developmental stage in the life cycle.

When married patients are concerned, the anorexia nervosa or bulimia often serves as a means of bridging the gap between the spouses — hence temporarily hiding marital discord (see Chapter 17). The occurrence of an eating disorder in a married patient is often linked, in our experience, to an overinvolvement of the family of origin (of one or both spouses) in the marital relationship. Most

Table 1. Basic Interventions in Broken Home Situations

- Provide extra-support for the single-parent family.
- Promote and encourage clear intergenerational boundaries.
- Assess the function of the eating disorder against the background of the deceased or absent parent.
- Help the (ex)-marital partners and/or single parent family to deal with the unresolved marital conflicts and the emotionally unfinished marriage or divorce (when indicated).
- Help the family system and/or single parent to deal with the repressed feelings of grief and the working through of the abnormal mourning process (when indicated).

married patients, when confronted with a decision regarding divorce and separation, indeed return "back home" toward their own parents and become overprotected and isolated from the outside world, while blaming their ex-husband for having caused the divorce!

Interventions

Although family treatment in single-parent families follows the same phases as described in Chapter 15, some additional interventions need our special attention (see Table 1).

Provide extra-support for the single parent: The custodial parent mostly feels isolated, depressed, helpless and alone. The therapist must therefore try to join as soon as possible the single parent, aiming at ventilating their distress and feelings of loneliness. We often meet the parent in individual sessions and further try to encourage him or her to search for support outside the family. In our experience, these individual sessions, first aimed at providing support to the single parent, often evolve toward an intensive individual psychotherapy which commonly deals with issues such as the importance of: independence from the family of origin, separation and distancing from the daughter (patient), growing individuation and autonomy, grief and acceptance of loss of the partner, fear and ambivalence toward engaging in a new relationship, etc.

Promote and encourage clear intergenerational boundaries: This is necessary in order to strenghten the parental subsystem and leadership and, therefore, deserves therapeutic priority. The parents often present with depression or passivity and give little evidence of being responsible for carrying out the executive duties of the family (Frey, 1984). The loss of control and absence of adequate executive functioning, a common characteristic in eating disorder families, are often more pronounced in single-parent families. The therapist must teach the parents — in some cases we even have to force the parents — to take over responsibility and set limits on the patient's behavior. The parent should make clear his or her desire that the patient gain weight and improve psychologically (Sargent & Liebman, 1985). Individual sessions may help to create boundaries between the parent and the eating disorder patient regarding the differentiation between those issues which are family matters and those which are the private, personal matters of the parent alone. By making a strong bond with the parent, the therapist can temporarily function as a buffer between the parent and the patient. The same applies to the parent's family of origin, since single parents usually become very dependent upon their own parents. In the case of married patients, this intergenerational-boundary setting, especially toward the family of origin of one or both spouses, is often of crucial importance. The therapist must therefore be very attentive to undo the attempts and efforts of the patient to involve the family of origin in separation and divorce issues.

Assess the function of the eating disorder against the background of the deceased or absent parent: As mentioned earlier, a detailed functional analysis may reveal whether or not the eating disorder does have a special function within the family system as to the deceased or absent parent. The therapist must, therefore, explore the family's feelings concerning the loss of the parent.

> *Example:* Linda, a 23-year-old student, developed severe anorexia nervosa, shortly after the death of her mother five years before. At the time of admission to our hospital the functional analysis showed that Linda did replace her mother and played a co-parental role with her father. The anorexia nervosa appeared to help the family in evading the painful confrontation with the loss of their mother. As soon as Linda started to improve in the hospital, her father suddenly forced her to stop the treatment, against medical advice.

Help the (ex-)marital partners and/or single-parent system to deal with the unresolved marital conflicts or the emotionally unfinished marriage (when indicated): When the functional analysis reveals hidden marital conflicts and/or unresolved emotional issues concerning the separation and divorce of the parents, the therapist must try to bring these issues into the open in separate individual sessions with the single parent. The eating disorder may function as a "lightning conductor" that is frequently used by the parents as a means of evading the confrontation with the hidden feelings and conflicts. In some cases it is important to invite the absent parent and try to incorporate him or her in the treatment process (see also Schneider, 1981). In (ex-)married patients, it is our experience that the eating disorder often functions as a means of repressing the threat of separation.

> *Example:* Nora, a 28-year-old divorced woman, developed anorexia nervosa soon after her separation, when she was living again in her family of origin. During the middle phase of the treatment, at the moment she was confronted with her stagnating weight curve, Nora discovered her repressed feelings about her separation from her husband and how her eating disorder was detouring that painful experience: she was fleeing back into the role of the "ill" child instead of coping with the situation of being a divorced woman.

Help the family system and/or single-parent system to deal with the repressed feelings of grief and the unfinished mourning process (when indicated): The therapist must carefully prepare the family to deal with acceptance of the loss of the partner. This can be done more easily when the eating disorder itself has improved and, hence, may no longer function to hide an unfinished mourning process. In many cases it is up to the therapist to introduce the issue of death and loss into the therapeutic scene, sometimes by prescribing a grief ritual (see Van der Hart, 1983).

Example: Judy's father suddenly died from a heart attack, actually five years before she was admitted to our hospital for a complicated anorexia nervosa (at the age of 22). Before the death of her father, Judy was behaving "extremely difficult, having frequent temper tantrums," as her mother pointed out. After the loss of her father, she became very silent and started her self-starvation. Ever since, it seemed as if time had stopped for this family. Mother isolated herself from the outside world and went on behaving as if her husband were still alive. She talked with him from the morning till the evening and cried every day for several hours. Only after several months of intensive treatment did we carefully plan a farewell-ritual for mother (in individual sessions) to pass through the pathological mourning process (the important element was the writing of a farewell letter to her deceased husband).

TRANSGENERATIONAL ISSUES

In the family therapy literature as well as in our own everyday practice with the families of eating disorder patients, we are more and more confronted with transgenerational issues. Therefore, we want to explore more in detail this rather "new" issue, one that offers a widened perspective on the therapeutic work with these families.

Several authors (e.g., Boszormenyi-Nagy & Spark, 1984; Bowen, 1976; White, 1983) propose to examine transgenerational issues as factors that have a possible influence on the onset and maintenance of psychological or psychopathological problems.

The classic family therapy was concentrated on working with the nuclear (two-generational) family: the father, the mother and the child(ren). This approach results in a momentary cross-sectional view of the family system and neglects influences from and interactions with the extended family; in addition, it overlooks the consideration of the longitudinal family development, the so-called family life cycle. There is a growing awareness that the idea of the nuclear family as a static entity or isolated social island is a myth.

A nuclear family always starts with two partners becoming parents. These parents themselves are the children of their parents, the products of the families they were raised in. Each marriage incorporates the intersection of two

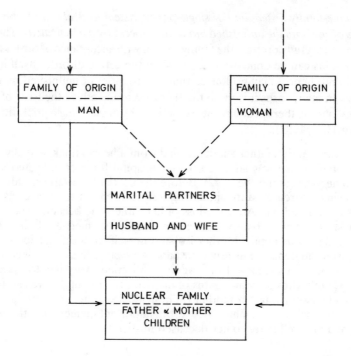

Figure 1: Direct, actual influence (—) and indirect, transgenerational influence (-----) of the grandparental systems on the current parental system.

different families. These families of origin have a direct and an indirect, transgenerational influence on the nuclear family (see Figure 1). The *direct* influence is the actual, present impact the grandparents (and the in-laws) as real persons have on the nuclear family. The *indirect* transgenerational influence refers to the totality of introjects (see Sperling, 1985) a person builds up during his childhood years and carries on with him: ideas, values, myths, beliefs, roles, interaction patterns etc. It is the nonsubstantial legacy from the previous generations of his family. In the everyday reality of a family, these two types of influence cannot be separated or even clearly distinguished because of their mutual reinforcement and interplay.

Clinical Impressions

Regarding the literature on family therapy with anorexia nervosa patients, we see that the few publications about these transgenerational issues deal with clinical impressions of these indirect influences. White (1983) suggests that there is a link between the condition of anorexia nervosa and *certain rigid and implicit family beliefs,* that are transmitted from one generation to the next and have a very constraining impact on the autonomy development of all family members. These beliefs or introjects restrict the range of choices available to the family members by limiting their forms of interaction both with each other and with others outside the family, and by prescribing specific roles to certain daughters making them vulnerable to anorexia nervosa.

A first component of these family beliefs is *the loyalty* to other family members and to the family tradition. Any behaviors that do not measure up to this standard of loyalty are considered as acts of selfishness or betrayal, and trigger transactions that induce guilt and promote conformity within the family system. White (1983) states that it is apparent that food functions as an important vehicle for the transmission of this currency of guilt in these families.

A second component is *the specific role prescription* for women in these families: they are expected to be sensitive, devoted and self-sacrificing. These expectations are most strongly and specifically applied to certain daughters, who are the ones most likely to become anorexic.

Finally, a third component is the reality construction by *insightfulness,* that exists in anorexic families. Their members believe they can see into themselves and others and know the true motivations and intentions behind all behavior.

> These members seem unable to recognize the existence of relatedness and its bearing upon behavior. Individual integrity is evaluated according to the interpretation of one's intentions, the nature and quantity of one's feelings, the degree of sensitivity to the comfort of others, and the level of understanding of needs of others. Usually there exists an adequacy/inadequacy continuum, and each member is rated by others and rates self and others, according to this continuum. (White, 1983, p. 258)

Conrad (1977) described another transgenerational influence in anorexia nervosa families, namely a process of *transgenerational emotional deprivation.* Conrad emphasizes that it is vital to understand the development of anorexia nervosa within the context of the total, extended family. The anorexic child may be the spokesman for the emotional deprivation and starvation of her parents. By means of her symptoms, the patient provides her parents with some nurturance: in fact, the whole family is emotionally hungry and the anorexic child translates the family's affective hunger into starvation, thereby concealing at the same time the more fundamental needs of her family members.

Sperling and Massing (1972) report both an indirect and a direct transgenerational influence. They suppose that anorexia nervosa families have a typical sociodynamic constellation that differs from average families: they are dominated by *a pronounced ascetic achievement and promotion ideology, related to anxiety about sensuality.* The authors state that these characteristics are frequently modeled by a dominating mother or grandmother and that the mothers of anorexics work outside the home to enable the family—and especially the fathers—to live according to a high prestige standard. Thus, what they call the "neurosis of anorexia nervosa" (*Magersuchtneurose*) is transmitted by the pathogenic ideology of a female person of the previous generation. The fathers, on the other hand, are often suffering from chronic diseases (and especially alcoholism) or they died early. They often occupy a special "privileged" position in the family and in the cases where the grandmother lives within the family, she is the one that encourages this position of the father (Sperling & Massing, 1972).

More recently, Slade (1984) has suggested that anorexia nervosa is a condition that appears to develop in families that have had to cope with premature loss, with personal disability and with the stressing effects of changes in social status, economic pressure, often in successive generations. A transgenerational perspective would clarify the way in which *the stress of loss* (as a result of death, divorce or desertion) *and of personal disabilities* (such as a permanent physical handicap, a mental illness or a drinking problem) *among the male members* (grandfathers, fathers) in these families, *has fallen disproportionally onto the women*. Consequently, the maternal as well as the paternal grandmothers of anorexics can be seen as women who lived in (marital) situations where difficulties and deprivations were often quite severe. With a partner who was contributing little or nothing to the security or status of the family as a whole, many raised their children and provided the main source of income by working outside the home. They had a great impact on their children — i.e., the generation that became parents of anorexics — especially regarding themes such as achievement. The maternal grandmothers nurtured beliefs and attitudes in their daughters (the anorexics' mothers) somewhat in conflict with those conventionnaly expected in women: for instance, that security is not to be taken for granted, and that male support is not to be relied upon. On the contrary, their experience and their personalities nurtured the great impact that themes such as achievement and self-improvement have in the anorexics' families.

The high incidence of permanent disability or absence among anorexics' fathers might suggest that all these beliefs and attitudes have been reinforced in the parents' generation. Slade (1984) notes that, while there may be good reasons to believe that the attitudes and the behavior of the anorexics' mothers may be judged as anxious, overcontrolling, overprotective etc., it is also important to appreciate the extent to which their behavior manifests values and aspirations that have grown out of their own life experiences, and out of the experiences of the women in preceding generations, where *a culture of survival* is to be found. The option of conforming entirely to the female role may never have been available to them; and like any other mothers, they transmit their life experience and their culture to their children, the anorexia nervosa patients (Slade, 1984, p. 127). That is the reason why this author emphasizes the necessity of the individualizing explanations of anorexia nervosa: what does it mean for this person, with this family history at this particular development stage, referring to the patient's own life experience within and outside the home?

Case Examples

Case 1

Some of the previously noted clinical impressions of transgenerational issues can also be found in the few case reports available in the anorexia nervosa literature where transgenerational influences are stressed. The most remarkable example we found is given by Conforto and Maura (1972). They describe the (indirect) internal dynamics and (direct) interactions in the extended family of a 16-year-old anorexic patient. They characterize this type of family constellation as a "superego matriarchate" (in an Italian society!): the mother (and usually the grandmother) plays a central role, while the father (also the grandfather) is a background figure. The patient was hospitalized because of a severe anorexia nervosa that began two years ago. Through interviews and home visits, the authors could develop a detailed view of the familial structure and dynamics.

In this family, three generations are living together: the maternal grandparents, the parents and the patient. They have not had any contact for the last eight years with the relatives of father, namely his mother and his sister, although they live in the same city (his father died long ago). As a matter of fact, the paternal grandmother is blamed as the cause of the anorexia nervosa, because she continuously warned her granddaughter that her condition would get worse if she kept on being so selective about her food.

The family is socially very isolated: they have no friends, no membership of any kind, no contact with neighbors or family; the outside world is experienced as threatening and dangerous. The maternal grandmother is the undisputed leader of the family: very autoritarian and inflexible, with very strong ties to her daughter and granddaughter, and overtly disapproving toward the father. Four months after the birth of the patient, the grandmother left the conjugal room to sleep with the future patient, and this situation changed only very recently. Although the mother behaves extremely passively and dependent toward her own mother, there seems to exist a comfortable and strong feeling of unity and complementarity between them. The father of the patient is rather unstable, vulnerable and addicted to alcohol, like his father-in-law (the maternal grandfather). He feels incapable of intervenetion in the relationship between his wife and his mother-in-law, who form a coalition against him that strengthens their tie. He attributes his impotence to the fact that the house they live in, is the property of his mother-in-law.

This is the psychological environment the patient was raised in: always satisfied in all her needs on a level of extremely primitive functions (such as hunger, cold, physical health) but in reality she is estranged from "real" maternal affection because her mother, who still is herself a dependent daughter, is unprepared for her maternal role and experiences herself as an incapable mother, which makes her feel very guilty toward her daughter. Every possible, corrective influence that the patient's father could exercise is systematically boycotted; because of his job (as an emanation of the outside world) he is disapproved of by his mother-in-law and his wife. Their attitude toward him is an obstacle for the patient to find some comfort with her father and to experience him as a valuable identification model.

In order to survive, the patient had to choose the only role that her mother allowed her: that of a person without a will, without any independence or autonomy. But the choice she actually finally made is very ambivalent: by becoming anorexic, in fact, she rejects this pseudo-love in a very aggressive manner (Conforto & Maura, 1972).

The authors remark that the therapy they applied was unsuccessful because the dynamics in this family remained unaltered and impenetrable by every attempt at "intrusion." In fact, we have the impression that the grandmother and especially the mother have been scapegoated in their treatment (for example, only the father was allowed to have contact with the hospitalized patient). Meanwhile, it is conceivable that the father (and maybe also the grandfather) had some benefit from the existing situation and that the patient herself was not merely a victim. We think that an attempt to involve all parties concerned (maybe even the paternal grandmother) into the treatment might have given a much better chance for change in this family system.

Case 2

We will now discuss a case from our own clinical practice. We chose this example for several reasons: first, it is a clear illustration of some characteristics described above; second, it describes several practical problems in the management of such difficult cases; third, in contrast with the experience of Boszormenyi-Nagy and Spark (1984), we do not have the impression that the grandparents are always so willing or even eager to join the family therapy sessions; in the following case, we noted a subtle but strong resistance on their part.

Peggy was 14 years old at her first admission to our hospital because of severe anorexia nervosa problems with a marked emaciation (from 60 kg to 37 kg for 1m61), vomiting, amenorrhea, abuse of laxatives, hyperactivity and a complete social isolation. When Peggy was 11 years old, the family life was totally disrupted by the sudden death of her father due to a heart attack. He was a 42-year-old manager who was running the company owned by the family, together with his brother-in-law (his only sister's husband). His wife was at that time 38 years old and left her job as a teacher to become involved in the family business. Peggy herself reacted very coolly to her father's death, despite the fact that she was his favorite child (she has a brother Sven who is 3 years younger than she is). Her mother was in mourning and developed a very strong emotional tie with Peggy, with whom she discussed all her personal problems. But that mourning stopped at once when her own mother (patient's grandmother) told her — for an unkown reason — that she knew that her late husband was adulterous and regularly visited prostitutes. Now Peggy's mother began to go out and met her actual partner, Francis, a 38-year-old divorced employee of a rival company. Almost a year after their first contact, he came to live in with the family in mother's villa. That is the time the anorexia nervosa problems emerged: neither Sven nor Peggy could accept his arrival in the family. Especially Peggy manipulated and blackmailed her mother and became so unmanageable that the latter — completely at her wit's end — decided to send her to a boarding school, where she ran away after a few days. When her mother welcomed her back home, the situation got out of hand very quickly and became complete chaos. Peggy's mother was not capable of managing either her household or her position in the company (where her brother-in-law took serious advantage of the situation, a fact the mother realized only much later). In the meantime, Francis, mother's friend, was not accepted by her family because of the business circumstance, and he seemed to withhold himself from becoming involved in the entire situation.

During the treatment, Peggy continued to be the "naughty child" and refused to engage herself in any therapy. The family therapy sessions were focused upon building up a joint authority of both parental figures and on introducing some basic rules at home. But these attempts were soon and unexpectedly interrupted when mother *together with the grandmother* came to tell us that they wanted to take Peggy home and stop the treatment. Six months later, the mother called us. She was very upset and asked for a new hospitalization because Peggy was in an even more critical somatic condition than the first time (33 kg and a serious hypokalemia). We agreed to a second admission on the condition that the grandparents (mothers' parents) would join the family sessions, since apparently the grandmother played an important role in the crucial instance of breaking off the previous treatment. They all agreed and, in the beginning, Peggy showed a positive evolution.

In the three-generational family sessions (without mother's friend), we noticed that the grandmother completely dominated her daughter (Peggy's mother), who behaved very obediently and passively, agreeing with all of her mother's statements. The grandfather just sat there, letting his wife control the situation. When a problematic issue was discussed, grandmother let us know that her husband was a cardiac who could not stand any tension ("His heart, you know!"). After a month, Peggy's mother told us that her parents had left for a vacation of six months in Spain. Because they had not announced this, and since our inpatient treatment has a maximum time limit of six months, we considered this as an ultimate escape on the part of the grandparents. But, at the same time, we felt this was a good opportunity to strengthen mother's position in the absence of her parents. We therefore started an individual therapy in order to work through her own separation problems regarding her mother. Meanwhile, the nuclear family was seen together to build up a joint parental authority. This goal, however, was seriously hampered by the mother's ambivalent relationship with Francis who kept playing the role of an outsider. Though Peggy's condition evolved in such a way that she could be discharged from the hospital, she continued trying to profit from this unstable parental dyad. Therefore, we decided, in agreement with mother and Francis, that Peggy would return to the boarding school. She did so, but after a month — at the moment the grandparents returned from their holidays! — she ran away and mother kept her at home against our advice. In the meantime, Peggy also lost weight again (probably also started binge eating and vomiting) and broke off the outpatient group therapy, another maneuver the mother seemed to accept, so-called, against her will! So, apparently, we are back again in the chaotic situation and treatment impasse from which we started one year before.

A Transgenerational View on Anorexia Nervosa

In our opinion, the heart of the matter in transgenerational issues deals with the acquiring of autonomy, the balancing of old roles or loyalties and new relationships (Boszormenyi-Nagy & Spark, 1984), the working through of one's "roots" while developing at the same time one's own "wings" (Sperling, 1985). The clinical impressions reported in the literature, our own clinical experience as well as the findings from our explorative study (see Chapter 7), all point to the same direction: the detachment process of the parents is reflected in the detachment process of the anorexic child.

As a synthesis of the different sources we utilized, we can build up an hypothesis about the family structure of three generations which, among other factors, contributed to the development or maintenance of an eating disorder in one member of the third generation. We want to emphasize that this is only a speculative exploration, based upon assumptions that have to be investigated in a more systematic manner. An important issue here is the question of whether characteristics are significantly more pronounced in the families of anorexia nervosa patients than in the general population. But as we noted in Chapter 7, the transgenerational perspective certainly merits further (ideally longitudinal) research. The following considerations may inspire this type of investigation.

The grandmothers (most often the maternal!) of anorexics are described as dominating women, married to "missing" men whose absence might appear to be psychological (e.g., by illness, alcoholism) or on the reality level (due to death, divorce, regular separation). Those grandmothers are generally very involved onto their daughters, the mothers of anorexics who themselves are described as passive, dependent or dominating women, married to a man with a striking resemblance with their absent fathers.

It is possible that, just because of this absence of the males over several generations, the grandmothers and the mothers transmit their specific reality construction to their children in general and *their image of what it means to be a woman* to their daughters in particular. In the literature, we find contradictory statements about the transgenerational role expectations for women in anorexia nervosa families. White (1983) states that the women are expected to be sensitive, devoted and self-sacrificing, i.e., the traditional (rather extreme) female role. On the other hand, Slade (1984) and Sperling and Massing (1972) stress the importance of an achievement ideology in these families. According to Slade (1984), it is based upon their life histories: socio-economic circumstances have forced the women into a survival culture, whereas Sperling and Massing (1972) related it to their anxiety about sexuality. The males (grandfathers, fathers), then, are supposed to be unable to exert a corrective influence on this feminine image because of their own (pathological) insecurity or because they may profit from it (or perhaps both).

The result of these transgenerational introjects is that the adolescent daughter of the actual generation is hampered in her development of autonomy this legacy of cognitions and by the processes families use to make their members conform to their ideas. When the youngster starts dieting (for whatever reason), she may then discover — without being fully aware of it — the counter-controlling power of self-starvation which allows her to obtain a certain (though pseudo-) autonomy without violating the rules of loyalty, since as a sick girl she must be taken care of by the family. Moreover, the self-starvation is an unusually exacting performance and as such a caricature of — and thus also a protest against — the achievement ideology in the family. The anorexic stance is the acme of loyal stubbornness or submissive revolt, a subtle but influential form of passive aggression the patient's mother possibly had dreamed of without daring to put it into practice against her own mother. This might explain the anorexic's mother's mixture of feelings — admiration, anger, helplessness — resulting in an inconsistent reaction toward her daughter. But this attitude, in turn, reinforces the anorexic behavior etc.

Treatment Considerations

The implications of the aforementioned ideas regarding therapy are rather scarce in the literature. Several authors stress the importance for the therapist to adopt a transgenerational viewpoint when gathering information about the family history. White (1983) calls it "the construction of a genogram" that will help the therapist focusing on transgenerational material in the therapy. In a similar way, Kramer (1985) states that the therapist has to pay specific attention to the *transgenerational diagram* of the family.

> The process of diagramming is a mutual exploration of transgenerational issues, giving the therapist an opportunity to highlight interfacing parallels easily missed in verbal history-taking. Children may know very little about their family history and often enjoy the process. When a child is the identified patient (as it is the case with anorexia nervosa), diagramming shifts the focus to the parents and their view of the larger

system, often providing clues as to how one specific child has been identified as special. Such a child may feel relief as the parent focuses on unresolved family of origin issues, easing the downward pressure.
(Kramer, 1985, p. 34)

A next stage in therapy is to invite (or, in some cases such as the one we describe, to suggest that) the grandparents to join some or all family sessions. The
observation of the way in which the grandparents interact with their grandchil-
dren (the patient) and children (the patient's parents) can reveal important information to the therapist. Boszormeyi-Nagy and Spark (1984) present some
techniques and comments regarding the *inclusion of grandparent(s) in the treatment.* They state it is important for therapists to glean the principles of credit-
debit accounting (cf. loyalties) between the generations. This may consist of a.o.
the (re)clarification and modification of certain fixed attitudes, but the most important goal is the modification of the behavior itself. With respect to the anorexia nervosa condition, White (1983) states that the major goal in treatment is
to help the family members, and especially the anorexic patient, to leave the role
of "victim of tradition." The therapist has to challenge the constraining influence of the family's rigid system of implicit beliefs. Because direct attempts
to contest such beliefs tend to intensify their constraining nature, such a challenge should preferably be indirect.

As a final remark, we would like to warn against the possible pitfall that
adopting a transgenerational viewpoint in a narrow-minded way may convey the
wrong message that grandparents are the real cause of the problem. This would
mean that the scapegoat role is shifted to the grandparental generation (in particular, from mother to grandmother). Needless to say that such an attitude on
the part of the therapist would induce unjustified guilt feelings and undermine
the treatment itself. As soon as a courtroom atmosphere slips into the therapeutic approach, treatment is doomed to fail.

CONCLUSION

We propose a widened perspective in the family approach to eating disorders,
especially a transgenerational view on these problems. The issue of finding a
way out of the attachment-autonomy or loyalty-individuation conflicts goes beyond the classical two-generational viewpoint. The attention paid to these transgenerational issues is relatively recent, and we must be aware that changes in
theoretical orientations are not yet readily transmitted into therapeutic practice or systematic research. The cases of chronic eating disorders in adults or
broken-home situations often force us to place the anorexia or bulimia against
the background of family dynamics, regardless of the generation which is placed
in the therapist's focus.

REFERENCES

Andrews, T.J. & Irwin, M. (1985), Anorexia nervosa: The role of divorce. *BASH Newsletter*, 4(7):9-10.

Bowen, M. (1976), An interview with Murray Bowen (by David Berenson). *The Family*, 3:50-62. Reprinted in: Bowen, M., *Family Therapy in Clinical Practice*. New York: Jason Aronson, 1978, pp. 389-411.

Boszormenyi-Nagy, I. & Spark, G. (1984), *Invisible Loyalties. Reciprocity in Intergenerational Family Therapy*. New York: Brunner/Mazel (original edition: Harper & Row, 1973).

Bruch, H. (1973), *Eating Disorders. Obesity, Anorexia Nervosa, and the Person within*. New York: Basic Books.

Conforto, C. & Maura, E. (1972), Dinamiche familiari in un caso di "anorexia mentale" (Family dynamics in a case of anorexia nervosa). *Rivista Sperimentale di Freniatria*, 96:143-152.

Conrad, D.E. (1977), A starving family: An interactional view of anorexia nervosa. *Bulletin of the Menninger Clinic*, 41:487-495.

Frey, J. (1984), A family systems approach to illness maintaining behaviors in chronically ill adolescents. *Family Process*, 23:251-260.

Hall, A. (1982), Deciding to stay an anorectic. *Postgraduate Medical Journal*, 58:641-647.

Hsu, L.H.G. & Lieberman, S. (1982), Paradoxical intention in the treatment of chronic anorexia nervosa. *American Journal of Psychiatry*, 139:650-653.

Kesmet, J.K. & Mirkin, M.P. (1985), Troubled adolescents in divorced and remarried families. In: Mirkin, M.P. & Koman, S.L. (Eds.), *Handbook of Adolescents and Family Therapy*. New York: Guilford Press, pp. 273-293.

Kramer, J.R. (1985), *Family Interfaces: Transgenerational Patterns*. New York: Brunner/Mazel.

Morawetz, A. & Walker, G. (1984), *Brief Therapy with Single-Parent Families*. New York: Brunner/Mazel.

Sargent, J. & Liebman, L. (1985), Eating disorders. In: Henao, S. & Grose, N.P. (Eds.), *Principles of Family Systems in Family Medicine*. New York: Brunner/Mazel, pp. 213-242.

Schneider, S. (1981), Anorexia nervosa: The "subtle" condition. *Family Therapy*, 8:49-54.

Sperling, E. (1985), Der Mehrgenerationenaspekt in der Familiendynamik (The multigenerational aspect in family dynamics). In: Ermann, M. & Seifert, T. (Eds.), *Die Familie in der Psychotherapie. Theoretische und Praktische Aspekte aus Tiefenpsychologischer und Systemtheoretischer Sicht*. Berlin: Springer-Verlag.

Sperling, E. & Massing, A. (1972), Besonderheiten in der Behandlung der Magersuchtfamilie (Particularities in the treatment of the anorexia nervosa family). *Psyche*, 26:357-369.

Sperling, E., Massing, A., Georgi, H., Reich, G. & Wöbbe-Mönks, E. (1982), *Die Mehrgenerationen-Familientherapie* (The Multigenerational Family Therapy). Gottingen: Vandenhoeck & Ruprecht.

Taipale, V., Tuomi, O. & Aukee, M. (1971), Anorexia nervosa: An illness of two generations? *Acta Paedopsychiatrica*, 38:21-25.

Tseng, W.S. & McDermott, J.F. (1979), Triaxial family classification: A proposal. *Journal of Child Psychiatry*, 18:22-43.

Vandereycken, W. (1988). Anorexia nervosa in adults. In: Blinder, B.J. et al. (Eds.), *The Eating Disorders. Diagnosis, Treatment, Research*. New York: PMA Publishing Corp.

Van der Hart, D. (1983), *Rituals in Psychotherapy. Transition and Continuity*. New York: Irvington.

White, M. (1983), Anorexia nervosa: A transgenerational system perspective. *Family Process*, 22:255-273.

Chapter 17

Eating Disorders in Married Patients: Theory and Therapy

Stephan Van den Broucke and Walter Vandereycken

INTRODUCTION

While the vast majority of eating disorder patients are adolescents who are not married, eating disorders may also be observed in married subjects. In fact, as the average age at onset in the patient population appears to be gradually increasing (Garfinkel & Garner, 1982), the number of married women treated for anorexia nervosa or bulimia has increased progressively over the last decade (Dally, 1984). In spite of their growing importance, however, research with reference to this patient group has thus far remained very scarce. More specifically, the connection between eating disorders and marital relations has grossly been neglected in the literature. Marriage is a basic social institution which to a great extent determines the lifestyle and health of an individual, but as far as we know, no researcher or clinician has systematically addressed the following questions: What is the impact of the disorder on the relationship between the patient and her spouse? What is the role of the relationship in the development and/or maintenance of the disorder? The limited information that is available about this issue is mostly based on single case reports and on impressionistic observations, rather than on systematic assessment and methodologically sound research.

The present chapter is intended to provide specific information regarding this patient group, particularly regarding the characteristics of their marital relationship. First, we will document the incidence, the clinical features and the prognosis for married patients as inferred from case descriptions reported in the literature. Current theories, based on clinical impressions, about the marital relationship of these patients will then be discussed briefly. These views are substantiated by the findings of recent surveys which cast some light on the specificity of this patient group and on aspects of their marital relationship. Finally, some information is provided with regard to the therapeutic approach to these patients and their spouses.

INCIDENCE, CLINICAL FEATURES, AND PROGNOSIS

The precise percentage of married subjects among the population of eating disorder patients is unknown, and even a rough estimate is difficult to make. While most clinicians acknowledge that the number of married women seeking treatment for anorexia nervosa or bulimia is increasing, no prevalence studies of these disorders according to marital status have yet been reported to confirm this intuitive impression.

In our own sample, which is described elsewhere (Vandereycken & Pierloot, 1983), the average number of married cases among the hospitalized anorexia nervosa patients has increased significantly since 1979 (33% at one point). Yet at the same time there was also an increase of the average age of our patients, as well as a tendency toward more complicated eating disorders, i.e., bulimia with vomiting/purging (Vandereycken, 1988). Thus, it is conceivable that the prevalence of married eating disorder patients is contaminated by other factors such as age, chronicity or type of the disorder. For example, Garfinkel and Garner's (1982) series of 193 patients contained 33 married ones, or 17% of their subjects. Their sample, however, was one made up rather chronically ill patients, and may therefore give an inaccurate estimation of the actual share of married patients in the population. On the other hand, chronic illness itself often goes unnoticed in married patients (Hall, 1982), so the percentage of married women in the subpopulation of chronic patients may in fact be much greater than these figures suggest.

Marriage also appears to be more common among bulimic patients than among abstainers. Huon's (1985) group of bulimia patients contained 15% married subjects and 4% divorced or separated ones. In Garfinkel and Garner's sample, the ratio of married patients in the bulimic group to the abstaining patient group is almost two to one (22.7% bulimics versus 11.5% abstainers). This is in accordance with the finding by Beumont et al. (1976) that all the vomiters/purgers in their series had regular boyfriends, compared with 53% of the abstainers. As to the age factor, Dally and Gomez (1979, p. 136) reported that 40% of their older patients, who developed the disorder at 19 years or later, were married. The same authors also state that women with anorexia tardive (or late-onset anorexia nervosa) are almost invariably married (Dally & Gomez, 1979, p. 155). In view of these observations, an estimation of the global incidence of eating disorders in married patients based on their prevalence in research groups seems unwarranted.

A similar problem arises with regard to the clinical characteristics of the disorder as presented by married patients. Since most information is based on descriptive case reports, general conclusions about their clinical features must be regarded as tentative. In the more than 60 case reports of married eating disorder patients which we traced in the literature, the presenting age varied from as young as 22 years to 60 years and older. The same applies to the age of onset and the duration of the illness. Elkaim (1979) has described a woman who became anorexic at the age of 15, and whose weight problems continued for over 30 years, lasting through most of her married life. Several other authors (Brusset, 1977; Maillot et al., 1979; Vecht-van den Bergh, 1979; Oyewumi, 1981) have also reported cases of middle-aged married women with anorexia nervosa or bulimia which had developed during their adolescence. In other instances, however, the onset of the disorder is situated later in life, i.e., in middle age or even after the menopause. When occurring at a later age, the eating disorder sometimes represents a relapse into a condition that had previously existed on a subclinical level. Wells (1980), for example, has described a case of a married woman who developed anorexia nervosa following pregnancy at the age of 28, but who had been preoccupied with her weight since the age of nine. A similar case has been reported by Thomas and Harris (1982), who documented the development of anorexia nervosa following termination of pregnancy in a 38-year-old mother of three children, who had experienced an untreated episode of bulimia 18 years before, at the time of her first pregnancy.

Among the factors eliciting the eating disorder in married life, pregnancy or childbirth are not uncommon. Several authors, including Dally and Gomez (1979), Wells (1980) and Jonas et al. (1984) have documented such cases. Evidently, the changing body image or the typical cravings for food during pregnancy may induce a fear of losing control of the self-regulation of food intake and weight (Vandereycken, 1982). Also, the fear of future pregnancies or the resentment that "the child has taken something from me," i.e., the husband's attention, may be present. Other factors which have been mentioned as provoking the disorder include marital conflicts, discovering an extramarital affair of the husband, the growing up of teen-aged children, and retirement. In the few cases of anorexia nervosa in married males reported in the literature, an unsuccessful marriage (Palmer, 1980) and detachment from the parental home (Kwee & Duivenvoorden, 1985) seemed to have triggered the disorder.

In general, the eating disorder symptoms manifested by married anorexia nervosa patients (emaciation, severe weight loss and amenorrhea) are identical to those observed in adolescents. Although these symptoms are often more serious, they may last for a long period of time without being noticed. Amenorrhea, for instance, may be masked by the use of oral contraceptives (Elkaim, 1979). Behavioral features associated with anorexia nervosa, such as dieting, secreting food, gorging and self-induced vomiting, laxative abuse and hyperactivity, are also often found. For example, the well-known case described by Kellet et al. (1976) concerned a 54-year-old woman who was referred to the hospital with a three-year history of increasing weight loss totalling 17 kg (or 35% of her ideal weight), avoidance of carbohydrates, and the use of "slimming" tablets and purgatives. She had been seen to make herself vomit, and experienced her body as being too fat. Levitan (1978) mentioned that his 40-year-old married patient evidenced a grossly inaccurate conception of her body image. The latter feature was also reported by other authors (Vecht-van den Bergh, 1979; Thomas & Harris, 1982, Böning, 1984).

Well-documented case reports of married bulimia (nervosa) patients have been given by Madanes (1981), Jonas et al. (1984), Haley (1984), and Andersen (1985). As in adolescent bulimics, these patients' weight losses were less dramatic, whereas binge eating accompanied by frequent vomiting were the most prevalent behavioral characteristics.

It is probable that the occurrence of an eating disorder in a married woman is associated with a poor outcome. Seidensticker and Tzagouris (1968) and Crisp (1977) have mentioned marriage among the factors affecting the outcome. Hsu et al. (1979) state that being married while ill with anorexia nervosa is associated with a poor prognosis, although they presume that this may also be related to the later age of onset in this group. Although in some instances, successful clinical remission has been attained in married anorexics (Crisp et al., 1977; Fishman, 1979; Oyewumi, 1981), or in bulimic patients (Madanes, 1981; Jonas et al., 1984), the course of the illness in these patients often becomes chronic, or may show frequent and severe relapses.

CLINICAL CONSIDERATIONS ABOUT THE MARITAL RELATION

Married anorexia nervosa patients naturally divide into two groups: those whose illness was present at the time of their marriage and those whose eating or weight problems occurred afterward. Drawing from their own clinical experience, several authors have accordingly identified different types of relationships in these couples.

If a patient was already anorexic before she married, the marriage is embedded in the strong neurotic needs of both partners, and the existence of the eating disorder is crucial to the stability of the relationship. As Crisp (1980, p. 81) puts it, "a man who marries an anorectic is marrying...someone who presumably meets his own needs for a barren and usually nonexistent sexual relationship, and who may be concerned primarily in feeding him up." In a similar vein, Andersen (1985, p. 142) states that a patient "may marry a man whom she would not marry if she were not ill, because she feels she doesn't deserve anyone better," while the well spouse may marry an anorexic patient "to fulfil his fantasies of helping or rescuing her." At first, such a relationship may have a mutually sustaining aspect, but it usually becomes increasingly unsatisfactory for both partners. When the illness persists, the initial willingness of the husband to improve his spouse may over time lead to a sense of failure, and subsequently to separation or divorce. Sometimes the development of a marital conflict represents the incentive for seeking treatment. In other instances, however, the stabilizing effect of the illness on the marital relationship results in an opposition to treatment on the part of the husband.

When anorexia nervosa occurs after the marriage, it often represents a recurrence of a previous episode that had taken place before the marriage (Andersen, 1985), or it is rooted in unresolved adolescent developmental conflicts. According to Dally and Gomez (1979), these patients have transferred their adolescent conflicts and problems onto their husbands. They expect their spouses, who are often sexually immature themselves, to be strong, protective, understanding, loving and undemanding partners. Any discordant event affecting the functioning of the marital unit, such as a marital crisis, pregnancy, the birth of a child or social or professional pressure, may then trigger the disorder. Unable to communicate their true feelings to their husbands, the patients-to-be retreat to starvation and emaciation in order to protect themselves and their marital status. Fishman (1979) has pointed out that the anorexic symptoms thus serve a homeostatic purpose for the functioning of the marital unit. An eloquent example of how the symptoms may foster an extreme collusion between the spouses has been provided by Love et al. (1971). When the medical team planned to inspect the feces of one anorexia nervosa patient for signs of laxative abuse, the patient managed to smuggle her stools out of the hospital, and convinced her husband to smuggle in his own feces in order to replace hers!

In addition to the dynamics mentioned above, the themes pervading the marital relationship of a bulimic patient and her spouse are secrecy and power. Andersen (1985) states that most bulimics feel guilty about their practice and persistently try to hide the bingeing and purging from their partners. According to Hall (1982), the most chronic cases of bulimia may occur in married women who seem otherwise well adjusted and keep their secret from their husbands. Similarly, Boskind-White and White (1983, p. 117) report that "unbelievable as it may seem, bulimarexics have managed to keep their behavior a total secret from husbands and other loved ones for as long as ten to fifteen years." When the eating problems are finally revealed, the husband may at first feel relieved, as a "food problem" seems rather insignificant as compared with what he may have suspected, e.g., an extramarital affair. However, as the symptoms remain present, bewilderment, suspicion and anger gradually take over. At this stage, the balance of power in the marriage is strongly influenced by the disorder. While the vomiting increases the patient's weakness in relation to her husband, it may simultaneously give her power over her spouse, who cannot control the vomiting (Madanes, 1981).

It is evident that the findings thus far reported may not be generalized across all married anorexia nervosa and bulimia patients, as they are based on clinical observations of limited numbers of patients. We will now report the findings of the few recent studies in which the connection between the eating disorder and the marital relationship was investigated more systematically.

SYSTEMATIC INVESTIGATION OF THE MARITAL RELATION

Lafeber (1981) has investigated the connection between the course of anorexia nervosa and the relationship with a partner in 60 patients, 23 of whom were married. Her findings indicate that a recovery from the disorder often triggers a relational crisis: in two thirds of the cases where treatment had been reasonably successful, relational problems occurred afterward. These crises typically reflected the patients' fear of psychological and physical maturity, and could further be subdivided into (1) problems associated with sexual intercourse, birth control, pregnancy, childbirth, motherhood, etc.; (2) problems resulting from delayed oedipal conflicts, involving an inability to combine nonerotic feelings of respect and erotic love for the husband (substituting for the father); and (3) problems arising when the patient's newly developed interests and personality collide with those of the spouse. In addition, it was pointed out that recovery from anorexia nervosa is very unlikely if the spouse himself evidences a clear psychological disturbance. In such cases, the patient's improvement is thwarted by the spouse, for whom the physical and mental health of the patient appears to be intolerable.

In order to study the part played by the husband and the patient in late-onset anorexia nervosa, Dally (1984) has conducted a survey of the backgrounds and personalities of 50 married anorexics and their spouses. His patients were divided into four groups: (1) those who developed anorexia nervosa during the engagement period leading up to marriage; (2) those who developed the disorder during marriage but before any pregnancy; (3) those who developed it within three years of childbirth; and (4) those who developed the disorder at or after the menopause. His findings suggest that, in the first three groups, anorexia nervosa developed as a maladaptive solution to a growing marital crisis in women who had not successfully coped with the developmental conflicts of adolescence. When the eating disorder began during engagement or during marriage before pregnancy it typically represented a reaction to a growing disappointment and anxiety with the marital relationship after the initial "childlike closeness" between the partners had been abandoned. When the disorder developed following childbirth, it reflected the patient's fear of the responsibility of being a good mother and her resentment of a marital bond in which mutual understanding and warmth were missing. In postmenopausal patients, on the other hand, the syndrome appeared to be secondary to a depression. Here, the anorexia usually arose in response to an actual or threatened loss (e.g., death or illness of the husband, marriage or children) in a setting of long-standing tension and dissatisfaction, while the desire for thinness was less apparent. So, whereas adolescent anorexia nervosa and the condition occurring during the engagement period or during marriage form a continuum, postmenopausal anorexia nervosa may constitute a different entity.

In general, the husbands in this study were immature men whose personality mirrored that of their wives. They doubted their own ability to satisfy and retain the affection of their partners and held unrealistic expectations regarding marriage. Three types of husbands were identified: (1) an emotionally and sexually dependent type who avoids open confrontation with his wife and accepts her illness as a way to secure a mutual dependency; (2) a type who is more capable of growth and change, and who detaches himself from his wife's illness by taking up a relationship with another woman or by putting all his energy into his work; and (3) a type who does not allow his wife to live an independent life and who expects her to be an extension of himself if they are to live in harmony. The latter type is usually considerably older than his wife and may have been married before. According to Dally, the character of the husband is an important prognostic factor, for "the weak, passive man (type 1) invariably establishes a strong neurotic centre to the marriage, which renders the outcome less favorable" (Dally, 1984, p. 427).

Evidently, the findings of this survey to a great extent corroborate the impression that the relationship between an anorexic patient and her husband mostly represents a neurotic bond, which is essential for the development and maintenance of the disorder. It appears, however, that different patterns of relationships must be distinguished according to the type of husband.

Although Lafeber's (1981) and Dally's (1984) findings are based on a relatively large number of patients, and as such, add to the understanding of the role of the marital relation in the development of anorexia nervosa, they are still of a descriptive kind. In order to identify the specific characteristics of the disorder as presented by married subjects, a systematic comparison with a representative group of unmarried patients is necessary. Moreover, quantifiable methods measuring the quality of the relationship must be used in order to investigate its impact.

A comparison of demographic and clinical features in comparable samples of married and single patients is described elsewhere in this volume (see Chapter 10). The results indicate that from the clinical point of view married and single patients are strikingly similar, yet for the married ones the disorder appears to be more serious, has a longer duration and a worse prognosis. Furthermore, despite the tendency of the married patients to be underweight beforehand, the actual onset of the problems is at a comparatively late age. These findings, together with the corroborating results of a cluster analysis, suggest that the relationship with a partner probably influences the onset and/or the course of the eating disorder.

In an attempt to further investigate this connection we performed an exploratory study of the relationship qualities and the interaction structure of ten couples of which one partner had developed an eating disorder (see Chapter 10). The findings indicate that, in general, these couples considered their marriage as satisfactory and that the interaction was predominantly cooperative. A closer inspection of the interaction data, however, revealed a mutual reinforcement of the wife's role as a dependent patient and of the husband's role as protective caretaker, respectively. Furthermore, it could be argued that cooperative interaction only existed on a superficial level, while the partners were unable to communicate about more intimate matters. A similar interdependency and impairment of the intimate communication between the spouses had also been inferred from clinical case studies (see above). However, because no clear hypotheses regarding the latter issue guided our study, further reseach is necessary to substantiate this post hoc consideration.

THERAPEUTIC CONSIDERATIONS

Because most research with reference to the relationship between eating disordered patients and their (marital) partners is relatively recent, it is not surprising that its implications for therapy have remained virtually unexplored. Like the theoretical considerations concerning these patients' marriages, information regarding the treatment of married anorexia nervosa or bulimia patients is mostly based on clinicians' experience with the treatment of isolated cases. Despite these limitations, several authors have offered specific guidelines for treatment, which cover a variety of approaches including concomitant therapy for the spouse as well as marital and sex therapy.

Treatment and subsequent improvement of an eating disorder may severely challenge the marital relationship (Dally & Gomez, 1979; Crisp, 1980; Lafeber, 1981). Some of the most common problems resulting from improvement include: (a) an increased assertiveness on the part of the ill spouse, which threatens the stability of the relationship; (b) a sudden discharge of long-repressed anger by the patient, effecting a counterreaction by the well spouse, who feels unappreciated; (c) expressions of anger by the well spouse, who had previously stored up his feelings out of fear of harming the ill spouse; and (d) demands for separation or divorce by either partner (Andersen, 1985).

In order to curb these effects and to use them for enhancing growth in both partners, a concomitant *support program* for the husband may provide a useful adjunct to the patient's therapy. Such a program may fulfil the husband's need for information and may help him to ventilate his feelings of frustration, guilt, anger, anxiety and isolation. Provided that the marital bond is sufficiently strong and that the well spouse is willing to explore change, this support may take the form of a group program (comparable to the parent-counseling groups described in Chapter 18). An outline of such a program as well as its benefits and limitations have been presented by Leichner et al., (1985).

In other cases, especially those where the illness serves a clear hemostatic role in the marriage, more persuasive approaches are recommended. According to Crisp (1980), it is important to involve the husband, even if he opposes change and if the motivation for therapy is mainly the patient's. In such cases, the husband must be helped to engage in psychotherapy without impairing his self-esteem. Dally and Gomez (1979) suggest that, from the outset, while the therapist explores the problem and develops rapport with the patient, the husband must be interviewed by a co-therapist. Later, joint interviews can be set up with the patient, the spouse and the two therapists, during which the child-like manipulation of each partner by the other is pointed out. The couple is then encouraged to recognize each others needs and to improve their communication of feelings.

Depending on the role the illness serves in the relationship, *marital therapy* may be indicated in addition to the individual inpatient or outpatient program for the ill spouse. Andersen (1985) has listed the principles of marital therapy for anorexic and bulimic patients as follows:

1. The patient should be fully evaluated, especially with regard to her social and marital functioning.
2. The nature of the disorder must be reviewed with the couple from a factual, nonblaming standpoint. Couples are urged not to blame themselves or each other.
3. The couple must be asked what goals they have for treatment, both individually and as a couple. Among the areas that often require treatment are: communication skills, sexual functioning, expectations, behavioral norms, eating patterns and parenting abilities.
4. The couple is urged to see the focus of the treatment as an improvement of the marital relatioshipn rather than as treatment of an identified patient, with a passive stance allowed to the other.
5. Specific goals must be determined, to be achieved over a fixed number of sessions. Ideally, improvement in the individual's treatment program is paralleled by progress in the marital relationship.

The prognosis for marital therapy with eating disorder patients depends on the degree and the stage of the illness, the length of the preceding stable marital relationship and the maturity of the partners. The longer the illness or the more unstable the relationship. and the more immature the partners, the less likely is the chance that improvement of the disorder will also lead to a strengthened marital bond.

As to the contents of the marital therapy, several therapeutic models may be adopted. Beeren (1979) has described the course of marital therapy along *analytic* lines, aimed at providing the couple with insight into the unconscious internal conflicts influencing their relationship. More specifically, the partners' collusive defense systems with regard to eating, sexuality, and passivity/activity, establishing an overcompensatory and a regressive attitude of the husband and the wife, respectively, must be exposed and worked through.

An example of directive *behavioral* marital therapy with a bulimic patient has been provided by Joele (cited in Vandereycken, 1981). Here, the focus of the therapy was the secrecy of the bingeing and purging, and the lack of trust on the side of the husband. The patient was accordingly instructed to monitor the frequency of her bingeing and to vomit only twice each day, at designated times, and in the presence of her spouse. The husband's controlling behavior was re-labeled as an exaggerated form of concern, which reinforced his wife's lying about her symptoms. Consequently, a behavioral contract was drawn up, through which the husband was forbidden to ask questions about his wife's eating behavior, provided that she would tell him about it spontaneously. This procedure resulted in a quick extinction of the symptoms and in an improvement of this couple's relationship.

A *directive-strategic* therapeutic approach involving both partners has also been advocated by Haley (1984). In an illustrative case report of a married bulimic patient, the author describes how, during the initial sessions, the couple's cooperativeness was tested by way of demanding their compliance with minor tasks. For instance, the husband was instructed to weigh his wife on a daily basis without telling her how much she weighted, and to keep a log of how many times each day she vomited. In addition, the consequences of the wife's recovery for both partners were elaborately discussed. Once their commitment to the therapy had been fully established, an "ordeal" was set up and introduced as a guaranteed cure. Each time the patient vomited, both partners were to pay a rapidly increasing amount of money to the therapist, the idea being that the couple thus had to comply with a task that was far worse than the symptom itself. As predicted, the symptoms quickly disappeared. A similar strategy has been followed successfully by Madanes (1981). In this case, the couple was instructed to throw away food every time the wife felt the urge to vomit. Thus, a substitute behavior was created, which, like the vomiting (but without its determinental effects), provided the wife with a means to restore the equilibrium of power in the relationship with her husband.

Finally, since sexuality proves to be one of the key problems in these couples, *sex therapy* is often indicated. Several authors (Crisp et al., 1977; Andersen, 1985) have therefore included a form of specific therapy for sexual dysfunctions in their treatment program for married patients.

CONCLUSIONS

The therapeutic approaches discussed above are for the most part extensions of existing treatment modalities for individuals or families. Evidently, more research is required in order to evaluate their applicability to the treatment of marital units. Furthermore, treatment interventions should ideally link up with research findings concerning the connection between anorexia nervosa or bulimia and the patient's marital relationship. Although the current state of the research with regard to married anorexics does not allow such an approach, the outline presented above does contain a few provisional cues. In the first place, it appears that, irrespective of age, the marital relationship does affect the course of the disorder. This implies that, when treating married patients, attention must be paid to the characteristics of the relationship, including the relationship between the onset of the disorder and the timing of the marriage. Second, the strength of the mutual interdependency of both partners (and thus the prognosis for treatment) seems to vary according to the type of husband concerned. Assessment of the husband's personality and of the communication between the spouses seems a useful step in planning the treatment program. Finally, because the spouses apparently are unable to communicate about intimate matters, they may benefit from communication-skills training as part of the treatment program. This last aspect, however, certainly requires more specific research regarding the interaction between the patients and their spouses. Such research, which should imply the use of direct-observation techniques in order to study the interaction on a microanalytic level, may then substantiate whether these interaction patterns are specific and abnormal, and how they are related to the development and/or the maintenance of the eating disorder.

REFERENCES*

*Andersen, A.E. (1977), Atypical anorexia nervosa. In: Vigersky, R.A. (Ed.), *Anorexia Nervosa.* New York: Raven Press, pp. 655-673.

*Andersen, A.E. (1985), Family therapy and marital therapy of anorexia nervosa and bulimia. In: Andersen, A.E., *Practical Comprehensive Treatment of Anorexia Nervosa and Bulimia.* Baltimore: Johns Hopkins University Press, pp. 135-148, 160-164.

*Beeren, J. (1979), Ervaringen met een partner-relatie-therapie on analytic lines bij een anorexie-patiënte en haar echtgenoot (Experiences with a partner relation therapy on analytic lines with an anorexia nervosa patient and her husband). *Tijdschrift voor Psychiatrie,* 21:489-506.

Beumont, P.J.V., George, G.C.W., & Smart, D.E. (1976), "Dieters" and"vomiters and purgers" in anorexia nervosa. *Psychological Medicine,* 6:617.

*Böning, J. (1983), Psychogene Essstörungen und Anorexie in Senium (Psychological eating disturbances and anorexia in later age). *Praxis der Psychotherapie und Psychosomatik,* 28:170-180.

*Böning, J. (1984) Primäre Spätanorexien. Ueberlegungen zu einer integrativen Psychopathologie (Primary late-onset anorexia nervosa. Considerations of an integrative psychopathology). *Psychotherapie und Medizinische Psychologie,* 34:97-105.

*Boskind-White, M., & White, W.C. (1983), *Bulimarexia: The Binge/Purge Cycle.* New York-London: W.W. Norton & Company, pp. 116-127.

*Brink, T.L. (1979). *Geriatric Psychotherapy,* New York: Human Sciences Press, pp. 130, 170-173.

*Brusset, B. (1977), *L'Assiette et le Miroir. L'Anorexie Mentale de l'Enfant et de l'Adolescent* (The plate and the mirror. Anorexia nervosa in the child and the adolescent). Toulouse: Privat, pp. 151-155.

Crisp, A.H., Kalucy, R.S., Lacey, J.H., & Harding, B. (1977), The long-term prognosis in anorexia nervosa: some factors predictive of outcome. In: Vigersky, R.A. (Ed.), *Anorexia Nervosa.* New York: Raven Press, pp. 55-65.

*Crisp, A.H. (1980), *Anorexia Nervosa: Let Me Be.* London-New York: Academic Press-Grune & Stratton, pp. 71-72.

---

* The references with an asterisk contain one or more case reports on married patients with an eating disorder.

*Dally, P., & Gomez, J. (1979), *Anorexia Nervosa.* London: W. Heinemann Medical Books, pp. 100-101, 153-155.

*Dally, P., & Gomez, J. (1980), *Obesity and Anorexia Nervosa. A Question of Shape.* London-Boston: Faber and Faber.

Dally, P. (1984), Anorexia tardive. Late onset marital anorexia nervosa. *Journal of Psychosomatic Research,* 18:423-428.

*Elkaim, M. (1970), Une approche systémique de quelques cas d'anorexie mentale (A systemic approach to a few cases of anorexia nervosa). *Revue d'Action Sociale,* 2:22-37.

*Fishman, H.C. (1979), Family considerations in liaison psychiatry. A structural family approach to anorexia nervosa in adults. *Psychiatric Clinics of North America,* 2:249-263.

*Florin, I. (1982), Therapie einer bulimischen Anorexie (Therapy of a bulimic anorexic). In: Fiegenbaum, W. (Ed.), *Psychologische Therapie in der Praxis.* Stuttgart: W. Kohlhammer, pp. 11-39.

Garfinkel, P.E., & Garner, D.M. (1982), *Anorexia Nervosa. A Multidimensional Perspective.* New York: Brunner/Mazel.

*Hall, A. (1982), Deciding to stay anorectic. *Postgraduate Medical Journal,* 58:641-647.

*Haley, J. (1984), *Ordeal Therapy. Unusual Ways to Change Behavior.* San Francisco-London: Jossey-Bass, pp. 47-58.

Hsu, L.K.G., Crisp, A.H., & Harding, B. (1979), Outcome of anorexia nervosa. *Lancet,* 1:62-65.

Huon, G.F. (1985), Bulimia: Therapy at a distance. In: Touyz, S.W., & Beumont, P.J.V. (Eds.), *Eating Disorders: Prevalence and Treatment.* Sydney: Williams & Wilkins, pp. 62-65.

*Jonas, J.M., Harrison, G.P., Hudson, J.I., & Satlin, A. (1984), Undiagnosed vomiting in an older woman: Unsuspected bulimia. *American Journal of Psychiatry,* 141:902-903.

*Kellett, J., Trimble, M., & Thorley, A. (1976), Anorexia nervosa after the menopause. *British Journal of Psychiatry,* 128:555-558.

*Kwee, M.G.T., & Duivenvoorden, H.J. (1985), Multimodal residential therapy in two cases of anorexia nervosa (adult body weight phobia). In: Lazarus, A.A. (Ed.), *Casebook of Multimodal Therapy.* New York-London: Guilford Press, pp. 116-138.

*Laboucarié, J., Rascol, A., Karkous,E., Queritet, M.-C. & Philip, B. (1966), L'anorexie mentale: Données résultant d'une experience clinique et thérapeutique de 173 cas (Anorexia nervosa: Data from the clinical and therapeutic experience with 173 cases). *Revue de Médicine de Toulouse,* 2:193-210.

*Lafeber, C. (1971), *Anorexia Nervosa.* Leiden: Stafleu, pp. 79-80.

*Lafeber, C. (1981), Wisselwerking tussen herstel van anorexia nervosa en de partnerrelatie (Interaction between recovery from anorexia nervosa and marital relation). *Tijdschrift voor Psychiatrie,* 23 (Suppl.):97-103.

*Launer, M.S. (1978), Anorexia nervosa in late life. *British Journal of Medical Psychology,* 51:375-377.

Leichner, P., Harper, D., & Johnston, D. (1985), Adjunctive group support for spouses of women with anorexia nervosa and/or bulimia. *International Journal of Eating Disorders,* 4:227-235.

*Levitan, H.L. (1978), Implications from an unusual case of multiple psychosomatic illness. *Psychotherapy and Psychosomatics,* 30:211-215.

*Love, D.R., & Brown, J.J. (1971), An unusual case of self-induced electrolyte depletion. *Gut,* 12:284-290.

*Lützenkirchen, J., & Böning, J. (1976), Anorektisches Syndrom und Depression: Ueberlegungen anlässlich einer Kasuistik (Anorexic syndrome and depression: considerations in the light of a case study). *Schweizer Archiv für Neurochirurgie und Psychiatrie,* 118:175-184.

*MacLeod, S. (1981), *The Art of Starvation.* London-New York: Virago-Schocken Books.

*Madanes, C. (1981), *Strategic Family Therapy.* San Francisco-Washington-London: Jossey-Bass, pp. 39-48.

*Maillot, S., Pras, B., Pelol, J.-Y., François, M., & Porot, M. (1979), Une anorexie mentale à l'âge de la ménopause (Anorexia nervosa at the age of menopause). *Annales Médico-Psychologiques,* 137:519-523.

*Mester, H. (1981), *Die Anorexia Nervosa.* Berlin-Heidelberg-New York: Springer Verlag, pp. 68-83.

*Meyer, B., & Weinroth, L. (1957), Observations on psychological aspects of anorexia nervosa. *Psychosomatic Medicine,* 19:389-398.

*Oyewumi, L.K. (1981), Is anorexia nervosa a disease of all ages? *Psychiatric Journal of the University of Ottawa, 6:39-42.*

*Petzold, E. (1979), *Familienkonfrontationstherapie bei Anorexia Nervosa.* (Family confrontation therapy in anorexia nervosa). Göttingen: Verlag für Medizinische Psychologie im Verlag Vandenhoeck & Ruprecht, pp. 175-179.

*Palmer, R., (1980), *Anorexia Nervosa. A Guide for sufferers and their families.* London: Penguin Books.

Seidensticker, J.F., & Tzagouris, M.G. (1968). Do anorectics get well? Current research and future needs. *American Journal of Psychiatry,* 138:319-323.

*Selvini-Palazzoli, M. (1974), *Self-Starvation. From the Intrapsychic to the Transpersonal Approach to Anorexia Nervosa.* London: Chaucer, pp.119-120.

*Smith, S.M., & Hanson, R. (1972), Failure to thrive and anorexia nervosa. *Postgraduate Medical Journal,* 48:382-384.

*Thomas, C.S., & Harris, B. (1982), Anorexia nervosa following termination of pregnancy. *British Journal of Psychiatry,* 141:428.

*Vandereycken, W. (1981), Eetstoornissen (Eating disorders). In: Orlemans, J. (Ed.), *Handboek voor Gedragstherapie* (Handbook of behavior therapy). Deventer: Van Loghum Slaterus, pp. C4-3, 32-35.

Vandereycken, W. (1982), Uncommon eating/weight disorders related to amenorrhea, infertility and problematic pregnancy. In: Prill, H.J., & Stauber, M. (Eds.), *Advances in Psychosomatic Obstetrics and Gynecology.* Berlin-Heidelberg: Springer-Verlag, pp. 124-128.

Vandereycken, W. (1988), Anorexia nervosa in adults. The influence of age and chronicity on the clinical picture of eating disorders. In: Blinder, B.J., Chaitin, B.F., & Goldstein, M. (Eds.), *The Eating Disorders.* New York: PMA Publications.

Vandereycken, W., & Pierloot, R. (1983), Long-term outcome research in anorexia nervosa. The problem of patient selection and follow-up duration. *International Journal of Eating Disorders,* 2(4):237-242.

*Vecht-van den Bergh, R. (1979), Anorexia nervosa op oudere leeftijd (Anorexia nervosa at older age). *Nederlands Tijdschrift voor Geneeskunde,* 123:105-108.

*Weeda-Mannak, W. (1981), Het belang van vroege herkenning van anorexia nervosa (The importance of early recognition of anorexia nervosa). *Tijdschrift voor Psychiatrie,* 23(Suppl.):5-12.

*Wells, L.A. (1980), Anorexia nervosa: An illness of young adults. *Psychiatric Quarterly,* 52:270-282

Chapter 18

Counseling Groups for Parents of Eating Disorder Patients

Ellie Van Vreckem and Walter Vandereycken

I n the previous chapters we plead for a constructive and flexible attitude toward the families of eating disorder patients. We emphasized repeatedly how important it is to enhance a positive parental involvement in the residential treatment of anorexia/bulimia nervosa patients and to help the parents cope with ambivalent feelings aroused by the problems with their children as well as by the hospitalization itself. Parent-counseling groups have proved to constitute such a valuable alternative to the more traditional approaches that we consider it worthwhile to pay special attention to this method.

SPECIFIC ADVANTAGES

Parent-counseling groups have some advantages above individual contacts with parents (in this text, individual contacts refer to separate sessions with the parent couple or a single parent). Besides the fact that groups are more economical in view of the increasing number of patients, they are in the first place aimed at reducing the feelings of isolation in parents, spouses or other family members. Many of them are convinced that the problems encountered with an anorexic or bulimic relative reflect unique and shameful family circumstances. In the counseling group, they feel a sense of relief when they discover that similar problems exist in other families. Most of them had frustrating experiences with other parents, family members, close friends or acquaintances who seemingly did not understand the situation and indirectly blamed the parents by giving them advice about how to educate their children and how to handle the problem. Few parents felt they were understood and supported by their social network, and now they meet people with the same feelings of guilt and helplessness. Most of them are thoughtful, respectable, and engaging people they can easily identify with.

347

A second important potential of the group situation is a modification of the parental attitude toward the therapists. In individual contacts, their feelings of shame, submission and despair, as well as revolt, ambivalence and jealousy toward the therapists can be very intense. The therapist may be seen as an omnipotent figure (a "super-parent"), or as a rival snatching away their children from them, or as a judge condemning and punishing them for their failures. In the group they feel reassured by the presence of the other parents: the fact they now constitute the majority in front of the therapist(s) makes them considerably less vulnerable (Jeammet, 1984). Individual therapeutic contacts with the parents may fuel sometimes rather problematic attitudes. Doumic (1962), for example, emphasized feelings of rivalry in the mother of an anorexic girl toward a female therapist. Jeammet and Gorge (1980) mentioned two possibly alternating types of parental reactions: (1) idealization of the therapist in case of depressive parents with predominant feelings of culpability and inferiority, and (2) vindictiveness and hostility in case of very sensitive and narcissistically vulnerable parents (especially the fathers would show the latter reaction in the beginning of the therapeutic contact). The counseling group provides an opportunity to make these feelings more tolerable, and to avoid direct and painful confrontations with the therapists, by bringing instead the interactions with other group members to the foreground.

It is both interesting and noteworthy that neither those who work with these groups nor the parents themselves experience the feelings that the very existence of such a parent-counseling group might be viewed as an indirect implication of blame or accusation of the "failing" parents. In fact, most parents feel guilty anyway. No doubt they are quite sensitive about being rejected as a scapegoat (the "bad" parents as cause of the disorder). On the part of the therapists, interventions can now be orientated to the group as a whole and, hence, are less likely to be seen as accusations. In our own group we prefer to introduce a difficult theme in a rather indirect and seemingly didactic way, for example: "In many cases we discovered that anorexia or bulimia means a crisis in the child's maturational process." Such a statement in the group induces various reactions and meanings, often resulting in lively and enriching discussions.

As have other authors (Hauer, Janzing and Zantvoort, 1985), we noticed that parents are more convinced or impregnated by information given in the group than in individual contacts. During and after the group sessions we often see parents illustrating and exchanging our information with each other. We then pay special attention to the right moment for didactic explanations: parents questioning each other about some issues are also open to some information from the therapist regarding that issue.

Last but not least, in individual contacts parents often maintain an asking and waiting stance, or keep focusing on "the illness" (or its evolution) instead of on their own reactions to their children. Sharing the experiences of other parents (spouses or family members), the group members themselves progressively take over more active roles: they give advice, reconstruct past experiences, and gain insight into their own problems, disagreeing or sympathizing with their "fellows" in the group (Jeammet & Gorge, 1980). Defeated, depressive and guilty, but also oppositional and vindictive parents may change into active group members who are gaining self-confidence and self-respect while trying to understand and help others.

The formal characteristics of parent-counseling groups may vary considerably. The group described by Jeammet and co-workers in France (Jeammet et al., 1975; Jeammet & Gorge, 1980), who were the first to report on such procedure for anorexics' parents, meets once every three weeks for an hour and a half; it is an open group of 8 to 15 parents, with mothers outnumbering fathers by two to one. In Canada, Rose and Garfinkel (1980) reported on a group for parents of hospitalized anorexia nervosa patients: ten sets of parents met bi-weekly for 18 months and the sessions lasted for 90 minutes; a successfully treated anorexia nervosa patient was engaged as a volunteer co-therapist.

In our own treatment setting at the University Psychiatric Center in Kortenberg, the second author (W.V.) started in 1977 with a parent counseling group for hospitalized anorexia nervosa patients. From the beginning, the group was structured and intended to provide a supportive, nonjudgmental and educational setting which focused on the shared experience of parenting an anorexic adolescent now admitted to an inpatient treatment program (see Vandereycken & Meermann, 1984). Usually 16 to 30 parents meet every two weeks for one hour. Occasionally other family members, relatives, spouses, friends or acquaintances may attend the meetings. The group is conducted by both of us, the second author (W.V.) being the coordinator and supervisor of the total inpatient treatment without direct involvement or individual contacts with either patients or families, unlike the first author (E.V.V.), who, besides her acting as a co-therapist in the counseling group, is one of the central therapists in the inpatient program. Hence, as a co-therapist couple we may represent the complementary partnership between a more distant observing "father" and a more emotionally involved "mother."

We neither select the group members nor require participation in the parent group as a prerequisite for treatment, but we are persistent in inviting and encouraging the parents to join the group while emphasizing its importance both for them and the hospitalized patient. Moreover, we reinforce participation in the counseling group in a way which proved to be very efficient and rewarding, especially in the beginning of treatment: immediately after each meeting the participants are allowed an extra hour for visiting their hospitalized relative, regardless of the latter's evolution and related privileges (even if no other visits are allowed).

In our setting each parent couple or single parent has additional individual contacts with one of the psychotherapists of our team, in order to work through some themes on a more concrete and personal level, as explained before (see

Chapter 14). Other authors (e.g., Rouam, 1984) appear to confirm our positive experience with combining different forms of therapeutic contacts with parents: they are not only complementary to each other, but also allow flexibility in both the focus (group meetings, individual contacts with parents, family session) and the content (from indirect educational advice to direct therapeutic intervention) of our approach, taking into account the needs and capacities of each family.

DIFFERENT GOALS

With regard to the aims and goals of parent groups, we found in the literature different forms of parent groups according to the therapeutic model the authors worked with. Jeammet and co-workers (Jeammet et al., 1971; Jeammet & Gorge, 1980; Jeammet, 1984) describe psychoanalytically oriented groups for parents of hospitalized anorexia nervosa patients. Their groups are aimed predominantly at helping parents to *facilitate the separation-individuation process* of their children. They certainly are not considered as personal psychotherapy for the parents but rather as a type of indirect family therapy, insofar as they attempt to improve the functioning of the whole family system. Without being physically present in the group, patients are strongly alive in the feelings and thoughts of their parents. In contrast with individual fámily sessions together with all the children, parents usually express in the groups, spontaneously and freely, their — often narcissistic — fantasies about their children. And this is the very material Jeammet intends to work with. Parents must first learn to express their feelings and ideas about their ideal parental role in comparison with the ideals of their own parents, and then to express their transferential emotions, especially the ones involving conflict, toward the therapists. The experience that criticism is allowed and accepted by therapists, but handled within certain limits, is fundamental for therapeutic groups. Parents may learn that criticism does not destroy relationships in the group and that defense mechanisms can be reduced without feeling threatened.

Jeammet and Gorge (1980) describe the last phase in the parent group as the emergence of reminiscences of one's own youth. The therapists attempt to raise the parents' feelings of attachment to — but also disillusionment with — their own parents. Working through these feelings, parent groups can finally stimulate the process of differentiation between parents and children. Therefore, problems of the children must be separated from those of the parents (Jeammet & Gorge, 1980).

Within the same psychoanalytic frame of reference, Rouam (1984) points out that parents themselves have to determine the level of their engagement in the group. This implies that the therapists have to take seriously into account the psychological capacities and limitations of each parent couple before starting a transferential process. Some couples are not prepared for it. Probably in order to avoid strong transferential processes, most authors do not want to use the parent group as an intensively therapeutic instrument, but rather limit its goals to the level of parent counseling: it combines then a mixture of supportive, didactic and exploration, insight-oriented elements. The parent-counseling group of Rose and Garfinkel (1980) was composed of parents who were considerated not suitable for family therapy but who were in search of support and help for the education of their child. Evaluating the group, the therapists had the impression that insight about family dynamics was rather poor and infrequent. This can be attributed, according to the authors, to a cautious approach of the group leaders and to the open structure of the group (regular addition of new members).

Though Rossman and Freedman (1982) worked with parents of hospitalized disturbed adolescents, their findings do not differ essentially from our experiences with parents of eating disorder patients. They structured their group to provide a *task-oriented, supportive and educational* setting. Many interventions by the group leaders are designed to minimize the level of anxiety in the group. Parents are not encouraged to express feelings related to personal past experiences. The expression of anger is actively discouraged in the group. The group leaders assume the position that the parents must relinquish their understandable wishes to find someone or something to blame for previous family predicaments. Moreover, the expression of ambivalent feelings concerning the marital relationship is redirected toward conjoint marital sessions.

In the same sense, Lewis and MacGuire (1985) advise individual marital therapy at the very moment parents are able to move toward looking at common problems reflected in the other parents, and to use this observation in order to gain insight into some of their own family dynamics. Mostly, however, parents see the child's illness as contributing (in a linear-causal sense) to their marital difficulties, with the rift between them widening as their daughter demanded more and more attention. It may require, then, a positive working alliance and nonthreatening atmosphere in the group, before therapists can help parents to realize that the illness may have served the purpose of uniting both of them through their shared anxiety over their child (Lewis & MacGuire, 1985).

We experience in our group that parents are able to gain further insight in their own functioning throughout the group process, but we do not intend to go as far as Jeammet and Gorge (1980), who directly analyze personal matters such as the parents' past and their relation with the grandparents. We prefer to focus on these issues in separate family or couple sessions. We emphasize in our group a *future-oriented and reeducative* attitude. Because we know that mothers and fathers usually have not created a good balance in their mutual care about their child—the mothers being often overinvolved and the fathers at too great an emotional distance, or vice versa—we insist upon the presence of both parents in our group to create a new equilibrium in their future education, without paying too much attention to past "errors."

As mentioned in Chapter 14, we insist upon establishing an "adequate joint authority" in the education of the children. We pay much attention to the role of the father and his importance for his daughter, with whom he seems to avoid an overtly emotional contact (Verbeek & Verbeek, 1977). Fathers are encouraged in our group to intervene more directly, to make closer contact and to accept conflicts with their daughters in order to learn to set and maintain limits. The fathers' participation in the counseling group is a clear sign of their involvement and it is, practically always, much appreciated by their daughters as well as by their wives (see also Jeammet and Gorge, 1980).

We address ourselves to the parents (or spouses or relatives) as *co-therapists:* we ask their explicit cooperation and support (e.g., by respecting the therapeutic contract) in order to guarantee, reinforce and consolidate the impact of the treatment. We insist upon their co-responsibility in the treatment and, thus, indirectly in the separation-individuation process of their daughters. In the counseling group, we reinforce the co-therapist role of the parents by sharing information regarding the treatment program (see also Appendix of Chapter 13) and by didactic explanations of common family problems (e.g., the "empty nest" syndrome) and possible meanings of anorexic or bulimic behavior. Time and again we emphasize our need to be supported and trusted by the patients' family.

A final remark regarding a formal aspect of the counseling groups. In the case of married patients we invite the spouses to attend the group. But, though their need for support and information is similar to the parents', their relationship with the patient is a different one and may certainly not be addressed as a parent-child interaction (though it frequently looks like this!). The major advantage of mixing up parents and spouses (or boyfriends) in the same group is that the latter can point out the marital difficulties arising from the patients' continuing dependence on their parents. A husband provoked a deep silence in one of our group sessions when he described how the past and actual spoiling of his wife by her parents resulted in her suppression of even the slightest frustration, which she apparently released through extremely frequent bulimia and subsequent vomiting, a behavior he had to keep secret from her parents on her request! Having spouses and their parents-in-law meet each other in the counseling group is a difficult situation for both of them. Spouses are most of the time silent, as if they were tangled between two fires: their wife and her parents, and now even the hospital staff too. Furthermore, while parents have to work through a separation process, spouses have to find a new equilibrium in a relationship based on equality. For these reasons and since the number of married eating disorder patients is steadily increasing, we prefer to form a *separate group for spouses* (or partners living together with the patient), as has been described by Leichner et al. (1985). Though the patients' marriage requires specific attention (see Chapter 17), one must keep in mind that their emotional ties with their parents most often remain very strong (see Vanderlinden & Vandereycken,

1984) so that involvement of the parents still may be a crucial element in the treatment process.

GROUP THEMES

Looking over our long experience with parent-counseling groups, we encountered several recurring themes, many of which are also reported by other authors. We highlight the most important ones.

Guilt, Anger, and Frustration

We noticed in our group an initial cathartic stage in which parents tell of their experiences living with an anorexic or bulimic daughter. They compare their difficulties and discuss the similarities and differences of the patient's past and current behavior. Most parents come to the group feeling primarily bewilderment and dismay. They express their despair and anger over their frustration in coping with their problematic child. Very often they ventilate an understandable indignation regarding a general practitioner who completely denied or minimized the problem, or an internist who just pumped in some weight by tube feeding. Many parents initially derive support from sharing these common problems (Rose & Garfinkel, 1980). With regard to the ever-recurring question about the "cause" of the eating disorder, we immediately translate this issue into the real question: "Are we guilty?" We then attempt to relieve guilt feelings, first and foremost, by encouraging them to verbalize their feelings of demoralization, helplessness and ambivalence (Vandereycken & Meermann, 1984). We stress that these feelings in fact, reflect their wish to become involved constructively in the treatment of their daughters. It is this involvement, this positive concern and sense of responsibility which we would like to use now as a "therapeutic instrument" for the *future*. So, we relabel in terms of a constructive and future-oriented attitude.

> *Example:* A mother told us she thought the eating problems of her daughter started when the mother had to be hospitalized for a very serious operation. Her daughter was terrified by the idea that her mother could die. One of our reactions was to ask the mother how she could help her daughter in future experiences of mourning, for instance, when a beloved animal dies or a friendship is broken.

Rossman and Freedman (1982) pay specific attention to the complexity of guilt feelings. In their groups, the therapists simply accept parental expressions of guilt and anxiety, while indicating that the meetings can help parents to learn new behaviors that will leave them feeling less helpless and unhappy. But, as the authors underline, parental guilt feelings often serve varying defensive functions. Self-criticism can be understood as a way of forestalling anticipated criti-

cal comments from the leaders or other group members. Guilt feelings sometimes conceal underlying anger toward the adolescent patient or reflect parental ambivalence in providing realistic behavioral limits (Rossman & Freedman,
1982). Jeammet and Gorge (1980) stress that guilt feelings already exist before
the illness of the child and are connected with unresolved conflicts and feelings
of ambivalence toward their own parents. Moreover, parents are sometimes
more willing to speak and think about their "errors" than accept the more frightening idea of "losing" their child through the normal developmental process of
separation and individuation.

When all this seems unbearable, parents are eager to designate a scapegoat,
which can be any of various events or persons: past therapists, a certain lifestyle,
the society, other family members, the educational system of the school, the present treatment and finally the patients themselves. Parents can be quite aggressive toward their otherwise "sick" children, but this often reflects their helplessness and impotence. Some authors (Rouam, 1984; Jeammet & Gorge, 1980) interpret this aggression as oriented toward their own inner parental images and
norms. Sudden shifts in extreme feelings from admiration and mothering into a
total rejection of the child are not uncommon. Rouam (1984) emphasizes the
parents' fascination elicited by the determination, will-power and obstinacy of
the anorexic girl. These feelings prevail when parents compare their daughters
as if they want to know "who has the thinnest one" (Rouam, 1984, p. 2166).

Jeammet and Gorge (1980) notice that the expression of ambivalence in the
group, often happens in the form of either criticism or admiration toward the
therapists. After a while and with the help of the group, parents come to realize that these conflicting feelings are rooted in the past, mirroring the ambivalence toward their own parents. Time and again, we notice that these ambivalent feelings are worked through once parents realize that nobody requires
them to be perfect and irreproachable.

Envy and Competitiveness

Sometimes parents have difficulties with the special attention their children
receive in the hospital. These feelings are difficult to admit and express in the
group, but are not infrequent. The envy and resultant competitiveness is sometimes expressed through anxiety about the adolescent's attachment to the hospital, or concern that the staff offers a more gratifying parental model (Rossman
& Freedman, 1982). Therefore, we present our counseling group as "a special
time for parents (or relatives) alone," and underscore that the content of the
meetings will be kept confidential. This seems a difficult point since patients are
very eager to know what is said in the parent group, and they try to control all
interactions in the same way as at home. And parents, on the other hand, are so
willing to please their children! Because parents have to learn to set healthier
limits, this confidentiality can be taken as a concrete opportunity for learning

to delimitate "private territory." Nevertheless the long-term effect on the patients of this "special group for relatives" has proved to be positive: patients feel relieved, less responsible for the well- being of their family and less guilty about the attention and support they receive from the therapists and nursing staff.

The Victimized Family

Another cluster of themes consists of explanations and explorations of distorted family functioning in confrontation with the eating problems. Parents report a considerable change in the family's eating pattern, which has been repeatedly adapted in futile efforts to keep the anorexic eating (Lewis & Mac Guire, 1985). We frequently hear stories of mothers cooking special meals at impossible hours, dieting themselves or eating large portions on demand of the daughter. Anorexics insist on eating less than everyone else at the table and they have frightening fantasies of losing control over eating. In many families the patients no longer eat at usual times and places (together with the rest of the family). For this reason, parents became reluctant to invite friends for a dinner or to celebrate family events. In the group, parents realize how strange or abnormal their habits have become and they are encouraged to reintroduce firm, healthy eating rules and to restore the mealtimes as socially agreeable events.

In our treatment program patients eat at fixed hours. Parents often report conflicts arising during the first weekends at home about the eating hours: patients want their meals at exactly the same time as in the hospital. In the beginning this can be viewed as a need for a mainstay, but later on this control has to be given up. The family members are encouraged to express very clearly their own wishes, and the parents are stimulated to find some realistic arrangements: strict rules in chaotic families and flexible ones in cases of rigid family functioning.

Parents are concerned with the impact of the patient's illness on the rest of the family, particularly the siblings (Lewis & MacGuire, 1985). They apprehend that the attention given to the anorexic or bulimic girl was at some cost to the other children. Senior group members may explain how this period of hospitalization can afford parents a concrete opportunity to find a new equilibrium with the other children.

Attachment and Separation

A lack of boundaries between the anorexic/bulimic girl and the parental subsystem is a frequent observation (see Chapter 2). Lewis and MacGuire (1985) emphasize the closeness between mothers and daughters. Jeammet and Gorge (1980) called it "the fusion of generations."

Examples:

- We often hear mothers proudly explaining how they relate to their daughters as being their best friend!
- In some cases we know they sleep in the same room, while father is excluded.
- A mother frequently makes a slip in the group, while talking about the family, in the sense of "my brother (father)" instead of "her brother (father)."
- Mothers can narcissistically admire their child: "My daughter dares to do (can do) what I can't."
- Others denigrate her: "She is a failure like me. My mother told me I wasn't a good wife or mother, and my daughter won't be either."
- Sometimes the anorexic/bulimic daughter takes the place of the grandmother, and is allowed to criticize, judge and control the whole family.

In these cases, mother and father apparently do not function as an intimate couple. The father is excluded from the mother-daughter union or is considered as (behaves himself as) another child. Negative attitudes toward the father are frequently reported, sometimes to the extent that the patient will not stay in the same room with him. But the opposite may exist too: a more or less erotization of the contact between father and daughter. These parents are no longer able to impose any rules and set limits (Jeammet & Gorge, 1980). They no longer function as a point of reference against which the girls can rebel without losing contact. These parents need their children too much for their own emotional equilibrium; some tend to speak without knowing whose feelings they are expressing.

Example: A mother clearly stated in the group that her daughter would not accept a school far from home. Many group members, however, immediately understood that the mother was the one who could not bear the separation.

A most important theme is that of separation-individuation and subsequent feelings of depression. Unresolved separation issues are a fundamental and common problem in families with anorexic/bulimic adolescents. Parents as well as children experience differentiation or individuation as a destruction of the familial relationships, engendering threatening feelings of loss, loneliness and failure. Conflicts have always been avoided in order to keep the illusion of the "one united family" intact. The anorexic/bulimic symptom is the unifying issue which allows family members to speak about everything except for becoming autonomous.

The depressive feelings of the parents we deal with in the counseling groups are usually associated with their helplessness regarding the eating disorder. Other authors focus on the underlying fear of losing the special ties with the children. Some therapists (Jeammet & Gorge, 1980; Rouam, 1984) intend to work directly with these underlying feelings of the parents. Others (Rossman &

Freedman, 1982) intervene more indirectly, and deliberately center the discussion on the adolescents' problem with separation so that parental anxieties are not intensified through the direct analysis of their unresolved ties. A discussion of the youngsters' problem in having to grow up and leave home — viewing the hospital separation as a practice for later — enables parents to recognize this conflictful issue and to help their children in coping with the normal separation process.

Control and Responsibility

All parents or relatives report having difficulties with control issues regarding the eating behavior of the patients. Spouses as well as parents often vacillate between periods of intrusive, controlling involvement and periods of emotional detachment (Leichner et al., 1985). Group members usually recognize the necessity of encouraging the patients to take their own responsibility for their health and their life in general, but they find this difficult, at the same time, as if they are afraid that the patient would "abuse this freedom."

Example: In the second phase of our inpatient treatment program (Vandereycken, 1985) the patient receives a set portion of food in the dining room where she eats together with other patients and under the supervision of a nurse. Sometimes parents propose to do the same at home during the first weekend. Only an open discussion can clear up the hidden motives: e.g., Does this proposition come from the girl or the mother? Is it intended to set new and healthier limits or to continue the old habit of controlling each other?

Parents are encouraged to tell in the group about their experiences of the first weekends, how it feels eating again with the whole family together.

Example: A mother told that her daughter refused to have dinner with the rest of the family on Sunday evening before returning to the hospital. She did not know how to react ("Do I have to force her or just neglect her behavior?") and finally chose to talk for five minutes with her daughter who was able then to express her sadness about having to leave the family and return to the hospital. The mother returned to the other family members at the dinner table, and after a few moments the daughter joined them and ate normally. We congratulated the mother in front of the other parents with the way she handled that situation, and we explained that by enabling the patient to share her feelings, she no longer needed her anorexic behavior at that moment.

The Hidden Issue: Sexuality

A last theme we like to mention is one parents almost never speak about spontaneously, neither in the group nor individually: sexuality. This is all the more surprising because the anorexic behavior very often stands for the inexpressible fear of the sexual transformations of the pubertal body, for the fear of the necessity to make a sexual choice (Rouam, 1984). This silence of the parents can only be understood as the expression of their own fears or insecurity regarding sexual issues. Jeammet and Gorge (1980) said that in their groups only the fathers ever speak about sexual matters, often with a lack of control in telling personal feelings or intimate events. In contrast, the mothers keep always silent on these matters in the group.

Leichner, Harper and Johnston (1985) report that in their group for spouses, husbands agree that they felt their wives did not like physical closeness or sexual contact, but they seem to have accepted this aspect in their relationship. They are reluctant to discuss these issues with their wives because of their fears that this might further aggravate their eating disorder. We encountered similar resistance in our group and noticed, in some cases, a strong coalition between the mother and the patient's boyfriend, provoking feelings of rivalry, guilt and further rejection of sexuality in the patient. The patient does not understand why her cool and distant mother suddenly becomes gentle and flexible toward her boyfriend and she is puzzled by their seemingly compliant behavior to each other.

Finally, the symptom of amenorrhea, which all mothers are worried about, is a typical issue for fruitful discussion in the group: it appears to be neutral as a topic and is therefore easy to speak about, but it allows, at the same time, to introduce the theme of sexuality. As in the case of eating, where we underline the social and interactional meanings, we stress that menstruation is more than just a physical phenomenon, and that it incorporates psychological aspects of womanhood and sexuality.

THE GROUP PROCESS

Regarding the group process, we distinguish, with the length of stay of each parent couple in the group, an evolution in the group themes we have discussed so far, as well as in the group dynamics.

From Restraining Observers to Active Participants

In the beginning of a group or when newcomers are added, parents initially seek information about the illness of their daughter, and direct their questions to the therapists. They often ask for solutions as to how they should respond to certain problems. Some group leaders take a very active stance (Rossman & Freedman, 1982), others are more withdrawn, but they always pay attention to encouraging the interactional group process. Parents or relatives are actively invited to share their common experiences. The therapists withhold from giving specific suggestions and instead guide the group in exploring the various feelings of the persons involved. As many issues recur in many different forms, it becomes increasingly obvious to the group members that there are no right answers that the therapists alone can give.

Jeammet and Gorge (1980) report that especially the fathers are very narcissistically vulnerable and insist upon receiving clear answers. They need an "idealizing tranference" with the male therapist. Feelings of parental frustration and disappointment about the therapists' attitudes are counterbalanced by the stimulation of a strong group cohesion. In a group situation of benevolent concern, parents will discover their "peers" (mostly mothers seek contact with each other). Some authors (Rossman & Freedman, 1982; Leichner et al., 1985) encourage informal and supportive contacts between the parents beyond the group sessions (e.g., making phone calls or speaking to one another between meetings when difficulties arise) in order to strengthen the group cohesion.

Therapists encourage the group members to take over the educative role. We repeatedly stress that parents have much more to learn from each other than from us, because they are directly and emotionally involved, whereas we observe things from a more neutral and distant point of view. In an ongoing group, an informal subsystem of "senior parents" usually evolves. Parents, especially those with authority conflicts, are more likely to accept support, direct confrontation and reinterpretation from each other than from the group leaders. Similarly, senior members are more convincing when they speak in defense of the therapeutic program and its rules or consequences for the family (prevention of drop-out from treatment; Vandereycken & Meermann, 1984) or when they plead for the girls' leaving home to live on their own in a selfsupporting way.

Jeammet and Gorge (1980) summarized the evolution in this therapeutic role as follows: parents first become co-therapists for the other parents, then for their children, and finally for themselves.

From Abandoned Parents to Creative Partners

Parallel to the evolution of the therapeutic role of the parents, there is an evolution in their process of working through various feelings aroused by the treatment as it becomes apparent in the evolution of the themes of these feelings. This process is sometimes strikingly similar to that of the patients in their group psychotherapy sessions (see Vandereycken et al., 1986). The first themes, as we described above, are the expression of guilt, shame, anger and ambivalence toward their children and the hospital team. By sharing their experiences in the group, parents receive support, reassurance and sympathy from their peer group members.

A following step is the working through of the separation process. As we know, anorexic/bulimic patients have strong ties with their families. When they are confronted with their feelings of dependence and the subsequent necessity of individuation, they are moving out of the eating-control phase into what appears to be a depressive, obsessional phase (Lewis & MacGuire, 1985). Parents are subject to the same process. The hospitalization itself and later on the realization that their children growing up, elicit a storm of feelings the group has to deal with. At this point in the evolution, the role of the therapists — balancing between support and confrontation — is very important for every participant. The leaders should point out the positive aspects of conflicts with the children so that separation issues can move out of the sphere of punishment into the realistic acceptance of the necessity, for all concerned, to take some distance from each other in order to reach a richer level of individuality (Rouam, 1984; Jeammet & Gorge, 1980).

Parents need much attention and concern now, and the group atmosphere ought to be safe and stimulating. Jeammet et al. (1973) describe this second phase as one in which parents do not any longer ask what to do, but are at least beginning to see their daughter as a distinct person struggling with her own internal conflicts and ambivalent feelings. For parents and children, the realization that they have to work through this process of individuation separately, on their own, is painful but essential. As Rouam (1984) points out: parents have to give up their fantasies of omnipotence and parental idealization, as much as their children have to give up the (would-be) omnipotence of their symptoms.

> *Example:* A bulimic patient stopped thinking she had to be perfect in order to make her mother feel she was a good mother and to give her father the love he missed. Hereafter, she could start for the first time a relationship with a boyfriend and could accept some love and criticism. Now the parents were able to question their conviction that their daughter could only get rid of her bulimic problems if she would come back home.

The question of leaving home is very often discussed in our counseling groups. Parents are frightened by the idea that everything is going to turn into a catastrophe. Knowing and feeling that we, as therapists, take these matters very seriously, together with our insistence on a well-planned and intensive aftercare program, will give them considerable confidence and relieve their anxieties about the future.

A final step in the evolution of the group process is the expression of the changes occurring in the parents' own lives. Gradually there is arising a psychological space for themselves and they finally can think again about their own past and future. Time and again, we consider this as the most touching moments in our group work: we hear parents planning new activities, pursuing again their favorite hobbies, and seeing old friends. After a period of surprise or even jealousy, patients are happy with this evolution and feel themselves released from the "responsibility" for their parents' happiness and from the guilt feelings that they caused them so much sorrow.

Example: In the beginning, parents do not even think about going on holidays without their hospitalized daughter ("leaving that poor girl"), but later on many will take this possibility seriously into consideration. Although few parents will accept a long vacation away from their hospitalized daughter, it may be initially a great step to take a whole weekend free for themselves.

It is important for parents to realize that they have the right and duty to live (again) as marital partners and to reshape their lives in accordance with this purpose.

CONCLUSION

Parent-counseling groups certainly have their limitations. One of the pitfalls might be that an existing fragmentation of the family is reinforced by using separate treatment modalities for the family's subsystems. Therefore, some practitioners prefer an alternative, integrating the dynamics of group therapy and family therapy: "multiple family therapy," i.e., the treatment of several (entire) families simultaneously through the vehicle of a group meeting led by therapists (see e.g., Koman, 1985; Mc Farlane, 1982). We, on the other hand, do not feel the need for this enlarged scope since our parent-counseling group fits better in the flexible approach we described in Chapter 14. Moreover, our primary goal is not to treat families, but to offer them guidance and support and to obtain their active participation in a collaborative working relationship during inpatient treatment.

"Regardless of the particular family treatment approach, parent counseling groups seem especially helpful in providing isolated, demoralized parents with the opportunity to experience gradual increments in self-esteem within a supportive treatment setting. The group offers a network of helping relationships within which the parents unburden themselves, obtain guidance and advice from both the other parents and the leaders, and in turn experience the gratification of having something to offer to others" (Rossman & Freedman, 1982, p. 404). In our experience (see also Vandereycken & Meermann, 1984), such a counseling group appears to be a useful treatment modality to aid parents in coping with ambivalent feelings about hospital treatment, to gain insight into the psychological and interactional meanings of the eating disorder, to realize the need of the family's participation in the change process, to strengthen collaborative relationships between parents and treatment staff, and to enhance motivation for engaging in family or marital therapy if necessary.

REFERENCES

Doumic, A. (1962), Aide à apporter aux parents d'adolescents atteints d'anorexie mentale (Helping parents of adolescents with anorexia nervosa). *Revue de Neuropsychiatrie Infantile,* 10:253-260.

Groen, J.J. & Feldman-Toledano, Z. (1966), Educative treatment of patients and parents in anorexia nervosa. *British Journal of Psychiatry,* 112:671-681.

Hauer, J., Janzing, C. & Zantvoort, F. (1985), Oudergroepen en residentiële psychosebehandel-
ing (Parent groups and residential treatment of psychotics). *Tijdschrift voor Psychiatrie,* 27:536-
551.

Jardin, F. (1973), La psychothérapie "institutionnelle" de l'anorexie mentale (The "institutional"
psychotherapy of anorexia nervosa). *Revue de Neuropsychiatrie Infantile,* 21:167-172.

Jeammet, P. (1984), Le groupe de parents: Sa place dans le traitement de l'anorexie mentale (The
parent group: Its place in the treatment of anorexia nervosa). *Neuropsychiatrie de l'Enfance,*
32:299-303.

Jeammet, P. & Gorge, A. (1980), Une forme de thérapie familiale: Le groupe de parents (A form
of family therapy: The parent group). *Psychiatrie de l'Enfant,* 23:587-636.

Jeammet, P., Gorge, A., Zweifel, F. & Flavigny, H. (1971), Etude des interrelations familiales de
l'anorexique mentale et d'un groupe de psychothérapie des parents (Study of family relations
in anorexia nervosa and of a psychotherapeutic group for parents). *Revue de Neuropsychiatrie
Infantile,* 19:691-708.

Jeammet, P., Gorge, A., Zweifel, F. & Flavigny, H. (1973), Le milieu familial des anorexiques
mentaux: Incidences sur le traitement (The family milieu of anorexia nervosa patients: Influences on the treatment). *Annales de Médecine Interne,* 124:247-252.

Koman, S.L. (1985), Conduct in short-term inpatient multiple family groups. In: Mirkin, M.P. &
Koman, S.L. (eds.), *Handbook of Adolescents and Family Therapy.* New York: Gardner Press,
pp. 173-191.

Leichner, P., Harper, D. & Johnston, D. (1985), Adjunctive group support for spouses of women
with anorexia nervosa and/or bulimia. *International Journal of Eating Disorders,* 4:227-235.

Lewis, H.L. & MacGuire, M.P. (1985), Review of a group for parents of anorexics. *Journal of
Psychiatric Research,* 19:453-458.

Mc Farlane, W.R. (1982), Multiple-family therapy in the psychiatric hospital. In: Harbin, H.T.
(ed.), *The Psychiatric Hospital and the Family.* Jamaica (N.Y.): Spectrum Publications, pp. 103-
129.

Rose, J. & Garfinkel, P. (1980), A parents' group in the management of anorexia nervosa. *Canadian
Journal of Psychiatry,* 25:228-232.

Rossman, P. & Freedman, J. (1982), Hospital treatment for disturbed adolescents: The role of
parent-counseling groups. *Adolescent Psychiatry,* 10:392-406.

Rouam, F. (1984), Réflexions sur un groupe thérapeutique de parents d'anorexiques (Considerations on a therapeutic group for parents of anorexics). *Semaine des Hôpitaux (Paris),* 60:2163-
2167.

Vandereycken, W. & Meermann, R. (1984), *Anorexia Nervosa. A Clinician's Guide to Treatment.*
Berlin-New York: Walter de Gruyter.

Vandereycken, W. (1985), Inpatient treatment of anorexia nervosa: Some research-guided
changes. *Journal of Psychiatric Research,* 19:413-422.

Vandereycken, W., Vanderlinden, J. & Van Werde, D. (1986), Directive group therapy for patients
with anorexia nervosa or bulimia. In: Larocca, F.E.F. (ed.), *Eating Disorders: Effective Care
and Treatment.* St. Louis: Ishiyaku EuroAmerica, pp. 53-69.

Vanderlinden, J. & Vandereycken, W. (1984), Directive family therapy in adult patients with
severe or chronic anorexia nervosa. *International Journal of Family Psychiatry,* 4:267-280.

Verbeek, N. & Verbeek, E. (1977), Anorexia nervosa: Karakteristiek en therapie van de driehoeksrelatie in het ouderlijk gezin (Anorexia nervosa: Characteristics and treatment of the
triangular relation in the family). *Tijdschrift voor Psychiatrie,* 19:685-703.

BIBLIOGRAPHY ON FAMILY ASPECTS OF EATING DISORDERS

This selective but almost exhaustive bibliography contains all the publications in the international literature (till the Summer 1987) which focus specifically on some family aspect of eating disorders. A translation of the title is added to each non-English publication. We have qualified each reference according to its main approach:

(G) = *General* article with an overview of various aspects and/or a review of the literature;

(P) = *Practice*-oriented article concerning management or treatment;

(R) = *Research* article describing a particular investigation;

(T) = *Theoretical* article with considerations or speculations.

Achimovich, L. (1985), Theory and research: Suicidal scripting in the families of anorectics. *Transactional Analysis Journal,* 15(1):21-29. (T)

Albert, E., Mouren, M.C. & Dugas, M. (1984), La famille dans l'anorexie mentale masculine (The family in male anorexics). *Neuropsychiatrie de l'Enfance,* 32:309-313. (T)

Alexander, N. (1986), Characteristics and treatment of families with anorectic offspring. *Occupational Therapy and Mental Health,* 6:117-135 (also in D. Gibson, ed., *The Evaluation and Treatment of Eating Disorders;* New York, Haworth Press, 1986). (P)

Amdur, M.J., Tucker, G.J., Detre, T. & Markus, K. (1969), Anorexia nervosa: An interactional study. *Journal of Nervous and Mental Disease,* 148:559-566. (R)

Andersen, A.E. (1985), Family and marital therapy. In: Author, *Practical Comprehensive Treatment of Anorexia Nervosa and Bulimia.* Baltimore: Johns Hopkins University Press, pp. 135-148. (P)

Andrews, T.J. & Irwin, M. (1985), Anorexia nervosa: The role of divorce. *BASH Newsletter,* 4(7):9-10. (T)

Aponte, H. & Hoffman, L. (1973), The open door: A structural approach to a family with an anorectic child. *Family Process,* 12:1-44. (P)

Baker, L.C. & Pontious, J.M. (1984), Treating the health care family. *Family Systems Medicine,* 2:401-408. (P)

Barcai, A. (1971), Family therapy in the treatment of anorexia nervosa. *American Journal of Psychiatry,* 128:286-290. (P)

Bartholomew, K.L. (1984), 'I would eat for her if I could': Guiding the paradox in an anorectic system. *Journal of Strategic and Systemic Therapies,* 3(1):57-65. (P)

Bauer, B.G., Anderson, W.P. & Hyatt, R.W. (1986), Family issues in therapy. In: Authors, *Bulimia: Book for Therapist and Client.* Muncie (Indiana): Accelerated Development Inc., pp. 123-144. (P)

Beckers, W. & Massing, A. (1974), Anorexia nervosa: Pubertätsmagersucht als Ausdruck einer Familien- Ideologie (Anorexia nervosa as expression of a family ideology). *Sexualmedizin,* 3:574-578. (T)

Beeren, J. (1979). Ervaringen met een partner-relatietherapie 'on analytic lines' bij een anorexia-patiënte en haar echtgenoot (Experience with a marital therapy 'on analytic lines' in an anorexia patient and her husband). *Tijdschrift voor Psychiatrie,* 21:489-506. (P)

Bemporad, J.R. & Ratey, J. (1985), Intensive psychotherapy of former anorexic individuals. *American Journal of Psychotherapy,* 39:454-466. (T)

Besançon, G., Deneux, A., Messiac, E. & Chiffolear, S. (1978), De l'anorexie mentale comme modèle psychopathologique dans une famille (Anorexia nervosa as a psychopathological model in a family). *L'Evolution Psychiatrique,* 43:583-596. (T)

Biederman, J., Rivinus, T., Kemper, K., Hamilton, D., MacFadyen, J. & Harmatz, J. (1985), Depressive disorders in relatives of anorexia nervosa patients with and without a current episode of nonbipolar major depression. *American Journal of Psychiatry,* 142:1495-1497. (R)

Bologna, N. (1983), Family therapy. In: Neuman, P.A. & Halvorson, P.A. (Eds.), *Anorexia Nervosa and Bulimia. A Handbook for Counselors and Therapists.* New York: Van Nostrand Reinhold, pp. 116-132. (P)

Boutonier, J. (1948), Le rôle de la mère dans la genèse de l'anorexie mentale. (The role of the mother in the development of anorexia nervosa). *Cahiers de Psychiatrie,* 2:3-9. (T)

Bruch, H. (1970), Family background in eating disorders. In: Anthony, I. & Koupernik, C. (Eds.), *The Child In His Family.* New York: John Wiley, pp. 285-309. (French translation of the same book published by Masson, Paris, 1970). (T)

Bruch, H. (1971), Family transactions in eating disorders. *Comprehensive Psychiatry,* 12:238-248. (T)

Bruch, H. (1973), Family frame and transactions. In: Author, *Eating Disorders. Obesity, Anorexia Nervosa, and the Person Within.* New York: Basic Books, pp.66-86. (G)

Bruch, H. (1978), Family disengagement. In: Author, *The Golden Cage. The Enigma of Anorexia\Nervosa.* Cambridge (Mass.): Harvard University Press, pp. 106-120. (Translation in Dutch: Baarne, In de Toren, 1979; French: Paris, Presses Universitaires de France, 1979; German: Frankfurt, Fischer Verlag, 1982). (G)

Buddeberg, B. & Buddeberg, C. (1979), Familientherapie bei Anorexia nervosa (Family therapy in anorexia nervosa). *Praxis der Kinderpsychologie und Kinderpsychiatrie,* 28:37-43. (P)

Caillé, P., Abrahamsen, P., Girolami, C. & Sorby, B. (1977), A systems theory approach to a case of anorexia nervosa. *Family Process,* 16:455-465. French version: Utilisation de la théorie des systèmes dans le traitement de l'anorexie mentale. *Evolution Psychiatrique,* 1978, 43:563-581 (reprinted in: *Cahiers Critiques de Thérapie Familiale et de Pratiques de Réseaux,* 1979, nr 1; also in: Caillé, P., *Familles et Thérapeutes.* Paris, E.S.F., 1985, pp. 94-107). (P)

Casper, R. & Jabine, J. (1986), Psychological functioning in anorexia nervosa: A comparison between anorexia nervosa patients on follow-up and their sisters. In: Lacey, J.H. & Sturgeon, D.A. (Eds.), *Proceedings of the 15th European Conference on Psychosomatic Research.* London: John Libbey, pp. 172-178. (R)

Ceaser, M. (1977), The role of maternal identification in four cases of anorexia nervosa. *Bulletin of the Menninger Clinic,* 41:475-486.

Collins, G.B., Kotz, M., Janesz, J.W., Messina, M. & Ferguson, T. (1985), Alcoholism in the families of bulimic anorexics. *Cleveland Clinic Quarterly,* 52:65-67. (R)

Collins, G.B., Kotz, M., Messina, M. & Ferguson, T. (1985), Affective disorder in bulimic anorexics and their families. *Cleveland Clinic Quarterly,* 52:399-401. (R)

Collins, M., Hodas, G.R. & Liebman, R. (1983), Interdisciplinary model for the inpatient treatment of adolescents with anorexia nervosa. *Journal of Adolescent Health Care,* 4:3-8. (P)

Combrinck-Graham, L. (1974), Structural family therapy in psychosomatic illness: Treatment of anorexia nervosa and asthma. *Clinical Pediatrics,* 13:827-833. (P)

Compernolle, T. (1981), Anorexia nervosa: Een eco-psycho- somatisch probleem waarvan de gezinsdysfunctie oorzaak en gevolg is en waarbij de autoriteit van de ouders een belangrijke rol speelt. (Anorexia nervosa: An eco-psycho-somatic problem of which the family dysfunctioning is both cause and consequence, and in which the parents' authority plays an important role). *Tijdschrift voor Psychiatrie,* 23(supplementum):80-86. (T)

Conforto, C. & Maura, E. (1972), Dinamiche familiari in un case di 'anoressia mentale'. (Family dynamics in a case of 'anorexia nervosa'). *Rivista Sperimentale di Freniatria,* 96:143-152. (T)

Conrad, D.E. (1977), A starving family: An interactional view of anorexia nervosa. *Bulletin of the Menninger Clinic,* 41:487-495. (T)

Cremer, J. (1980), Zur psychiatrische Betreuung von Kranken mit Anorexia-nervosa-Syndrom unter Berücksichtiging der Kommunikationsunterbrechung. (Psychiatric management of patients with anorexia nervosa: Interruption of Communication). *Praxis der Psychotherapie,* 25:259-267. (P)

Crémieux, A. & Dongier, M. (1956), Observations statistiques sur les familles où survient une anorexie mentale. (Statistical observations on families with anorexia nervosa). *Annales Méd-ico-Psychologiques,* 114(1):639-641. (R)

Crisp, A.H., Harding, B. & Mc Guinness, B. (1974), Anorexia nervosa. Psychoneurotic characteristics of parents: Relationship to prognosis. *Journal of Psychosomatic Research,* 18:167- 173. (R)

Crisp, A.H., Hall, A. & Holland, A.J. (1985), Nature and nurture in anorexia nervosa: A study of 34 pairs of twins, one pair of triplets, and an adoptive family. *International Journal of Eating Disorders,* 4:5-27. (R)

Dally, P.J. (1977), Anorexia nervosa: Do we need a scapegoat? *Proceedings of the Royal Society of Medicine,* 70:470-474. (R)

Dally, P. (1984), Anorexia tardive — late onset anorexia nervosa. *Journal of Psychosomatic Research,* 28:423-428. (R)

— Dare, C. (1983), Family therapy for families containing an anorectic youngster. In: *Understanding Anorexia Nervosa and Bulimia.* Columbus (Ohio): Ross Laboratories, pp. 28-37. (P)

— Dare, C. (1985), The family therapy of anorexia nervosa. *Journal of Psychiatric Research,* 19:435-443. (P)

Deegener, G. (1982), Oedipale Konstellationen bei Anorexia Nervosa. (Oedipal configurations in anorexia nervosa). *Praxis der Kinderpsychologie und Kinderpsychiatrie,* 31:291-297. (T)

Doerr-Zegers, O., Petrasic, J. & Morales, E. (1985), The role of the family in the pathogenesis of anorexia nervosa. In: Pichot, P., Berner, P., Wolf, R. & Thau, K. (Eds.), *Psychiatry, the State of the Art. Vol. 4. Psychotherapy and Psychosomatic Medicine.* New York: Plenum Press, pp. 459-465. (R)

Dongier, M. & Duchesne, A. (1966), Anorexie mentale et place dans la fratrie. (Anorexia nervosa and birth order). *Acta Psychiatrica Belgica,* 66:812-819. (R)

Doumic, A. (1962), Aide à apporter aux parents d'adolescents atteints d'anorexie mentale. (Helping parents of adolescents with anorexia nervosa). *Revue de Neuropsychiatrie Infantile,* 10:253-260. (P)

Edhouse, H. (1985), The child as the presenting symptom or the mother. Anorexia nervosa in a nine and a half year old child. *Australian Family Physician,* 4 (October):1-6. (T)

— Edwards, G. (1987), Anorexia and the family. In: M. Lawrence (Ed.), *Fed Up und Hungry: Women, Oppression and Food.* London: Women's Press, pp. 61-73. (T)

Ehrensing, R. & Weitzman, E. (1970), The mother-daughter relationship in anorexia nervosa. *Psychosomatic Medicine,* 32:201-208. (T)

Eisler, I., Szmukler, G. & Dare, C. (1985), Systematic observation and clinical insight — are they compatible? An experiment in recognizing family interactions. *Psychological Medicine,* 15:173-188. (R)

Ekberg, M. & Gilberg, C. (1977), (Family therapy in anorexia nervosa: An alternative treatment). *Läkartidningen,* 74:647-650. (P)

Elkaim, M. (1979), Une approche systémique de quelques cas d'anorexie mentale. (A systemic approach to some cases of anorexia nervosa). *Revue d'Action Sociale,* 2:22-37. (Reprinted in: *Cahiers Critiques de Thérapie Familiale et de Pratiques de Réseaux,* 1979, nr 1; *Feuillets Psychiatriques de Liège,* 1982, 15:252-265). (P)

Epple, H. (1984), Familientherapie bei Magersucht. (Family therapy in anorexia nervosa). In: Remschmidt, H. (Ed.), *Psychotherapie mit Kindern, Jugendlichen und Familien. Band 2.* Stuttgart: Ferdinand Enke, pp.71-76. (P)

Fagiani, M.B., Marocco, M.C. & Gianara, A. (1980), Dinamica di rapporto interpersonale tra le anoressiche e le famiglie. (The dynamics of the interpersonal relationship between anorexia women and their families). *Minerva Psichiatrica,* 21(1):25-44. (T)

Faltus, F. (1980), (Some of the pecularities of the family structure of patients with mental anorexia). *Ceskoslovenska Psychiatrie,* 76:228-234. (R)

Fishman, H.C. (1979), Family considerations in liaison psychiatry. A structural family approach to anorexia nervosa in adults. *Psychiatric Clinics of North America,* 2:249-263. (P)

Foster, F.G. & Kupfer, D. (1975), Anorexia nervosa: Telemetric assessment of family interaction and hospital events. *Journal of Psychiatric Research,* 12:19-35. (R)

Foster, S.W. (1986), Marital treatment of eating disorders. In: Jacobson, N.S. & Gurman, A.S. (Eds.), *Clinical Handbook of Marital Therapy.* New York: Guilford Press, pp. 575-93. (P)

Frazier, S.H., Faubion, M.H., Giffin, M.E. & Johnson, A.M. (1955), A specific factor in symptom choice. *Staff Meetings of the Mayo Clinic,* 30:227-243. (T)

Garfinkel, P.E. & Garner, D.M. (1982), The role of the family. In: Authors, *Anorexia Nervosa: A Multidimentional Perspective.* New York: Brunner/Mazel, pp. 164-187. (G)

Gensicke, P. (1979), Anorexia nervosa — ein familiales Socialisationsdefizit. (Anorexia nervosa — A deficit of the family's socialization). *Zeitschrift für Psychosomatische Medizin und Psychoanalyse,* 3:201-215. (T)

Gensicke, P. (1984), Die Anorexia-nervosa-Patientin und ihre Familie. (The anorexia nervosa patient and her family). *Aktuelle Ernährungs-Medizin,* 9(1):38-41. (G)

Gershon, E., Hamovit, J.R., Schreiber, J.L., Dibble, E., Kaye, W., Nurnberger, J., Andersen, A. & Elbert, M. (1983), Anorexia nervosa and major affective disorders associated in families: A preliminary report. In: Guze, S., Earls, F. & Barrett, J. (Eds.), *Childhood Psychopathology and Development.* New York: Raven Press, pp. 279-286. (R)

Gershon, E., Schreiber, J.L., Hamovit, J.R., Dibble, E.D., Kaye, W., Nurnberger, J.I., Andersen, A.E. & Ebert, M. (1984), Clinical findings in patients with 'anorexia nervosa' and affective illness in their families. *American Journal of Psychiatry,* 141:1419-1422. (R)

Giacomo, D. & Weissmark, M. (1985), An 'overweight' anorectic family. *Journal of Strategic and Systemic Therapies,* 4(1):61-68. (P)

⁓ Gilchrist, P.N., Mc Farlane, A.C. & Kalucy, R.S. (1986), Family therapy in the treatment of anorexia nervosa. *International Journal of Eating Disorders,* 5:659-668. (P)

Goldstein, H.J. (1981), Family factors associated with schizophrenia and anorexia nervosa. *Journal of Youth and Adolescence,* 10(3):385-405. (R)

Gowers, S., Kadambari, S. & Crisp, A.H. (1985), Family structure and birth of patients with anorexia nervosa. *Journal of Psychiatric Research,* 19:247-251. (R)

Groen, J.J. & Feldman-Toledano, Z. (1966), Educative treatment of patients and parents in anorexia nervosa. *British Journal of Psychiatry,* 112:671-681. (P)

Hall, A. (1978), Family structure and relationships of 50 female anorexia nervosa patients. *Australian and New Zealand Journal of Psychiatry,* 12:263-268. (R)

Hall, A. (1987), The patient and the family. In: Beumont, P.J.V., Burrows, G.D. & Casper, R.C. (Eds.), *Handbook of Eating Disorders. Part I: Anorexia and Bulimia Nervosa.* Amsterdam-New York-Oxford: Elsevier Science, pp. 189-199. (G)

Hall, A. & Brown, L.B. (1983), A comparison of the attitudes of young anorexia nervosa patients and non-patients with those of their mothers. *British Journal of Medical Psychology,* 56:39-48. (R)

Hall , A., Leibrich, J., Walkey, F.H. & Welch, G. (1986), Investigation of 'weight pathology' of 58 mothers of anorexia nervosa patients and 204 mothers of schoolgirls. *Psychological Medicine,* 16:71-76.

Halmi, K.A. & Loney, J. (1973), Familial alcoholism in anorexia nervosa. *British Journal of Psychiatry,* 123:53-54. (R)

Halmi, K.A., Struss, A. & Goldberg, S.C. (1978), An investigation of weights in the parents of anorexia nervosa patients. *Journal of Nervous and Mental Disease,* 166:358- 361. (R)

⁓ Harding, T.P. & Lachenmeyer, J.R. (1986) Family interaction patterns and locus of control as predictors of the presence and severity of anorexia nervosa. *Journal of Clinical Psychology,* 42:440-447. (R)

Harju, E. & Fried,R. (1982), Dysorexia as a family disorder: Three cases with an obese parent and an anorectic child. *La Clinica Dietologica,* 9:135-152. (T)

Harkaway, J. (1986), *Family Therapy and Eating Disorders.* Rockville: Aspen Systems Corp. (P)

Harper, G. (1983), Varieties of parenting failure in anorexia nervosa: Protection and parentectomy, revisited. *Journal of the American Academy of Child Psychiatry*, 22:134-139. (T)

Hedblom, J.E., Hubbard, F.A. & Andersen, A.E. (1981), Anorexia nervosa: A multidisciplinary treatment program for patient and family. *Social Work in Health Care*, 7(1):67-86. (P)

Hendrickx, J. (1981a), Gezinstherapeutische strategie in geval van anorexia nervosa. (Family therapeutic strategy in case of anorexia nervosa). In: van de Loo, K.J.M., Vandereycken, W. & Eykman, J.C.B. (Eds.), *Anorexia Nervosa: Diagnostiek, Behandeling en Onderzoek*. Nijmegen: Dekker & van de Vegt, pp. 134-150. (P)

Hendrickx, J. (1981b), De ontkenning van de interactionele context bij gezinnen met een anorectische patiënte. (Denial of the interactional context in families with an anorexic patient). *Tijdschrift voor Psychiatrie*, 21(Supplement):91- 96. (T)

Heron, J.M. & Leheup, R. (1984), Happy families? *British Journal of Psychiatry*, 145:136-138. (R)

Hodas, G., Liebman, R. & Collins, M.J. (1982), Pediatric hospitalization in the treatment of anorexia nervosa. In: Harbin, H.T. (Ed.), *The Psychiatric Hospital and the Family*. Jamaica (NY): Spectrum Publications, pp.131-141. (P)

Holland, A.J., Hall, A., Murray, R., Russell, G.F.M. & Crisp, A.H. (1984), Anorexia nervosa: A study of 34 twin pairs and one set of triplets. *British Journal of Psychiatry*, 145:414-419. (R)

Houben, M.E. (1981), Onderzoek naar enkele relatie- karakteristieken in gezinnen met een anorexia nervosa- patiënte. (Study of relation characteristics in families with an anorexia nervosa patient). *Tijdschrift voor Psychiatrie*, 23(Supplement):87-90. (R)

Hubschmidt, T. (1979), Zur strukturellen Familientherapie: Ein Fallbeispiel. (Application of structural family therapy: A case example). *Familiendynamik*, 4:173-184. (P)

Hudson, J., Pope, H., Jones, J. & Yurgulun-Todd, D. (1983), Family history study of anorexia nervosa and bulimia. *British Journal of Psychiatry*, 142:133-138; 428-429. (R)

Humphrey, L.L. (1983), A sequential analysis of family processes in anorexia and bulimia. In: *Understanding Anorexia Nervosa and Bulimia*. Report of the Fourth Ross Conference on Medical Research. Columbus (Ohio): Ross Laboratories, pp. 37- 46. (R)

Humphrey, L. (1986a), Family dynamics in bulimia. In: Feinstein, S.C. (Ed.), *Adolescent Psychiatry. Developmental and Clinical Studies. Volume 13*. Chicago: University of Chicago Press, pp. 315-332. (R)

Humphrey, L.L. (1986b), Structural analysis of parent child relationships in eating disorders. *Journal of Abnormal Psychology*, 95:395-402. (R)

Humphrey, L.L. (1987), Comparison of bulimic-anorexic and nondistressed families using structural analysis of social behavior. *Journal of the American Academy of Child Psychiatry*, 26:248- 255. (R)

Humphrey, L.L., Apple, R.F. & Kirschenbaum, D.S. (1986), Differentiating bulimic-anorexic from normal families using interpersonal and behavioral observation systems. *Journal of Consulting and Clinical Psychology*, 54:190-195. (R)

Huygen, F.J.A. (1976), Gezinsgeneeskundige colloquia, VII: Anorexia nervosa. (Conferences on family medicine, VII: Anorexia nervosa). *Huisarts en Wetenschap*, 19:57-60. (P)

Igoin-Apfelbaum, L. (1985), Characteristics of family background in bulimia. *Psychotherapy and Psychosomatics*, 43:161-167. (T)

Ishikawa, K. (1965), Ueber die Eltern von Anorexia-nervosa- Kranken. (About the parents of anorexia nervosa patients). In: Meyer, J.E. & Feldmann, H. (Eds.), *Anorexia Nervosa*. Stuttgart: Georg Thieme Verlag, pp. 154-155. (T)

Israel, L., Ebtinger, R., Bolzinger, R.M., Weil, J. & Wysoki, V. (1971), A propos des interventions inopportunes de l'entourage de l'anorexique. (About inappropriate interventions from the anorexic's milieu). *Revue de Neuropsychiatrie Infantile*, 19:639-643. (T)

Jardin, F. (1973), La psychothérapie institutionnelle de l'anorexie mentale. III. L'abord des familles au cours de l'hospitalisation. (Residential treatment of anorexia nervosa. III. Approach to the family during hospitalization). *Revue de Neuropsychiatrie Infantile*, 21:167-172. (P)

Jeammet, P, (1984), Le groupe de parents: Sa place dans le traitement de l'anorexie mentale. (The parent group: Its place in the treatment of anorexia nervosa). *Neuropsychiatrie de l'Enfance*, 32:299-303. (P)

Jeammet, P. & Gorge, A. (1980), Une forme de thérapie familiale: Le groupe de parents. (A form of family therapy: The parent group). *Psychiatrie de l'Enfant,* 23:587-636. (P)

Jeammet, P., Gorge, A., Zweifel, F. & Flavigny, H. (1971), Etude des interrelations familiales de l'anorexique mentale et d'un groupe de psychothérapie des parents. (Study of family relations in anorexia nervosa and of a psychotherapeutic group for parents). *Revue de Neuropsychiatrie Infantile,* 19:691- 708. (P)

Jeammet, P., Gorge, A., Zweifel, F. & Flavigny, H. (1973a), Incidences therapeutiques de l'étude psychodynamique de l'anorexie mentale et de son milieu familiale. (Therapeutic aspects of the psychodynamic study of anorexia nervosa and the family milieu). *Entretiens de Bichat-Psychiatrie,* 271-280. (P)

Jeammet, P., Gorge, A., Zweifel, F. & Flavigny, H. (1973b), Le milieu familial des anorexiques mentaux. Incidences sur le traitement. (The family milieu of anorexia nervosa patients. Influences on the treatment). *Annales de Médecine Interne,* 124:247-252. (P)

Jensen, L. (1968), Anorexia nervosa. *Acta Psychiatrica Scandinavica,* 44(Suppl.203):113-116. (T)

Johnson, C. & Connors, M.E. (1987), Family factors. In: Authors, *The Etiology and Treatment of Bulimia Nervosa.* New York: Basic Books, pp. 126-135. (G)

Johnson, C. & Flach, A. (1985), Family characteristics of 105 patients with bulimia. *American Journal of Psychiatry,* 142:1321-1324. (R)

Kagan, D. & Squires, R. (1985), Family cohesion, family adaptability and eating behaviors among college students. *International Journal of Eating Disorders,* 4:267-279. (R)

Kalucy, R.S. (1983), Family psychopathology and anorexia nervosa. In: Krakowski, A.J. & Kimball, C.P. (Eds.), *Psychosomatic Medicine. Theoretical, Clinical and Transcultural Aspects.* New York: Plenum Press, pp. 125-141. (T)

Kalucy, R.S., Crisp, A.H. & Harding, B. (1977), A study of 56 families with anorexia nervosa. *British Journal of Medical Psychology, 50:381-395. (R)*

Katz, R.L., Mazer, C. & Litt, I.F. (1985), Anorexia nervosa by proxy. *Journal of Pediatrics,* 107:247-248. (T)

Katz, S. (1985), Anorexia and bulimia support group helping victims' families. *Canadian Medical Association Journal,* 132:1077-1079. (P)

Keeney, B.P. & Ross, J.M. (1985), A structural family therapy case study of H. Charles Fishman. In: Authors, *Mind in Therapy. Constructing Systemic Family Therapies.* New York: Basic Books, pp. 177-204. (P)

Kerschner, H. (1980), Eating disorders in my family...A three-generational study. *The Family,* 8(2):98-108. (T)

Klessmann, E. & Klessmann, H.A. (1983), Anorexia nervosa: eine therapeutische Beziehungsfalle? Ein Fazit nach 13 Jahren ambulanter Therapie. (Anorexia Nervosa: A therapeutical double blind? A summary of 13 years of outpatient therapy). *Praxis der Kinderpsychologie und Kinderpsychiatrie,* 32:257-261. (P)

Koch, A. (1974), (Outpatient family therapy for a girl aged 14 years with anorexia nervosa). *Ugeskr. Laeg.,* 136:1031- 1033. (P)

Kog, E. (1987), Self-report family interaction in normal and eating disorder families. In: Huber, W. (Ed.), *Progress in Psychotherapy Research.* Louvain-la-Neuve: Presses Universitaires de Louvain, p. 394-406. (R)

Kog, E., Pierloot, R. & Vandereycken, W. (1983), Methodological considerations of family research in anorexia nervosa. *International Journal of Eating Disorders,* 2(4):79-84. (T)

Kog, E. & Vandereycken, W. (1985), Family characteristics of anorexia nervosa and bulimia: A review of the research literature. *Clinical Psychology Review,* 5:159-180. (G)

Kog, E., Vandereycken, W. & Vertommen, H. (1985a), Towards a verification of the psychosomatic family model. A pilot study of ten families with an anorexia/bulimia nervosa patient. *International Journal of Eating Disorders,* 4:525-538. (R)

Kog, E., Vertommen, H. & De Groote, T. (1985b), Family interaction research in anorexia nervosa: The use and misuse of a self-report questionnaire. *International Journal of Family Psychiatry,* 6:227-243. (R)

Kog, E., Vertommen, H. & Vandereycken, W. (1987a), Minuchin's psychosomatic family model revised: A concept-validation study using a multitrait-multimethod approach. *Family Process,* 26:235-253. (R)

Kog, E., Vertommen, H. & Vandereycken, W. (1987b), De Leuvense Gezinsvragenlijst: een nieuw gezinsdiagnostisch instrument. (The Leuven Family Questionnaire: a new instrument for family assessment). *Tijdschrift voor Psychiatrie,* 29:343-356. (R)

Koizumi, H. & Luidens, G. (1984), Cross-cultural issues in the treatment of intractable anorexia nervosa. *International Journal of Family Therapy,* 6:156-164. (P)

Kramer, S. (1987), Family structure and functional relationships. In: Blinder, B.J. (Ed.), *The Eating Disorders: Research, Diagnosis, Treatment.* New York: P.M.A. Publications. (G)

Krener, P.G., Abramowitz, S.I. & Walker, P.B. (1986), Relation of family factor to treatment outcome for bulimic patients. *Psychotherapy and Psychosomatics,* 45:127-132. (R)

Lafeber, C. (1981), Wisselwerking tussen herstel van anorexia nervosa en de partnerrelatie. (Interaction between recovery from anorexia nervosa and marital relationship). *Tijdschrfit voor Psychiatrie,* 23(suppl.):97-103. (R)

Lagos, J.M. (1981), Family therapy in the treatment of anorexia nervosa: Theory and technique. *International Journal of Psychiatry in Medicine,* 11:291-302. (P)

Launay, C., Trélat, J., Daymas, S., Tissot, A. & Jardin, F. (1965), Le rôle du père dans le développement de l'anorexie juvenile. (The role of the father in the development of anorexia nervosa). *Revue de Neuropsychiatrie Infantile,* 13:740-743. (T)

Lawrence, M. (1984), Anorexic women and their families. In: Author, *The Anorexic Experience.* London: The Women's Press, pp. 56-74. (G)

Leichner, P., Harper, D. & Johnston, D. (1985), Adjunctive group support for spouses of women with anorexia nervosa and/or bulimia. *International Journal of Eating Disorders,* 4:227- 235. (P)

Léger, J.M., Blanchinet, J. & Vallat, J.N. (1969), A la lumière de deux cas d'anorexie mentale du garon: peut-on faire jouer un rôle important à la personnalité du père dans la survenue de cette affection? (About two cases of anorexia nervosa in boys: Does the father's personality play an important role in the development of this disease?) *Annales Médico-Psychologiques,* 127(2):101-108. (T)

Levenkron, S. (1982), The family: source and resource. In: Author, *Treating and Overcoming Anorexia Nervosa.* New York: Charles Scribner's Sons, pp. 164-173. (P)

Lewis, C.R. (1982), Elisabeth Barrett Browning's 'family disease': Anorexia nervosa. *Journal of Marital and Family Therapy,* 8:129-134. (T)

Lewis, H.L. & MacGuire, M.P. (1985), Review of a group for parents of anorexics. *Journal of Psychiatric Research,* 19:453-458. (P)

Liebman, R., Minuchin, S. & Baker, L. (1974a), An integrated treatment program for anorexia nervosa. *American Journal of Psychiatry,* 131:432-436. (P)

Liebman, R., Minuchin, S. & Baker, L. (1974b), The role of the family in the treatment of anorexia nervosa. *Journal of Child Psychiatry,* 13:264-274. (P)

Liebman, R., Minuchin, S., Baker, L. & Rosman, B.L. (1975), The treatment of anorexia nervosa. In: Masserman, J.H. (Ed.), *Current Psychiatric Therapies. Volume 15.* New York: Grune & Stratton, pp. 51-57. (P)

Liebman, R., Sargent, J. & Silver, M. (1983), A family systems orientation to the treatment of anorexia nervosa. *Journal of the American Academy of Child Psychiatry,* 22:128- 133. (P)

Lockman, D. (1986), Rip-van-Winkle in 1986: Treatment phases for anorexia nervosa within a family systems model. *Journal of Strategic and Systemic Therapies,* 5 (1-2):A20-A27. (P)

Luton, J.P. (1984), La famille des anorexie mentales: le point de vue d'un somaticien. (The family in anorexia nervosa: the point of view of a somatic therapist). *Neuropsychiatrie de l'Enfance,* 32:305-307. (P)

Madanes, C. (1981), Case 2: Binge-eating and vomiting. In: Author, *Strategic Family Therapy.* San Francisco: Jossey Bass, pp. 39-48. (P)

Maloney, M.J. & Shepherd-Spiro, P. (1983), Eating attitudes and behaviors of anorexia nervosa patients and their sisters. *General Hospital Psychiatry,* 5:285-288. (R)

Manler, E. & Thomä, H. (1964), Ueber die simultane Psychotherapie einer Anorexia-nervosa-Kranken und ihrer Mutter. (About the simultaneous psychotherapy of an anorexia nervosa patient and her mother). *Jahrbuch für Psychoanalyse,* 3:174. (P)

Mester, H. (1981a), Die Familienstruktur. (The family structure). In: Author, *Die Anorexia Nervosa.* Berlin: Springer-Verlag, pp. 149-162. (G,R)

Mester, H. (1981b), Die unbewussten 'Spielregeln' innerhalb der Herkunftsfamilien. (The unconscious 'roles' in the families of origin). In: Author, *Die Anorexia Nervosa.* Berlin: Springer-Verlag, pp. 163-198. (T)

Miller, S.G. (1984), Family therapy of the eating disorders. In: Powers, P.S. & Fernandez, R.C. (Eds.), *Current Treatment of Anorexia Nervosa and Bulimia.* Basel: S. Karger, pp. 93-112. (P)

Minuchin, S. (1970), The use of an ecological framework in the treatment of a child. In: E. Anthony & C. Koupernik (Eds.), *The Child In His Family.* New York: John Wiley, pp. 41-57 (this book also appeared in a French translation: Paris, Masson, 1970). (P)

Minuchin, S. (1982), *Anorexia is a Greek Word* (film). Boston: Boston Family Institute. (P)

Minuchin, S. (1984), An anorectic family: Repatterning through therapy. In: Author, *Family Kaleidoscope.* Cambridge (Mass.): Harvard University Press, pp. 90-114. (P)

Minuchin, S., Baker, L., Liebman, R, Milman, L., Rosman, B. & Todd, T. (1973), Anorexia nervosa: Successful application of a family therapy approach (abstract). *Pediatric Research,* 7:294. (R)

Minuchin, S., Baker, L., Rosman, B.L., Liebman, R., Milman, L. & Todd, T.C. (1975), A conceptual model of psychosomatic illness in children: Family organization and family therapy. *Archives of General Psychiatry,* 32:1031-1038 (Reprinted in: Howells, J.G., ed., *Advances in Family Psychiatry. Volume I.* New York: International Universities Press, 1979, pp. 316- 338). (T,P)

Minuchin, S., Rosn, B. & Baker, L. (1978), *Psychosomatic Families: Anorexia Nervosa in Context.* Cambridge (Mass.): Harvard University Press (Dutch translation published by Van Loghum Slaterus, Deventer, 1983). (T,P,R)

Mirkin, M.P. (1983), The Peter Pan syndrome: Inpatient treatment of adolescent anorexia nervosa. *International Journal of Family Therapy,* 7:179-189. (P)

Mitchell, J.E., Hatsukami, D., Pyle, R.L. & Eckert, E.D. (1986), Bulimia with and without a family history of depressive illness. *Comprehensive Psychiatry,* 27:215-219. (R)

Moley, V.A. (1983), Interactional treatment of eating disorders. *Journal of Strategic and Systemic Therapies,* 2(4):10-28. (P)

Moore, A.J. & Coulman, M.U. (1981), Anorexia Nervosa: The patient, her family and key family therapy interventions, *Journal of Psychiatric Nursing,* 19(5):9-14. (P)

Morgan, H.G. & Russell, G.F.M. (1975), Value of family background a clinical features as prediction of long-term outcome in anorexia nervosa: Four year follow-up study of 41 patients. *Psychological Medicine,* 5:355-372. (R)

Moultrup, D. (1981), Composition and length of treatment in anorexia nervosa. In: Gurman, A.S. (Ed.), *Questions and Answers in the Practice of Family Therapy.* New York: Brunner/Mazel, pp. 133-137. (P)

Neal, J.H. & Herzog, D.B. (1985), Family dynamics and treatment of anorexia nervosa and bulimia. *Pediatrician,* 12:139-147. (G)

Norris, D.L. & Jones, E. (1979), Anorexia nervosa. A clinical study of ten patients and their family systems. *Journal of Adolescence,* 2:101-111. (R)

Oberfiels, R.A. (1981), Family therapy with adolescents. Treatment of a teenage girl with 'globus hystericus' and weight loss. *Journal of the American Academy of Child Psychiatry,* 20:822-833. (P)

Ordman, A.M. & D.S. Kirschenbaum (1986), Bulimia: Assessment of eating, psychological adjustment and familial characteristics. *International Journal of Eating Disorders,* 5:865-878. (R)

Overbeck, A. (1979), Zur Wechselwirkung intrapsychischer und interpersoneller Prozesse in der Anorexia Nervosa: Beobachtungen und Interpretationen aus der Therapie einer Magersuchtfamilie. (Reciprocity of intrapsychic disturbance and interpersonal processes in anorexia nervosa — Observed and explained within the setting of family therapy). *Zeitschrift für Psychosomatische Medizinund Psychoanalyse,* 25:216-239. (T)

Owen, S.E.H. (1973), The projective identification of the parents of patients suffering from anorexia nervosa. *Australian and New Zealand Journal of Psychiatry,* 7:285-290. (R)

Palmer, R.L., Marshall, P. & Oppenheimer, R. (1987), Anorexia and the family. In: Orford, J. (Ed.), *Coping with Disorder in the Family.* London: Croom Helm, pp 117-137. (G)

Papp, P. (1983), Case presentation: The daughter who said no. In: Author, *The Process of Change.* New York: Guilford Press, pp. 67-103. (P)

Parker, J.B., Blazer, D. & Wyrick, L. (1977), Anorexia nervosa: A combined therapeutic approach. *Southern Medical Journal,* 70:448-452. (P)

Peake, T. & Borduin, C. (1977), Combining systems, behavioral and analytical approaches to the treatment of anorexia nervosa: A case study. *Family Therapy,* 4:49-56. (P)

Perednia, C. & Vandereycken, W. (1987), Een transgenerationele visie op anorexia nervosa. (A transgenerational view on anorexia nervosa). *Kind & Adolescent,* 8:31-37. (T)

Perlman, L.M. & Bender, S.S. (1975), Operant reinforcement with structural family therapy in treating anorexia nervosa. *Journal of Family Counseling,* 3(2):38-46. (P)

Petzold, E. (1976), Thérapeutique de l'anorexie mentale. (Therapy with anorexia nervosa). *Médecine et Hygièn,* 34:154-155. (P)

Petzold, E. (1979), *Familien Konfrontationstherapie bei Anorexia Nervosa.* (Family Confrontation Therapy in Anorexia Nervosa). Göttingen: Vandenhoeck-Ruprecht. (P)

Petzold, E., Vollrath, P., Ferner, H. & Reindell, A. (1976a), Erfahrungsbericht über Familienkonfrontation bei Anorexia- nervosa-Patienten. (Report on the experience with family confrontation in anorexia nervosa patients). *Psychosomatische Medizin,* 6:207-212. (P)

Petzold, E., Vollrath, P., Ferner, H. & Reindell, A. (1976b), Familienkonfrontation — Beitrag zur Therapie der Anorexia- nervosa-Patienten. (Family confrontation — Contribution to the treatment of anorexia nervosa patients). *Therapiewoche,* 26:970-974. (P)

Pina Prata, F.X. (1980), Analyse differentielle du système rigide de l'anorexie mentale dans l'optique systémique de la thérapie familiale. (Differential analysis of the rigid system in anorexia nervosa from the systemic family therapy viewpoint). *Thérapie Familiale,* 1:145-164. (T)

Rabreau, J.P. (1984), Quelques théories familiales de l'anorexie mentale. (A few family theories of anorexia nervosa). *Semaine des Hôpitaux (Paris),* 60(30):2151-2160. (T)

Rakoff, V. (1983), Multiple determinants of family dynamics in anorexia nervosa. In: Darby, P.L., Garfinkel, P.E., Garner, D.M. & Coscina D.V. (Eds.), *Anorexia Nervosa: Recent Developments in Research.* New York: Alan R. Liss, pp. 29-40. (G)

Rampling (1980), Single case study. Abnormal mothering in the genesis of anorexia nervosa. *Journal of Nervous and Mental Disease.* 168:501-504. (T)

Rathner, G., Mangold, B. & Smrekar, U. (1987), Familientherapeutische Aspekte in der Behandlung von Anorexia nervosa. (Family therapeutic aspects in the treatment of anorexia nervosa). *Neuropsychiatrie,* 1:111-17. (P)

Rivinus, T.M., Biederman, J., Herzog, D., Kemper, K., Harper, G., Harmatz, J. & Houseworth, S. (1984), Anorexia nervosa and affective disorders: A controlled family history study. *American Journal of Psychiatry,* 141:1414-1418. (R)

Roberto, L.G. (1986), Bulimia: The transgenerational view. *Journal of Marital and Family Therapy,* 12:231-240. (P)

Root, M.P.P., Falloon, P. & Friedrich, W.N. (1986), *Bulimia: A Systems Approach to Treatment.* New York: W.W. Norton. (G,P)

Rose, J. & Garfinkel, P. (1980), A parents' group in the management of anorexia nervosa. *Canadian Journal of Psychiatry,* 25:228-232. (P)

Rosman, B.L., Minuchin, S., Baker, L. & Liebman, R. (1977), A family approach to anorexia nervosa: Study, treatment, and outcome. In: Vigersky, R. (Ed.), *Anorexia Nervosa.* New York: Raven Press, pp. 341-348. (P,R)

Rosman, B.L., Minuchin, S. & Liebman, R. (1975), Family lunch session: An introduction to family therapy in anorexia nervosa. *American Journal of Orthopsychiatry,* 45:846-853 (German translation in: *Familiendynamik,* 1976, 1:334-347). (P)

Rosman, B.L., Minuchin, S., Liebman, R. & Baker, L. (1976), Input and outcome of family therapy in anorexia nervosa. In: J.L. Claghorn (Ed.), *Successful Psychotherapy.* New York: Brunner/Mazel, pp. 128-139 (Reprinted in: S.C. Feinstein & P.L. Giovacchini (Eds.), *Adolescent Psychiatry. Developmental and Clinical Studies. Volume V.* New York: Jason Aronson, 1977, pp. 313-322). (P)

Rouam, F. (1984), Réflexions sur un groupe thérapeutique de parents d'anorexiques. (Considerations on a therapeutic group for parents of anorexics). *Semaine des Hôpitaux* (Paris), 60:2163-2167. (P)

Rouam, F., Basquin, M. & Duché, D.J. (1984), Deux anorexiques sur une seule balance: La tara et le contrepoids. (Two anorexic sisters on one scale: the weight and the counterweight). *Neuropsychiatrie de l'Enfance,* 32:316-319. (T)

Rudolph, E. (1981), Anorexia nervosa. Some multigenerational hypotheses. *The Family,* 9(1):43-45.(T)

Sargent, J. & Liebman, R. (1985), Eating disorders. In: Henao, S. & Grose, N.P. (Eds.), *Principles of Family Systems in Family Medicine.* New York: Brunner/Mazel, pp. 213-242. (G)

Sargent, J., Liebman, R. & Silver, M. (1985), Family therapy for anorexia nervosa. In: Garner, D.M. & Garfinkel, P.E. (Eds.), *Handbook of Psychotherapy for Anorexia Nervosa and Bulimia.* New York: Guilford Press, pp. 257-279. (P)

Schepank, H. (1983), Anorexia nervosa in twins: Is the etiology psychotic or psychogenic? In: Krakowski, A.J. & Kimball, C.P. (Eds.), *Psychosomatic Medicine.* New York: Plenum Press, pp. 1651-169. (T)

Schmidt, D. (1984), Paradoxe Verschreibung als einmalige familientherapeutische Kriseninter-vention im Verlauf einer Einzelbehandlung bei einer Patientin mit Magersuchterkrankung. (Paradoxical prescription as single family-centered intervention during an individual psycho-analytic therapy). *Psychotherapie und Medizinische Psychologie,* 34:232-236. (P)

Schmidt, G. (1985), Familientherapie bei Patienten mit Ess- Störungen, insbesondere bei Ano-rexia nervosa. (Family therapy in patients with eating disorders, in particular anorexia ner-vosa). In: Brakhoff, J. (Ed.), *Ess-Störungen: Ambulante und Stationäre Behandlung.* Freiburg: Lambertus Verlag, pp. 119-129. (P)

Schneider, S. (1981), Anorexia nervosa: The 'subtle' condition. *Family Therapy,* 8:49-54. (P)

Schwartz, R.C. (1982), Bulimia and family therapy: A case study. *International Journal of Eating Disorders,* 2(1):75- 82. (P)

Schwartz, R.D. (1982), Bulimia and family therapy: A case study. *International Journal of Eating Disorders,* 2(1):75- 82. (P)

Schwartz, R.C., Barrett, M.J. & Saba, G. (1985), Family therapy for bulimia. In: Garner, D.M. & Garfinkel, P.E. (Eds.), *Handbook of Psychotherapy for Anorexia Nervosa and Bulimia.* New York: Guilford Press, pp. 280-307. (P)

Scott, D.W. (1986), Anorexia nervosa: A review of possible genetic factors. *International Journal of Eating Disorders,* 5:1-20. (G)

Seltzer, W. (1984), Treating anorexia nervosa in the somatic hospital: A multisystemic approach. *Family Systems Medicine,* 2:195-207. (P)

Selvini Palazzoli, M. (1970), The families of patients with anorexia nervosa. In: E.J. Anthony & C. Koupernik (Eds.), *The Child In His Family.* New York: John Wiley, pp. 319-332 (this book was also translated in French: Paris, Masson, 1970). (T)

Selvini Palazzoli, M. (1972), La famiglia con paziente anoressica: Un sistema modello. (The family with an anorexic patient: A systems model). *Archivo di Psicologia, Neurologia e Psichiatria,* 33:311-344. (T)

Selvini Palazzoli, M. (1973), Cybernétique de l'anorexie mentale. (Cybernetics of anorexia ner-vosa). *Psychosomatische Medizin,* 5:33-41. (T)

Selvini Palazzoli, M. (1974), *Self-Starvation: From the Intrapsychic to the Transpersonal Approach to Anorexia Nervosa.* London: Chaucer-Human Context Books (American edition: Jason Aron-son, New York, 1978; German translation: Klett- Cotta, Stuttgart, 1982). (T,P)

Selvini Palazzoli, M., Boscolo, L., Cecchin, G. & Prata, G. (1976), Het gezin van de anorexia-patiënt en het gezin van de schizofreen. Een transactionele studie. (The family of the anorexia patient and the family of the schizophrenic. A transactional study). *Tijdschrift voor Psycho-*

therapie, 2:53-61 (French translation: *Actualités Psychiatriques,* 1982, 12:15-25; German translation: *Ehe,* 1975, 3:107-116: Italian version: *Terapia Familiare,* 1977, 1:29-42).

Selvini Palazzoli, M. (1977), Anorexia nervosa — Van individuele psychotherapie naar gezinstherapie. (Anorexia nervosa — from individual psychotherapy to family therapy). *Tijdschrift voor Orthopedagogiek en Kinderpsychiatrie,* 2:63-73.

Selvini Palazzoli, M. (1985), Anorexia nervosa: A syndrome of the affluent society. *Journal of Strategic and Systemic Therapies,* 4(3):12-16. (T)

Selvini Palazzoli, M., Boscolo, L., Cecchin, G. & Prata, G. (1977), Die erste Sitzung einer systemischen Familientherapie. (The first session of a systemic family therapy). *Familiendynamik,* 2:197-207 (French translation in: *Cahiers Critiques de Thérapie Familiale et de Pratique de Réseaux,* 1979, nr 1). (P)

Sichel, J.P. (1971), Considérations sur le rôle du père dans l'anorexie mentale. (Consideration on the role of the father in anorexia nervosa). *Revue de Neuropsychiatrie Infantile,* 19:651-654. (T)

Sights, J.R. & Richards, H.C. (1984), Parents of bulimic women. *International Journal of Eating Disorders,* 3(4):3- 13. (R)

Slive, A. & Young, F. (1986), Bulimia as substance abuse: A metaphor for strategic treatment. *Journal of Strategic and Systemic Therapies,* 5(3):71-84. (P)

Snakkers, J. (1984), Thérapie familiale et thérapie individuelle dans un case d'anorexie mentale. (Family therapy and individual therapy in a case of anorexia nervosa). *Neuropsychiatrie de l'Enfance,* 32:281-289. (P)

Sours, J.A. (1980), Families of anorexia nervosa patients. In: Author, *Starving to Death in a Sea of Objects. The Anorexia Nervosa Syndrome.* New York: Jason Aronson, pp. 317-330. (G)

Sperling, E. (1965), Die 'Magersucht-Familie' und ihre Behandlung. (The 'anorexia nervosa family' and its treatment). In: Meyer, J.E. & Feldmann, H. (Eds.), *Anorexia Nervosa.* Stuttgart: Georg Thieme Verlag, pp. 156-160. (T)

Sperling, E. & Massing, A. (1970), Der familiäre Hintergrund der Anorexia nervosa und die sich daraus ergebenden therapeutischen Schwierigkeiten. (The family background of anorexia nervosa and the related treatment difficulties). *Zeitschrift für Psychosomatische Medizin,* 16:130-141. (P,R)

Sperling, E. & Massing, A. (1972), Besonderheiten in der Behandlung der Magersuchtfamilie. (Particularities in the treatment of the anorexia nervosa family). *Psyche,* 26:358- 369. (P)

Sperling, E., Massing, A., Georgi, H., Reich, G. & Wöbbe-Mönks, E. (1982), Anorexie. In: Authors, *Die Mehrgenerationen-Familientherapie.* (The Multigenerational Family Therapy). Göttingen: Vandenhoeck & Ruprecht, pp. 124- 131. (T)

Steinhausen, H.C. (1981), Die Verhaltenstherapie und Familientherapie der Anorexia Nervosa — eine kritische Bestandsaufname. (Behavior therapy and family therapy in anorexia nervosa: A critical evaluation). In: Steinhausen, H.C. (Ed.), *Psychosomatische Störungen und Krankheiten bei Kindern und Jugendlichen.* Stuttgart: Kohlhammer, pp. 193-212. (G)

Stelzer, J. (1984), Point de vue psychoanalytique sur le traitement individuel et familiale l'anorexie mentale. (Psychoanalytic approach to the individual and family treatment of anorexia nervosa). *Neuropsychiatrie de l'Enfance,* 32:291-298. (P)

Stern, S., Whitake, C., Hagemann, N.J., Anderson, R.B. & Bargman, G.J. (1981), Anorexia nervosa: The hospital's role in family treatment. *Family Process,* 20:395-408. (P)

Stern, S.L., Dixon, K.L., Nemzer, E., Lake, M.D., Sansone, R.A., Smeltzer, D.J., Lantz, S. & Schrier, S. (1984), Affective disorders in the families of women with normal weight bulimia. *American Journal of Psychiatry,* 141:1224-127. (R)

Stierlin, H. & Weber, G. (1987), Anorexia nervosa: Family dynamics and family therapy. In: Beumont, P.J.V., Burrows, G.D. & Casper, R.C. (Eds.), *Handbook of Eating Disorders. Part I.* Amsterdam: Elsevier-Science, pp. 319-347. (T)

Strober, M., Morrell, W., Burroughts, J., Salkin, B. & Jacobs, C. (1985), A controlled family study of anorexia nervosa. *Journal of Psychiatric Research,* 19:239-246. (R)

Swift, W.J. (1982), Family therapy and anorexia nervosa: The hospital phase. In: Gurman, A.S. (Ed.), *Questions and answers in the Practice of Family Therapy, Volume 2.* New York: Brunner/Mazel, pp. 187-191.

Szmukler, G. (1983), A study of family therapy in anorexia nervosa: Some methodological issues. In: Darby, P.L., Garfinkel, P.E., Garner, D.M. & Coscina, D.V. (Eds.), *Anorexia Nervosa: Recent Developments in Research.* New York: Alan R. Liss, pp. 417-425. (R)

Szmukler, G., Eisler, I., Russell, G.F.M. & Dare, C. (1985), Anorexia nervosa, parental 'expressed emotion' and dropping out of treatment. *British Journal of Psychiatry,* 147:265-271. (R)

Taipale, V., Tuomi, O. & Aukee, M. (19), Anorexia nervosa: An illness of two generations? *Acta Paedopsychiatrica,* 38:21-25. (T)

Todd, T.C. (1985), Anorexia nervosa and bulimia: Expanding the structural model. In: Mirkin, M.P. & Koman, S.L. (Eds.), *Handbook of Adolescents and Family Therapy.* New York: Gardner Press, pp. 223-243. (P)

Vandereycken, W. (1980), Tussen mythen en feiten: Diagnose en behandeling van het zogenaamde anorexia nervosa gezin. (Between myths and facts: diagnosis and treatment of the so- called anorexia nervosa family). *Tijdschrift voor Relatieproblematiek,* 2:223-255. (G)

Vandereycken, W. (1985), Outpatient management of anorexia nervosa. *Pediatrician,* 12:118-125. (P)

Vandereycken, W. (1986), Participatie van het gezin in een residentiële behandeling van anorexia nervosa patiënten. (Participation of the family in an inpatient treatment of anorexia nervosa patients). *Gedragstherapie,* 18:315-322. (P)

Vandereycken, W. (1987), The constructive family approach to eating disorders: Critical remarks on the use of family therapy in anorexia nervosa and bulimia. *International Journal of Eating Disorders,* 6:455-467. (P)

Vandereycken, W. & Meermann, R. (1984), Has the family to be treated? In: Authors, *Anorexia Nervosa: A Clinician's Guide to Treatment.* Berlin, New York: Walter de Gruyter, pp. 151- 168 (revised German edition 1987). (P)

Vandereycken, W. & Perednia, C. (1986), La participation de la famille dans un traitement résidentiel de l'anorexie mentale. (The family's involvement in the inpatient treatment of anorexia nervosa). *Psychothérapies,* 6:191-195. (P)

Vandereycken, W. & Pierloot, R. (1981), Anorexia nervosa in twins. *Psychotherapy and Psychosomatics,* 35:55-63. (R)

Vanderlinden, J. & Vandereycken, W. (1984), Directive family therapy in adult patients with severe or chronic anorexia nervosa. *International Journal of Family Psychiatry,* 5:267-280. (P)

Vanderlinden, J. & Vandereycken, W. (1987), The effect of a residential treatment program on eating disorder patients and their families. In: Huber, W. (Ed.), *Progress in Psychotherapy Research.* Louvain-la-Neuve: Presses Universitaires de Louvain, pp. 407-420. (R)

van Strien, D.C., Hendrickx, J. (1985), Anorexia nervosa: Individuele en gezinsdiagnostiek. (Anorexia nervosa: Individual and family diagnostic approach). In: Ponjaert, I. & Vertommen, H. (Eds.), *Therapiegerichte Diagnostiek.* Leuven: Acco, pp. 335-346. (T)

Verbeek, N. & Verbeek, E. (1977), Anorexia nervosa: Karakteristiek en therapie van de driehoeksrelatie in het ouderlijk gezin. (Anorexia nervosa: Characteristics and treatment of the triangular relation in the family). *Tijdschrift voor Psychiatrie,* 19:685-703. (T)

Viret, C. (1985), Prise en charge hospitalière d'une psychotique anorexique mentale dans une optique contextuelle selon I. Boszorgmenyi-Nagy. (Inpatient approach to anorexia nervosa from a contextual perspective according to I. Boszorgmenyi-Nagy). *Archives Suisses de Neurologie, Neurochirurgie et de Psychiatrie,* 136(6):73-77. (P)

Weber, G. & Stierlin, H. (1981), Familiendynamik und Familientherapie der Anorexia nervosa Familie. (Family dynamics and family therapy of the anorexia nervosa family). In: Meermann, R. (Ed.), *Anorexia Nervosa: Ursachen und Behandlung.* Stuttgart: Ferdinand Enke, pp. 108-122. (T,P)

White, J.H. (1984), Bulimia: Utilizing individual and family therapy. *Journal of Psychosocial Nursing.* 22(4):22-28. (P)

White M. (1983), Anorexia nervosa: A transgenerational system perspective. *Family Process,* 22:255-275.(T)

Will, D. (1983), Some techniques for working with resistant families of adolescents. *Journal of Adolescence,* 6:12-26. (P)

Willenberg, H. (1986), Die Bedeutung des Vateors für die Psychogenese der Magersucht. (The significance of the father for the psychogenesis of anorexia nervous). *Materialien zur Psychoanalyse und Analytisch Orientierten Psychotherapie,* 12:237-277. (T)

Wilson, C.P. (1980), The family psychological profile of anorexia nervosa patients. *Journal of the Medical Society of New Jersey,* 77:341-344. (T)

Wilson, C.P. (1983), The family psychological profile and its therapeutic implications. In: Wilson, C.P., Hogan, C.C. & Mintz, I.L. (Eds.), *Fear of Being Fat. The Treatment of Anorexia Nervosa and Bulimia.* New York: Jason Aronson, pp. 29- 47. (T)

Winokur, A., March, V. & Mendels, J. (1980), Primary affective disorder in relatives of patients with anorexia nervosa. *American Journal of Psychiatry,* 137:695-698. (R)

Wold, P. (1973), Family structure in three cases of anorexia nervosa: The role of the father. *American Journal of Psychiatry,* 130:1394-1397. (T)

Wold, P. (1985), Family attitudes toward weight in bulimia and in affective disorder—a pilot study. *The Psychiatric Journal of the University of Ottawa,* 10:162-164. (R)

Yager, J. (1981), Anorexia nervosa and the family. In: Lansky, M.R. (Ed.), *Family Therapy and Major Psychopathology.* New York: Grune & Stratton, pp. 249-280. (G)

Yager, J. (1982), Family issues in the pathogenesis of anorexia nervosa. *Psychosomatic Medicine,* 44:46-60. (G)

Yager, J. & Strober, M. (1985), Family aspects of eating disorders. In: Hales, R.E. & Frances, A.J. (Eds.), *Psychiatry Update, Annual Review, Vol. 4.* Washington, D.C.: American Psychiatric Press, pp. 481-502. (G)

Zerbe, D.H. (1986), Countertransference, resistance and frame management in the psychotherapy of a 15-year-old anorexic and her mother. *Clinical Social Work Journal,* 14:213-223. (P)

INDEX